The HOLISTIC Guide for a HEALTHY DOG

Wendy Volhard

Kerry Brown, DVM

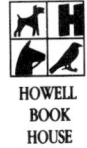

HOWELL
BOOK
HOUSE

Howell Book House
MACMILLAN
A Simon & Schuster Macmillan Company
1633 Broadway
New York, NY 10019

MACMILLAN is a registered trademark of Macmillan, Inc.

Library of Congress Cataloging-in-Publication Data

Volhard, Wendy.
Holistic guide for a healthy dog / by Wendy Volhard and Kerry L. Brown.
     p. cm.

Includes index.

ISBN 0-87605-560-9

1. Dogs—Nutrition. 2. Dogs—Food. 3. Dogs—Health.
4. Veterinary holistic medicine. I. Brown, Kerry L. II. Title.
SF427.4.V65 1995
636.7'0852—dc20 94-45507
   CIP
Manufactured in the United States of America

10 9   8   7   6

About the Authors

Wendy Volhard

Wendy is a member of the Animal Behavior Society, the United Kingdom Registry of Canine Behaviorists and the Advisory Board of the North American Wildlife Foundation. She gives seminars on behavior, instructing, training and nutrition and has lectured extensively all over America, Canada and the United Kingdom.

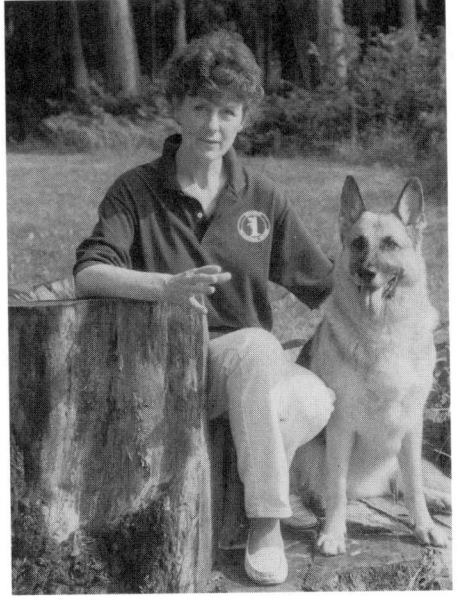

Wendy developed a system used worldwide for evaluating and selecting puppies. Her film *Puppy Aptitude Testing* was named Best Film on Dogs for 1981 by the Dog Writers' Association of America. Her four-part series "Motivating Your Dog for Competition," published by *Off-Lead* magazine, was named Best Series by the DWAA. She devised a Personality Profile for dogs that pinpoints what turns a dog on and off; it was published as a two-part article, "Drives—A New Look at an Old Concept," in the September and October 1991 issues of *Off-Lead* magazine, and it was named Best Article in a Specialty Magazine by DWAA.

She published *Back to Basics*, which features a balanced, home-made dog food, which she formulated. She is the co-producer of four videotapes on training and co-author of *Open and Utility Training—the Motivational Method* (Howell Book House, 1992), and the *Canine Good Citizen—Every Dog Can Be One* (Howell Book House, 1994).

Wendy is an active exhibitor who, together with her husband, Jack, has obtained over 40 Obedience titles, multiple High in Trial wins and Dog World Awards of Canine Distinction with her Landseer Newfoundlands, Yorkshire Terrier, Standard Wirehaired Dachshund, Labrador Retriever and German Shepherd Dog.

Over the past 28 years, through her training classes, lectures, weekend seminars, Holistic Study Group and five-day training camps, Wendy has taught more than 15,000 people not only how to communicate with their dogs and how to make training fun for both owner and dog, but also how to feed and keep dogs healthy and achieve mutually rewarding relationships.

Kerry L. Brown

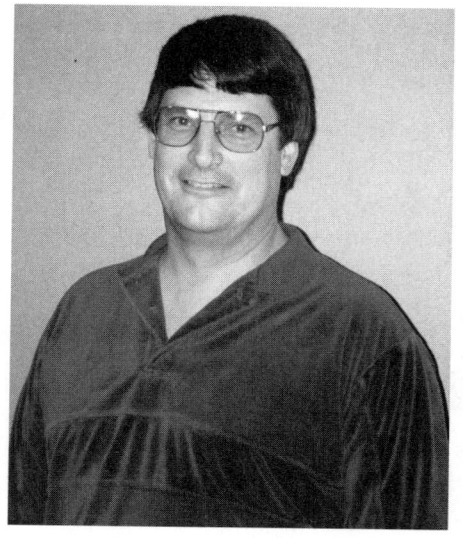

After graduating from Cornell Veterinary College in 1973, Kerry spent four years in a large and small animal practice before opening his own clinic in 1977. The Village Veterinary Hospital has grown from a one man practice to a facility with six veterinarians, all with various specialties in both large and small animals. This practice has become one of the most highly regarded animal hospitals in central New York and offers clientele up-to-date therapies in many fields.

Kerry has developed areas of expertise in surgery (both soft tissue and orthopedics) and internal medicine as well as in acupuncture, nutrition and reproduction. He has become a certified acupuncturist accredited by the International Veterinary Acupuncture Society.

Kerry and Wendy first worked together on the medical follow-up of natural diets in 1974. Since then, they have joined forces to investigate and search for ways to improve the health and lives of animal companions through the use of alternative therapies. Together they host a semiannual Holistic Study Group, which brings together experts in various alternative medicine fields to educate not only veterinarians but also other professionals in raising, training and working with dogs.

Contents

Acknowledgments

We want to thank our respective families, clients and students for their contributions and support. We are especially indebted to Sharee Curro for typing the medical manuscript; Diane Leadley, who drew the charts; and Karen Schlipf for all the illustrations and Brigitte Volhard for the photographs. A special note of gratitude to Sue Ann Lesser, DVM, for writing the chiropractic section and Meridy Milholland, M.Sc., who worked out the original Natural Diet charts. We also thank John Buser; Dr. Allen Kratz; Lucie Paradis, DVM; Jean Dodds, DVM; Mike Guerber; Mike Compton; and Sharon Sherman, who stood by with advice and encouragement.

My (Wendy) sincere thanks to Alan Otten who started it all, and to Andy Butler and Bill Phelps for taking such good care of my dogs while I was working on this project.

For both of us it has been a privilege to share our lives with our teachers—the dogs.

Preface

Purebred dogs are in trouble. Lifespans are getting shorter, diseases are becoming more prevalent, and unless something changes, the future looks bleak indeed.

There are four reasons that may have contributed to this state of affairs. **Breed selection** in some cases has progressed from function to form, thereby producing genetically weak individuals subject to debilitating diseases and poor quality of life. Environmentally created **stress** on the animal's immune system, principally the result of pollution, has further reduced the dog's vital forces. A rising number of **vaccinations**, from two in the first six months of life in the early 1970s up to as many as 45 today, has added to the attack on the puppy's immature immune system. **Diets**, insufficient to meet the nutritional needs of the dog or the increased stress levels, have contributed to an inability of the immune system to ward off and cope with disease. A frightening increase in autoimmune diseases and a virtual epidemic of cancer have been the result.

This book addresses the dog's nutritional requirements as they relate to health. In the first part, we present the facts that have led us to these conclusions. Serious deficiencies occur as soon as a puppy is weaned from mother's milk to a commercially prepared diet. Dog food is subjected to heat in manufacture when processed. Many vitamins and minerals are rendered useless and are not available to the dog through this food.

The recipes provided to the dog food industry by government agencies are not complete. Insufficient research has been done on many nutrients for some of the life stages of the dog, and virtually none on giant breeds. A majority of the protein contained in most of the foods comes from cereal grains. The dog is a carnivore (meat eater) who does not do well on this semivegetarian regimen. This lack of animal protein and sufficient amino acids from animal sources in the food is one of the biggest contributors to disease.

If dogs are not supplemented with products to make up for this lack of essential nutrients, they will show disease associated with these deficiencies. We have listed deficiencies associated with the lack of animal protein, vitamins and minerals. We have also provided an explanation of the testing procedures used by veterinarians on a sick dog, so the reader can interpret the results.

The second part of the book is devoted to a prevention program for raising dogs that counteracts these negative influences. This prevention program has been used successfully by us and hundreds of breeders and dog owners over the last 25 years. *Nothing has been included in this book that has not been subjected to thorough laboratory tests, including blood tests, fecal tests and urinalysis.* These tests have continued over a long period of time and over many generations of dogs.

There are plenty of good supplements that can be added to a dog's diet to improve health. We have worked with many over the years and have settled on those that we list because they work. These are the ones used in our tests.

This book will not give you all the answers, but it will empower you to improve your dog's health and longevity.

Chapter 1

Food—
What Difference
Does It Make?

The Foundation

In order to live, a dog must eat. How long the dog lives, as well as health, immune system, behavior and temperament, the ability to reproduce successfully and to recover from trauma, all depend on what is eaten. An animal that eats well lives a long life, coping with everyday stresses and strains. One that eats poorly is unhealthy and with age will begin to suffer from chronic diseases.

How is it possible that what we feed our dogs can make so much difference to their health? Think of the body as a house. If you build a strong foundation (pregnant mother's diet), the walls of the first story provide the support for the upper stories (puppyhood and adulthood). A roof that is made of the right materials and placed at the correct angles will be a protective covering over the whole house that will withstand even the most violent weather (immune system). Your house will outlast those around you that are built of less solid materials.

Building Blocks

In order to build a proper nutritional foundation, you need six building blocks: **protein, fat, carbohydrates, vitamins, minerals and water**. The quality of these building blocks and the ratio of one to another will determine how long your house will last.

Every cell in the dog's body needs fuel. Fuel comes from food, which is converted to energy. Energy produces heat, and how much heat is produced determines the ability of your dog to maintain and regulate body temperature. The quality and quantity of energy your dog needs to be able to run, play, work and live a long and healthy life depend on the quality and quantity of the fuel you provide. Nutritionists measure fuel in terms of how much energy it produces. They use the term *calories* to measure energy produced by individual foods. A dog will eat the quantity of food needed to meet individual caloric needs.

If the calories provided in dog food are sufficient, your dog's body will be able to produce energy for growth, maintenance, the production of enzymes and the ability to fight disease. Chemical reactions take place in the body that allow these enzymes to break down the food, making it available as a building block. The chemicals that are needed to trigger enzyme production come from the food the dog eats. If you provide a food with the correct amount of calories coming from *quality* sources mixed in the right proportions, your puppy will grow well. If the correct calories are not provided, you will produce an inferior dog, poor in health and short lived.

Growth

A puppy, during the first six months of life, increases birthweight anywhere from 15 to 40 times, depending on the breed. By one year of age birthweight will have increased up to 60 times. By contrast, humans reach maturity over a 20-year period. A dog, therefore, grows almost 12 times faster than a human, and if fed improperly as a puppy, even for a short while, may quickly exhibit symptoms of improper growth. A puppy needs almost double the amount of food of an adult—at times, even more than that.

Maintenance

As an adult, your dog needs a diet to maintain weight and provide enough energy to do the tasks you expect. A family pet, with no demands other than to play with the children and be a companion, needs a different diet than a dog who is used for hunting, showing or working.

With age, your dog's digestive system becomes less efficient, and you should make dietary changes that take aging into consideration.

Other factors that affect what your dog should eat are temperature and climate. If you live in a *cold climate*, your dog will require *more food* to maintain body heat calories than if you lived in a hot climate. Living in a hot climate often reduces hunger, but dogs burn up a lot of energy panting to stay cool. In the hotter climates, your dog needs a small amount of food that contains a lot of calories.

Food also has breed-specific results. *What produces energy or body heat in one breed may not in another.* A good example is a Border Collie whose ancestors were raised in Scotland. This breed has developed a digestive system that breaks down oats and lamb very well. A food made from chicken and corn may be digestible and turned into fuel, but the dog will need to eat more of this food in order to get the necessary nutrients.

Stress

A dog fed incorrectly will experience stress. That stress will manifest itself in the weakest part of the body. It may be runny eyes, ear infections, skin problems, crooked teeth or diseases of the bones and kidneys. Stress may manifest itself in an inability to breed, conceive, have a full-term pregnancy, whelp easily or make enough milk to feed puppies for several weeks. Dogs that are shy or afraid of thunderstorms or who show unprovoked aggression may also be exhibiting stress symptoms.

Dogs that are genetically sound, fed properly for the breed and the climate in which they live, and for the purpose they are being used, will be healthy animals.

Industry Controls

Where do you start when making the decision on what to feed your dog? There are two organizations that have researched this subject and control what is put into dog food. One is the National Research Council (NRC) and the other is the Association of American Feed Control Officials (AAFCO).

National Research Council

The NRC is composed of a body of scientists under the jurisdiction of the Food and Drug Administration and the Department of Agriculture. This body is responsible for supplying federal guidelines to the dog food industry. The research provided to the NRC comes from university studies and independent laboratories and covers the basic components of dog food, which are protein, fat, carbohydrates, vitamins and minerals. These studies are by no means complete and the guidelines abound with statements such as "remain to be determined," or "while histamine was reported to be an essential amino acid for the adult dog, no data were presented." These studies are incomplete in protein, carbohydrates, vitamins and minerals. The gaps are filled in by data based on theoretical knowledge and studies done on other species of animals. Some of the studies presented show clearly that certain breeds of dogs have different needs than others, but no

3

accommodation has been made for these breeds in the guidelines. There is no data available on the needs of giant breeds.

Association of American Feed Control Officials

AAFCO supervises the state regulation of pet foods. As of January 1994 the regulations stipulated by AAFCO have been followed by the dog food manufacturer rather than those guidelines determined by the NRC. AAFCO requires that certain testing procedures for dog foods be used in order to receive its stamp of approval. The testing is done in independent laboratories and the food must pass the labeling requirements.

For example, if a label states that a food is "complete and balanced" or is "nutritionally complete," or words to that effect, the food must go through certain feeding trials. These last from two to six weeks and ensure that the food does what the label states. If it says that the food is for puppies, or adult dogs, or all life stages, laboratory testing must prove that the food can indeed support life at those stages. The tests include blood plasma levels as well as fecal and urine analysis. When the test is completed satisfactorily, the AAFCO statement is placed on the label.

Two to six weeks is a short time frame to have a food tested, but at least the test is carefully controlled, and gross deficiencies of protein or other nutrients are revealed. It is one way for the consumer to be assured of the consistency of a product. Most foods today contain the AAFCO statement on the label.

AAFCO also requires the manufacturer to submit its food to be tested by an independent laboratory to ascertain what is in the finished product. If, for example, the product states it is 22 percent protein, the laboratory profile or assay, must support that assertion.

Labeling of dog food is strictly controlled. A company is told what can and cannot be put on the label. At present, a company that uses organically grown grains or superior sources of animal protein is unable to differentiate itself from a company that uses inexpensive, chemically laden ingredients. The consumer is left in the dark.

The dog food industry is in transition. There are no definite guidelines as to minimum amounts of nutrients required to keep dogs healthy in all life stages. In the meantime, the NRC guidelines printed in 1985, which list most of the minimum requirements of known nutrients, is one of the protocols that is followed. Another is a new concept of shared data from the Expert Committee on Nutrition. This committee is made up of dog food manufacturers.

The one "expert" that must be followed is the individual dog. Familiarize yourself with the information contained in the chapter on kinesiology and let your *dog* tell you what is right.

—Chapter 2—

The Ingredients of Dog Food

Most people have no idea what's in their dog's food. If their dogs pick at the food, people will change to another, trying to find the one just right for their dog. Feeding the correct food to a dog makes the difference between health and disease.

Dogs are carnivores, or meat eaters. Their teeth are formed to pull flesh apart. They have simple stomachs and a short digestive tract, ideal for digesting meat. Cereal and vegetable proteins are not as readily digested by the dog. While dogs have adapted somewhat to digesting these proteins, they have to eat a greater quantity of such foods to get the necessary nutrients. More food means more expense, as well as more voluminous stools. Dogs prefer a food high in animal protein, and it makes them healthier and perform better.

In order to choose a food that meets the nutritional needs of your dog, you need to understand something about protein, fat, carbohydrates, minerals, vitamins and water. These basic ingredients are the recipe for any food you feed a dog.

Protein—Amino Acids

At the very core of the dog's health and fitness are *amino acids*. Amino acids are the building blocks of protein and are necessary to life. If you are feeding an unsupplemented food high in cereal and vegetable proteins, chances are that your dog has an animal protein deficiency. Diseases that may result include:

- skin and chronic ear infections
- reproductive, heart, kidney, liver, bladder, thyroid and adrenal gland malfunctions
- some forms of epilepsy
- some kinds of cancer
- rage syndromes

- "spinning," or tail chasing
- lethargy
- aggression
- timidity
- lack of pigmentation
- inability to think and act clearly
- lack of appetite
- excessive shedding, as well as gastrointestinal upsets

Protein is composed of amino acids, of which 25 are presently known. Ten or 11, depending on the reference source you use, are essential and cannot be produced by the dog's body. The other 14 or 15 can be converted from the essential amino acids through a chemical chaining process taking place in the liver. These 10 or 11 essential amino acids can be obtained only through what the dog eats, and they must be consumed at the same meal in order to sustain a healthy life.

In a commercial dog food, protein is provided by combining animal sources, such as meat, byproducts, chicken, cheese, milk, fish, turkey or lamb, together with grain sources, such as corn, wheat, rice, soy and so on. The sum total of these proteins appears on dog food packages as **crude protein**. How these ingredients are arranged in the recipe and the quantity of those ingredients—whether the animal protein is listed first, third, or fifth—dictates the kind of protein available to the dog.

Amino acids are altered by heat, which in turn affects their bioavailability. Dry, semimoist or canned foods go through a heat process in manufacturing, and the finished product can be deficient in amino acids. Such a food, if fed without supplementation, can cause disease. Many amino acids are available only from animal sources, and if grains are the main source, a dog may develop one of the animal protein deficiency diseases listed above. Since amino acids are dependent on one another, a diet that contains too little of one will have a chain-reaction effect on the others and will reduce their utilization. To achieve the proper balance, it is necessary to combine foods with the correct amount of amino acids.

While the chemical composition of protein is similar for some grains and meat products, the bio-availability is different. Soy protein is used as a source of amino acids in food for animals that have complex stomachs, such as cattle and sheep, and as food for pigs, turkey and chickens. Some component parts of soy bind up their own nutrients and make them unavailable to the dog. *Young dogs and old dogs cannot utilize the amino acids from soy, hence it should be avoided.* Cottonseed meal falls into the same category.

The need for amino acids in the diet changes during differing life stages, climate and season changes, trauma or stress. When these stresses are experienced your dog's food should contain extra animal protein.

The National Research Council's findings showed that certain breeds of dogs, i.e., Labradors and English Pointers, had a greater need for amino acids from animal sources, than did Beagles. In our work, we have found there are many breeds of European origin whose requirements are similar to the Labrador. The content of dog food is made to accommodate the Beagle, not the Labrador.

The charts in Appendix I illustrate the food sources of amino acids and how they individually affect major organs in the body. They also show those diseases associated with deficiencies as well as the linkage with the other amino acids.

Physical Signs of Deficiencies

By observing your dog carefully, you can pick up signs of amino acid deficiencies. Many will be found on the feet and nails. Constantly biting or licking feet, crooked nails on one or more of the toes or toenails that are brittle can signal a protein deficiency. Pimples, skin discolorations and crooked whiskers are also deficiency signs. Look at the illustration of the Amino Acid Dog to see exactly where the deficiency points are. These are "indicator" points that can be checked using kinesiology. (See Chapter 13)

A Landseer Newfoundland we treated for many years had a pimple on the left side of her face in the middle of her whiskers. It was itchy and she would rub her face along the carpet and paw at it, sometimes breaking it open. The whisker coming out of this point was crooked and turned backward. The pimple was situated on the amino acid lysine point. Supplementing the dog's diet with an amino acid complex tablet containing lysine caused the pimple to disappear and the itching stopped.

For a list of animal protein sources commonly used in dog foods, see Chapter 19. For a charted explanation of all the amino acids and signs of deficiencies, see Appendix I and II.

Summary

1. FOOD PROTEINS ARE CONSIDERED COMPLETE ONLY WHEN THEY CONTAIN ALL THE ESSENTIAL AMINO ACIDS. Animal proteins are complete. Vegetable proteins are incomplete and unbalanced, but can be mixed with complete proteins to provide adequate amounts of EAAs.

2. DIETARY PROTEIN REQUIREMENTS ARE INFLUENCED BY VARIOUS FACTORS. These include digestibility, rate of protein synthesis, carbohydrate and fat levels in the diet and the timing of meals. Clinical factors can influence protein needs of the dog. These

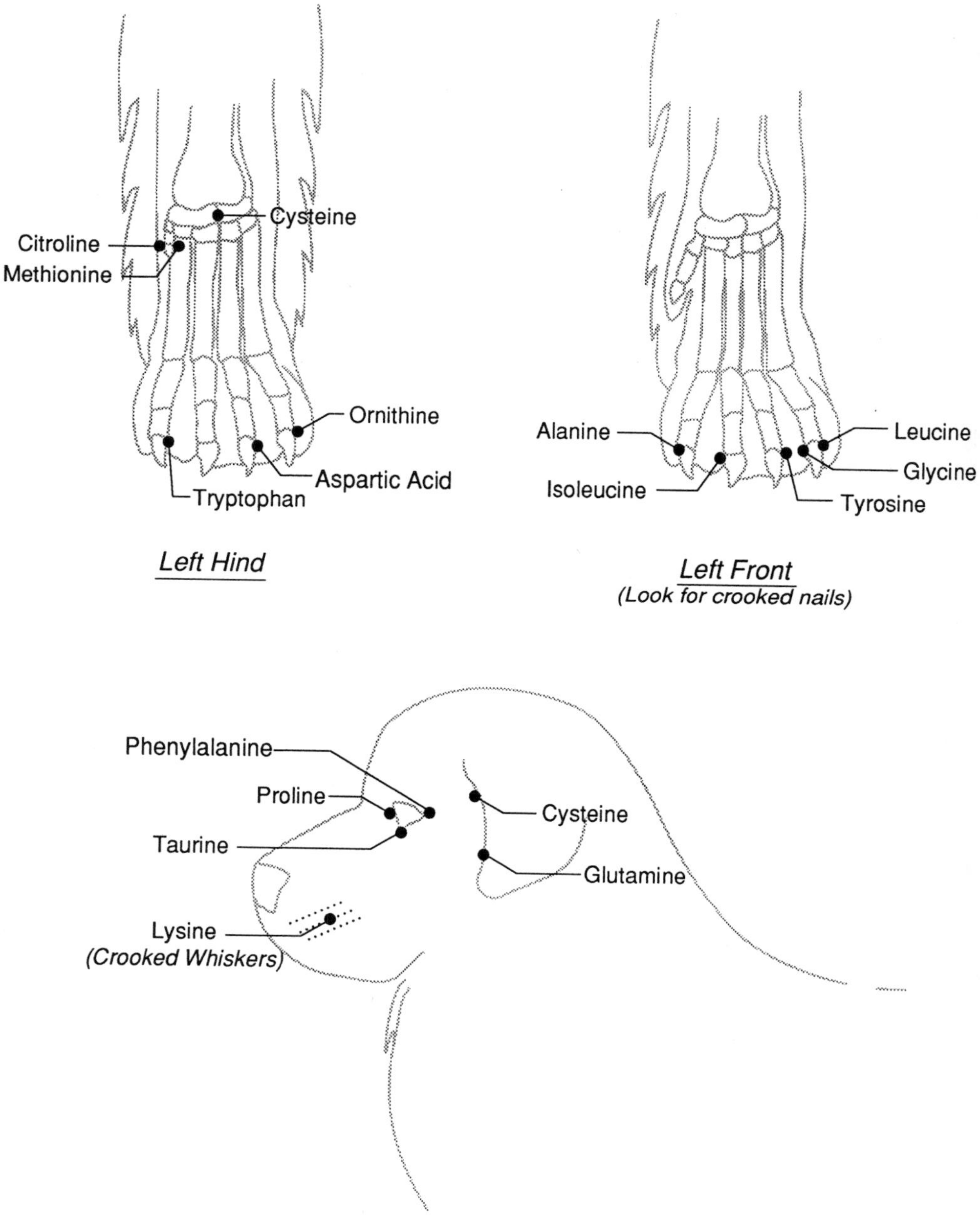

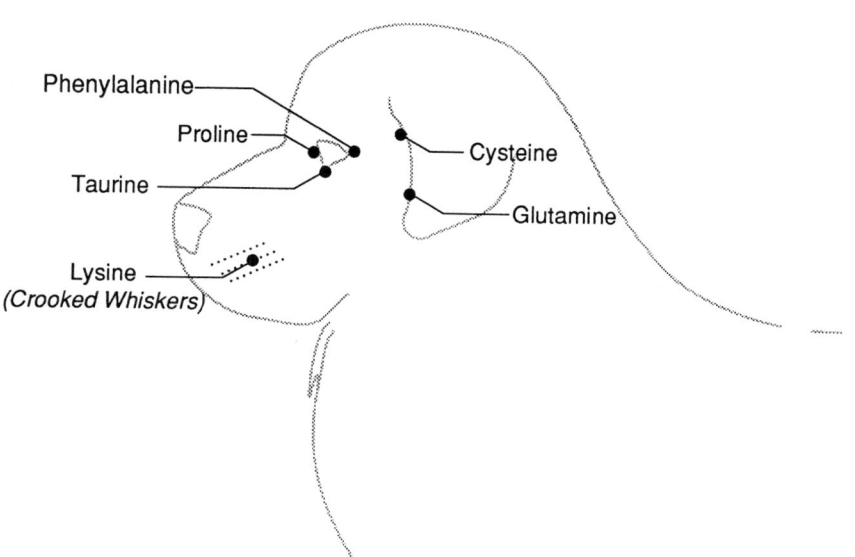

Left Hind

Left Front
(Look for crooked nails)

2-1: The Amino Acid Dog

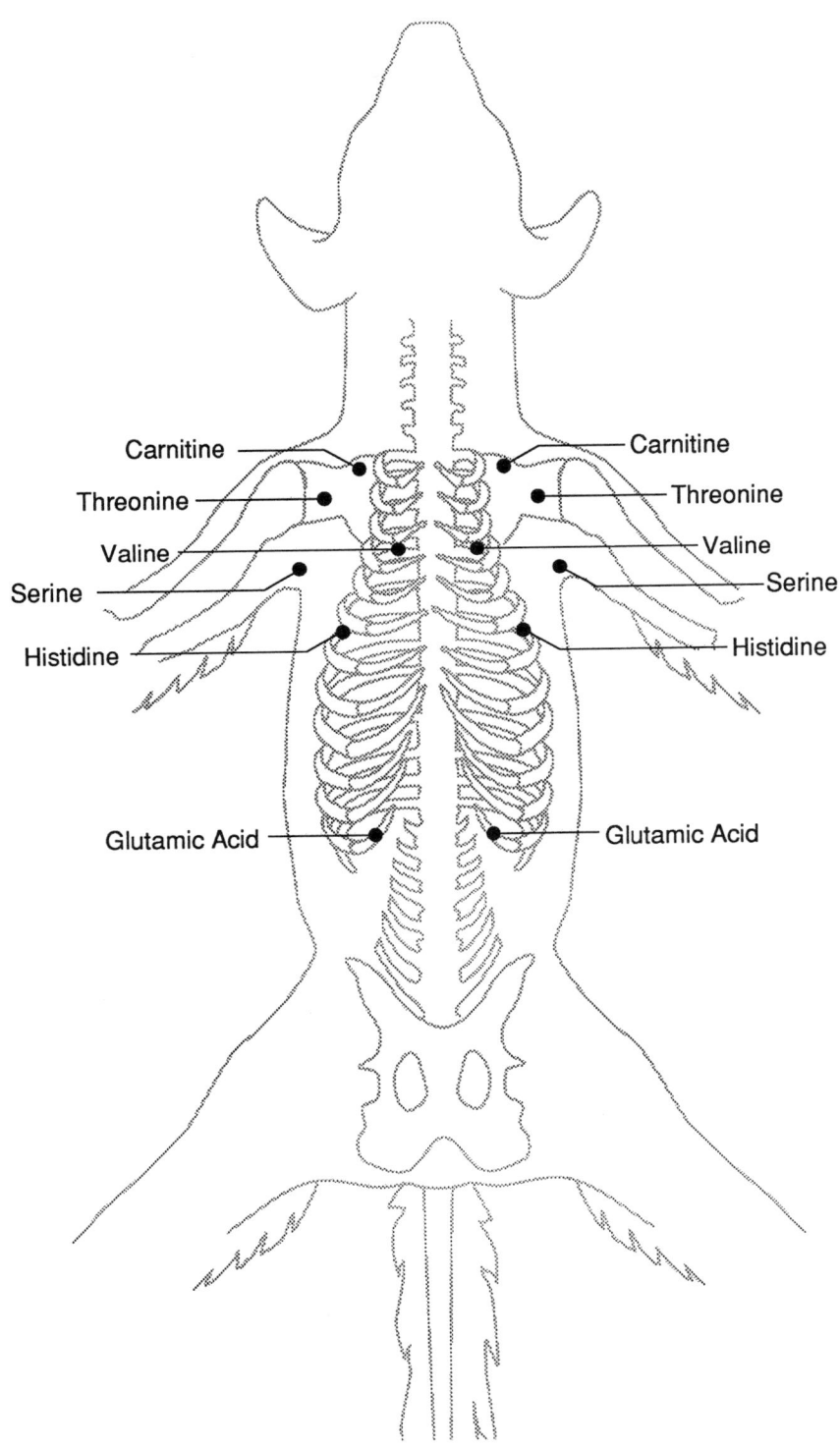

2-2: The Amino Acid Dog (underside)

include disease, medications and surgery or any other trauma to body tissue.

3. YOU CAN TEST TO SEE IF YOUR DOG IS DEFICIENT IN AMINO ACIDS. If you wish to supplement the dog's diet, test each of the following supplements to see what is best for your dog. Needs change with the seasons, so test several times during the year. Test procedures are outlined in Chapter 13 (Kinesiology).

Animal protein: Raw meat, raw liver, cooked meat (lamb, pork or venison), cooked chicken, cooked fish, milk, whole eggs (cooked for 5 minutes, plus shell), yogurt, kefir, cottage cheese, goats' milk. You can add a small amount of any of these proteins to your dog's diet. In total, supplementation should not exceed 10 percent of your dog's total diet.

Protein mixes: Test first. These can come from soy products to which many dogs are allergic.

Amino acid complex tablets. We like this form of supplement. The one that we use and that tests very well for most dogs comes from a milk (casein) base. This has not created allergies in the dogs we have tested. We prefer the complex tablet because without good reason it is unadvisable to isolate any of the amino acids when feeding dogs. Their interdependency is such that unless you have a degree in chemistry and understand fully how the isolated amino acid works, more harm can be done than good. Avoid supplementing with methionine alone if there is a history of liver disease. Too much methionine in relationship to other amino acids can cause coma and even death in dogs that have diseased livers. See Appendix I.

4. WHEN YOU SUPPLEMENT, MAKE SURE THAT THE DIET CONTAINS ADEQUATE VITAMIN C AND B COMPLEX, NECESSARY FOR PROTEIN DIGESTION.

5. MAGNESIUM MUST BE PRESENT IN THE DIET FOR THE EAAS TO WORK. A good vitamin-mineral mix such as that suggested in the Sources chapter would contain adequate amounts of minerals and vitamins B and C to complement the amino acids.

—Chapter 3—

Fat and Preservatives

Fat is necessary to provide energy as well as supple skin and a good hair coat. Fat is also needed in order for other nutrients to be absorbed. Every cell in the body contains fat, which transports the fat-soluble vitamins A, D, E and K through the body. It helps in the digestion of vitamin D, needed for the utilization of calcium in the body. Fats keep cells strong to protect them from invasion from microorganisms and damage by chemicals. They play an important part in the healthy functioning of the nervous system and in the manufacture of steroids and sex hormones. Cholesterol, the "good" kind, is responsible for some of the functions that support health of the brain, nervous system, liver, blood and skin. Internally, fat protects the vital organs from trauma and temperature change by providing padding and insulation. Fatty tissues even help to regulate body temperature.

Differences in Fats

There are two kinds of *fat*. One is the kind obtained *from animal tissues* (saturated fats) and the other *from plants* (polyunsaturated fats). Animal fat provides energy for the dog and is identified on the dog food package as poultry fat or beef tallow. Poultry fat from turkey or chicken is very digestible, and it also contains fatty acids necessary for a glossy coat. Beef tallow is less digestible and does not contain the same quantities of fatty acids.

Animal fats are the most concentrated form of energy (calories) that your dog can eat. Fats provide twice the energy of protein and carbohydrates. Still, a food that contains too much fat can be dangerous. A dog will eat less of a high-fat food and will subsequently suffer from deficiencies of other nutrients.

Fat from plants comes in the form of vegetable oils such as corn, wheat germ, sesame seed, lecithin, soybean and safflower oils. All contain the necessary ingredients for a **healthy coat** and soft, pliable skin.

The three ingredients in fat that contribute to **skin and hair coat** are **linoleic acid, linolenic acid and arachidonic acid**. These fatty acids are essential for a healthy life and are available only through what your dog eats.

When fats enter the stomach, they rise to the top and are therefore digested last. A meal high in fat causes the stomach to empty more slowly. When fats enter the small intestine, they are broken down further by bile that is secreted by the gallbladder. After this process, enzymes are released by the small intestine and pancreas so that the fatty acids can be released and used by the body. About 95 percent of the fat eaten by your dog is absorbed into the system, the rest is eliminated through the large intestine into the stool. Too much fat will make the stools shiny and has been related to high cholesterol, heart disease, mammary tumors in females and some forms of cancer of the colon.

The life stage of your dog will affect how much fat is needed. A young, growing dog needs fat in order to stimulate growth and to maintain healthy skin and coat. Puppies receiving too little fat have been shown to develop skin problems on the abdomen and thigh and between the shoulder blades. The skin becomes thickened and then ulcerated. Puppies fed a diet too high in fat fail to grow well, being deprived of the proper ratio of nutrients needed for correct growth.

Adult dogs that lead a sedentary life need less fat in their diet and quickly become obese if the diet is not adjusted to their needs. Working dogs, on the other hand, need a high-fat diet. Fat can be stored by the body and utilized when needed. A sled dog working in subzero temperatures will need a diet high in fat, just as will a hunting dog working in a hot, humid climate. Older dogs, because of their reduced exercise levels, will need less fat than younger dogs.

The best combination for your dog is a food that contains a mixture of animal fat and vegetable fat. Your dog gets energy and the essential fatty acids from both sources.

Fat found in dog food comes not only from animal fat and vegetable oils but many other ingredients as well. Cereal grains contain a certain percentage of fat. The fat listed on the dog food package is a combination of the fat in all of the ingredients.

If your dog's diet needs to be supplemented with fat, a **small** amount—1 teaspoon for dogs under 50 pounds and up to 1 tablespoon for larger dogs—of **cold** pressed safflower oil is probably the best. It has one of the highest linoleic acid contents, 95 percent to corn oil's 10 percent, and it has the least chance of causing an allergic reaction.

Fat in the food you feed your dog should constitute between 12 and 20 percent of the dry weight of the total diet.

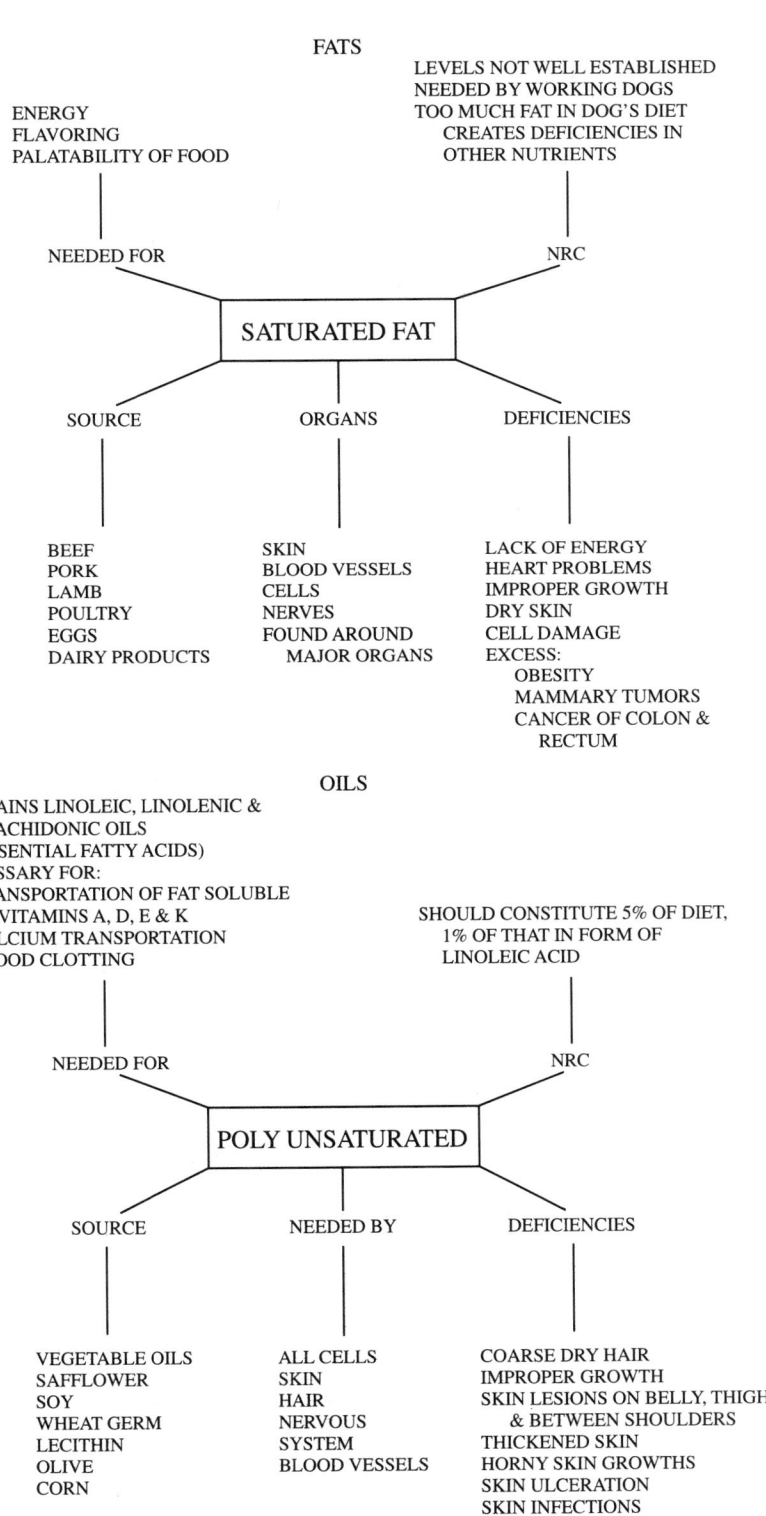

FATS

LEVELS NOT WELL ESTABLISHED
NEEDED BY WORKING DOGS
TOO MUCH FAT IN DOG'S DIET
CREATES DEFICIENCIES IN
OTHER NUTRIENTS

ENERGY
FLAVORING
PALATABILITY OF FOOD

NEEDED FOR

NRC

SATURATED FAT

SOURCE

ORGANS

DEFICIENCIES

BEEF
PORK
LAMB
POULTRY
EGGS
DAIRY PRODUCTS

SKIN
BLOOD VESSELS
CELLS
NERVES
FOUND AROUND
   MAJOR ORGANS

LACK OF ENERGY
HEART PROBLEMS
IMPROPER GROWTH
DRY SKIN
CELL DAMAGE
EXCESS:
   OBESITY
   MAMMARY TUMORS
   CANCER OF COLON &
     RECTUM

OILS

CONTAINS LINOLEIC, LINOLENIC &
   ARACHIDONIC OILS
   (ESSENTIAL FATTY ACIDS)
NECESSARY FOR:
   TRANSPORTATION OF FAT SOLUBLE
     VITAMINS A, D, E & K
   CALCIUM TRANSPORTATION
   BLOOD CLOTTING

SHOULD CONSTITUTE 5% OF DIET,
   1% OF THAT IN FORM OF
   LINOLEIC ACID

NEEDED FOR

NRC

POLY UNSATURATED

SOURCE

NEEDED BY

DEFICIENCIES

VEGETABLE OILS
SAFFLOWER
SOY
WHEAT GERM
LECITHIN
OLIVE
CORN

ALL CELLS
SKIN
HAIR
NERVOUS
SYSTEM
BLOOD VESSELS

COARSE DRY HAIR
IMPROPER GROWTH
SKIN LESIONS ON BELLY, THIGH
   & BETWEEN SHOULDERS
THICKENED SKIN
HORNY SKIN GROWTHS
SKIN ULCERATION
SKIN INFECTIONS
POOR BLOOD CLOTTING

3-1 and 3-2

Preservatives

It is not possible to talk about fat in the diet without talking about those substances that are used to preserve it. Vegetable oils become rancid quickly when exposed to even moderate temperatures and are vulnerable to heat, light and oxygen. Animal fats are a little more stable, but they also spoil quickly. Rancidity causes chemical chain reactions in the body that affect the utilization and absorption of other ingredients, often destroying joint fluids. Scientists think that lameness and arthritis in older dogs can come from the cumulative effect of feeding foods that have rancid fat.

Dog food manufacturers have a choice of which preservatives to use. They can use natural preservatives such as vitamins E and C, or they can use synthetic preservatives such as BHA, BHT or ethoxyquin. The natural preservatives do not change the food and become an integral part of it, allowing the cells of the body to become stronger and resist penetration. They have a shorter shelf life (6–8 months) than do foods preserved chemically (several years), and are only as good as the distribution system.

BHA and **BHT** are preservatives commonly used in animal food. It is how these preservatives are metabolized by the body and the changes that occur from using them that can be dangerous. These chemicals have been linked to depression of white blood cells and inhibiting the immune system as well as the absorption of glucose. Although strict regulation controls how much of these preservatives are used in prepared food for humans, there is less control in animal feeds.

Ethoxyquin has been the most debated preservative used in dog food. Since it was first added to dog foods, many breeders and pet owners have told stories of sterility and decreased fertility; deformed puppies; periodontal disease; precancerous lesions of the liver, kidney and bladder; vaccine failure; and increased incidence of cataracts. Ethoxyquin was originally approved by the FDA as a grain preservative intended for animals raised to be killed for food, and it was to be used no longer than 2 years. The safety of feeding it to dogs who live 10 to 12 years has never been proven, and the original studies run by the company who manufactured ethoxyquin were seriously flawed. Other countries have conducted studies on ethoxyquin and found it to be unsafe for long-term use in dog food. There is now a petition before the FDA to withdraw its use from the dog food market. Although ethoxyquin is still used as preservatives in some foods, the trend today is for more foods to be naturally preserved. It seems as if the marketplace is responding to dog owners' needs.

Foods that are naturally preserved have a short shelf life and need to be bought from a source that has a high turnover. If, when you open the package, the food smells rancid, return it. Always check the date of manufacture. If in doubt, call the manufacturer. Look in the chapter "Reading Labels" for information on reading the bar code dates on the package. Also, avoid foods where the fat has "bled" through the packaging. Foods containing BHA/BHT or ethoxyquin have longer shelf lives, but the continued feeding of these foods may cause long-term health problems for your dog.

Summary

1. FAT FROM ANIMAL SOURCES PROVIDES ENERGY FOR YOUR DOG AND CAN KEEP HIM WARM IN THE WINTER AND COOL IN THE SUMMER. Some animal fats have a small amount of essential fatty acids in them.
2. FAT FROM PLANTS IS A GOOD SOURCE OF ESSENTIAL FATTY ACIDS (EFAs), NECESSARY FOR GOOD SKIN AND COAT.
3. CLIMATE, BREED AND LIFE STAGE, AS WELL AS THE JOB YOUR DOG PERFORMS, WILL DICTATE NEEDS FOR FAT.
4. FATS SPOIL EASILY. If your dog food smells rancid, throw it away. Eating rancid food can cause your dog all sorts of health-related problems.
5. STORE DOG FOOD PROPERLY. If you buy in large quantities, take what you need for a few days and keep it in the refrigerator. The rest can be frozen and used as needed. This is crucial in hot weather.
6. LEARN TO READ LABELS. If your food contains ethoxyquin it has a great likelihood of causing long-term health problems for your dog and should not be used. If the food contains BHA/BHT, be aware that these preservatives have been linked to cancer in humans.
7. IF YOU ARE USING A DOG FOOD THAT IS PRESERVED WITH NATURAL VITAMINS, MAKE SURE THAT THE SOURCE FROM WHICH YOU BUY IT HAS A HIGH TURNOVER IN SALES. Natural foods have a short shelf life.
8. IF YOU ARE UNSURE WHETHER YOUR FOOD IS FRESH OR NOT, TAKE THE BAR CODE DATE AND CALL THE MANUFACTURER, WHO MUST, UNDER LABELING LAWS, LIST THE COMPANY PHONE NUMBER ON EVERY PACKAGE OF DOG FOOD. See the chapter on labeling for telephone numbers of manufacturers.

Canine Teeth

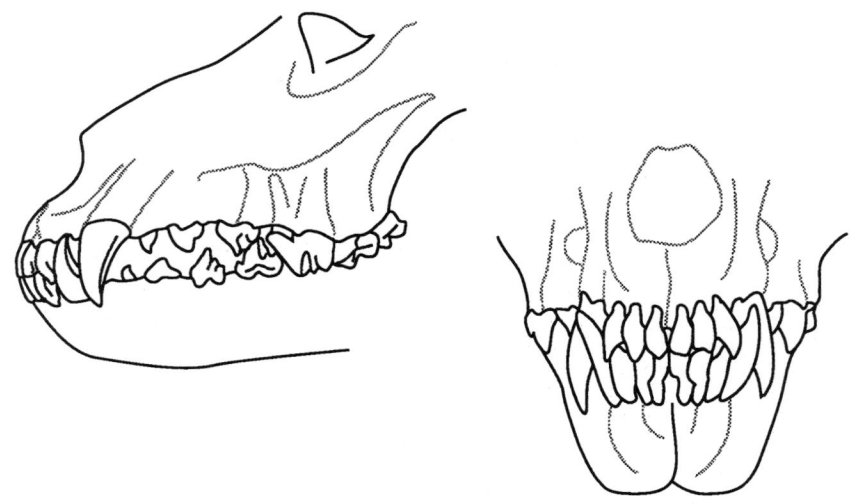

Human Teeth

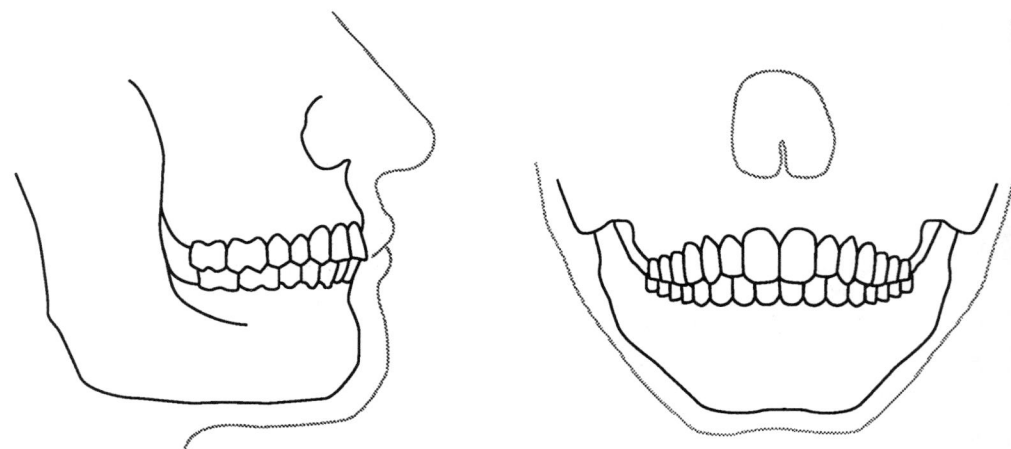

4-1: Comparison of Canine and Human Teeth

—Chapter 4—

Carbohydrates

There is a significant difference between humans and dogs in their need for carbohydrates and in their ability to digest them. The digestive tract of a human is longer than that of a dog, and the formation of jaws and teeth is entirely different. A dog's digestion starts in the stomach. Dogs' teeth— all 42 of them—are built to tear flesh apart. Dogs gulp their food as fast as they can, which then reaches the stomach with no digestion having taken place.

Human digestion starts in the mouth. A human chews food with 32 teeth, which have flat surfaces for grinding and breaking down food. Enzymes contained in the saliva contribute to this breakdown of the food, which is being digested before it reaches the stomach.

Carbohydrates come in two forms, simple and complex. Simple carbohydrates come from grains such as wheat, corn, rice, oats, soy and millet. They break down into starches and sugar when properly cooked. Complex carbohydrates come in the form of various fibers such as brans, hulls and peanut shells from the outside of plants plus pulps and pomaces from the inside of plants. A small amount is needed for proper digestion and stool formation. Nutrients are obtained from both sources, but most come from simple carbohydrates.

If carbohydrates are a major part of your dog's diet, the time and energy needed for digestion increase, the dog performs less well, large amounts of stool are produced, and a protein-deficiency disease may develop. Dogs have evolved as meat eaters and although they need some grains, their health and longevity will be better served on a diet containing more animal protein than protein from grains.

Think about the origin of the dog. It is unrecorded in history that wolves lit fires and cooked grains picked in fields! But there were whole carcasses available that contained everything needed for wolves to survive, including predigested vegetable matter in the intestinal tracts of their prey.

The reason the majority of dry dog foods contain such large amounts of cereal grains is that grains are a cheap source of nutrients. According to the NRC guidelines, "Carbohydrates provide an economical source of energy in the diet of dogs."

In a series of articles on nutrition in *Dog World* magazine in 1993, John Cargill writes that checking the package labels reveals the limited amount of animal protein in commercial dog food.

> [A] food label listed in order of weight; chicken, wheat, soy, corn and rice, might have the following percentages by weight: chicken—21 percent, wheat—20 percent, soy—20 percent, corn—20 percent, rice—10 percent. This is not a "chicken based" product. It is a cereal-based product with a ratio of cereal to chicken of 70:21 or 3.3:1. There is no way to tell from the labelling or from the advertising.

Allergic reactions to grains are common in dogs. The best diet for your dog matches that fed in the breed's country of origin as the breed developed. Each dog is an individual, and if yours refuses to eat his food, check the grains listed on the package. The dog may balk because of an allergy to one of the grains in the food.

Deficiency diseases can arise from using foods that are almost exclusively grain based. Usually they are the cheaper foods, which contain soy. Writing in January 1993 for *Good Dog!, The Consumer Magazine For Dog Owners*, Thomas Willard, a private consultant in the pet food industry, states

> . . . soybean meal, soy flour or corn gluten meal should never be the primary or even the secondary source of protein in a Super-premium or Performance food. Though these vegetable proteins are used in most animal feeds, they should not be used in the diets of carnivores such as dogs or cats. . . . soy is not an appropriate ingredient in dog food: It's one of the ingredients used in making pet foods that keep their nutrients "locked up." These are so poorly digested that the dog can't get enough to meet his daily requirements. . . . Soybean and cottonseed meals . . . contain anti-nutritional factors that Mother Nature put there to prevent digestion. . . . Soy and cottonseed meal should not be included in a puppy or senior diet. . . . These animals don't have the proper enzymes to "unlock" enough of these nutrients to grow or perform optimally.

A partial list put out by the AAFCO defining grains that are used in dog foods is in Appendix II. AAFCO allows a certain percentage of other grains to be included in the overall name of the grain. For example, a dog food listing an ingredient as "barley, 20 percent" may actually contain some corn. If your dog were allergic to corn you could come to the conclusion that he was allergic to barley!

Allergies to Grains
Most common: Corn, wheat, rice and rye
Least common: Oats, buckwheat, millet, quinoa

Acid, Alkaline Balance

Grains contain incomplete proteins, fat and various vitamins and minerals. They are divided into acid and alkaline. How acidic or alkaline those grains are will determine palatability and overall health of internal organs and skin. A diet too alkaline will tend to produce inflammation of the kidneys and urinary tract, resulting in diseases that produce stones or calculi and, more commonly, cystitis. A diet too acidic will produce mucousy stools, the coughing up of phlegm and runny eyes. Both can create vomiting and diarrhea.

Acid Base	Alkaline Base
Barley	Millet
Wheat	Buckwheat
Oats	Soy
Rye	Sprouted grains
Most breads	Quinoa

Grains in the Middle

Brown rice
  (leans more toward
  acid side of chart)
Corn (leans more toward
  acid side, depending on
  which part of the grain is used)

Determining which grain is acid based and which is alkaline based is confusing. For example, some sources state that corn is acid based and others that it is alkaline based. It is the same with barley and rice. We suspect that this relates to the part of the grain being used and where it was grown. The preceding chart is based on our own kinesiology testing results.

You can check to see if the food you are feeding your dog has the correct acid-alkaline balance. Put a pH strip into your dog's urine first thing in the morning. You can also test the dog's saliva. The pH of your dog's urine and saliva should be within the 6.2–6.5 range. If the result is substantially different from what it should be, you need to change your dog's diet.

The Digestive Tract

The digestive tract itself turns the food from an acid base in the stomach to an alkaline one in the intestines, and the balance changes as the food proceeds through the system. Wastes are excreted at the proper pH through either the bladder or bowels. It's a tricky journey, and to enjoy full health, your dog must have the necessary nutrients to make it all work properly. Feed correctly and the system works; unbalance it and the dog becomes ill.

Toxins Commonly Found in Stored Grains

Mycotoxicosis is the term used to describe the toxic effects of fungal growth in grains or other foodstuffs that have been exposed to moisture and heat. If present, *these toxins can be deadly* to your dog. Detectable only by laboratory analysis, they are not killed by heat.

University studies have shown that these toxins are capable of inducing cancer, mutations, suppressed immune functions, reduced response to vaccines and liver disease. Mostly found in grains grown in the southeastern states, these toxins have been responsible for many diseases found in dogs that were fed foods composed primarily of grains.

Aflatoxins are produced by aspergillus flavus and aspergillus parasitcus, which grow in corn, cottonseed and peanuts. They grow on the grains in the field, in storage and after processing. Feeding dogs from hoppers or feeding them outside, leaving the food exposed to the heat, light and air, produces aflatoxins in the food.

Another fungus, called **penitrem A**, is a common contaminant of household foodstuffs. Reports have shown that dogs ingesting moldy cheese or nuts thrown away in the garbage have exhibited muscle tremors, generalized seizures and nosebleeds, and in some cases they have died. Other fungi have been reported in Canadian wheat, oats, barley and rye. *If your dog food smells moldy or shows any kind of growth when you open the bag, throw it away or return it.*

It has been reported that contaminated cereal grains have been used in dog foods in the past. If your dogs refuse to eat a food they have previously enjoyed, pay attention! The food may be contaminated. If, after eating, your dog shows any signs of poisoning, go to a veterinarian immediately.

Summary

1. FOOD IS ETHNIC AND THEREFORE SHOULD BE BREED RELATED. Dog foods should contain cereals as close to those fed when and where the breed was developed.
2. DOGS ARE CARNIVORES, WHICH MEANS THEIR DIGESTIVE TRACT WAS DEVELOPED TO DIGEST A DIET CONTAINING *MORE MEAT THAN CEREAL GRAINS*. Some breeds have been able to adapt to a diet higher in cereal grains than animal protein; many breeds have not.
3. FOODS THAT LIST A LARGE NUMBER OF CEREAL GRAINS IN THEIR INGREDIENTS OFTEN ARE CEREAL-BASED FOODS EVEN IF THE FIRST INGREDIENT LISTED IS FROM AN ANIMAL PROTEIN.
4. CEREALS INDIVIDUALLY ARE DEFICIENT IN PROTEIN. They **do not contain all necessary amino acids**. Look for a mixture of grains on the label.
5. SOME CEREALS CAN CAUSE ALLERGIES IN CERTAIN BREEDS.
6. AMINO ACIDS FROM ANIMAL PROTEIN SOURCES COUNTERACT ALLERGIES TO GRAINS WHEN FED IN THE PROPER PROPORTION.
7. CEREALS PROVIDE AN ECONOMICAL WAY TO FEED DOGS.
8. MANY NUTRIENTS IN CEREAL ARE "BOUND UP" AND NOT AVAILABLE FOR THE DOG DURING THE DIGESTIVE PROCESS. This is especially true of soy and cottonseed.
9. GRAINS CONTAIN RESIDUES OF FERTILIZERS USED ON THE FIELDS WHERE THEY GROW AND INSECTICIDES SPRAYED ON THE PLANTS. These chemicals can induce allergies.
10. THE ACID/ALKALINE BALANCE OF THE BODY CAN BE AFFECTED BY THE GRAINS USED IN DOG FOOD. If your dog shows a lot of discharge (eyes, nose, penis, vulva) and mucousy stools, the diet *may* be too acidic. (These symptoms could also indicate infection—check with your veterinarian.) Look for a food with grains on the alkaline side of the chart. If your dog shows a tendency to urinary tract infections or itchy skin, the diet may be too alkaline. Look for foods that have a higher percentage of protein from animal sources and grains that fall on the acid side of the chart.

Excerpt on pg. 18 from Dog World *magazine reprinted with permission.*

Excerpt on pg. 18 from Good Dog!®, The Consumer Magazine For Dog Owners, *© 1993 Good Dog! (800) 968-1738. All Rights Reserved. Reprinted with Permission.*

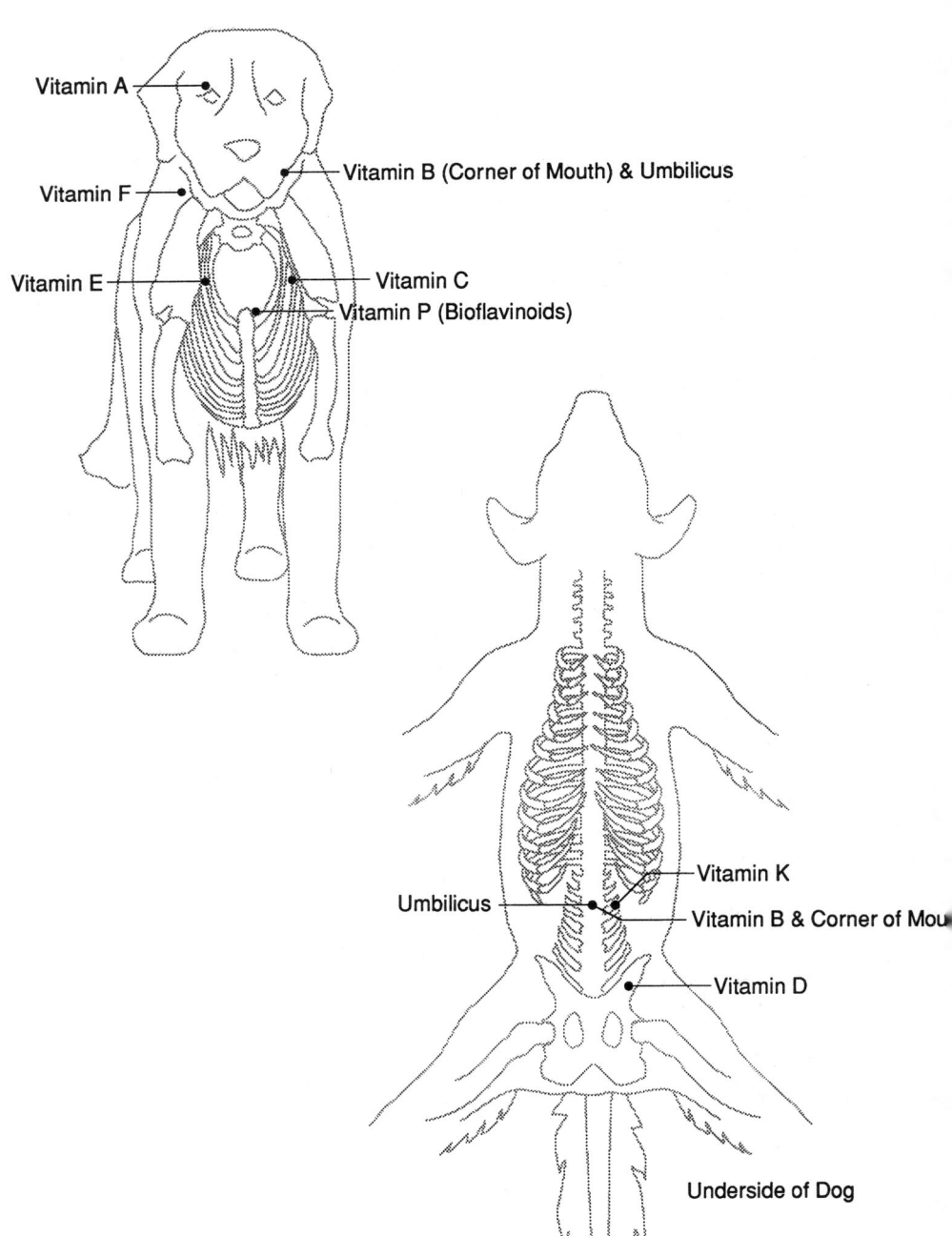

5-1: The Vitamin Dog

—Chapter 5—

Vitamins

Exciting research is being done all over the world on the influences of vitamins and minerals on health. Vitamins are essential to life and they contribute to good health by regulating the metabolism.

What Do They Do?

Vitamins release nutrients from ingested food and provide energy to the body. Some vitamins are fat soluble—vitamins **A**, **D**, **E** and **K**—and others are water soluble—vitamins **B** and **C**. Fat-soluble vitamins can be stored by the body in fatty tissue and the liver. Water-soluble vitamins are excreted daily and cannot be stored. Both types of vitamins are needed by the body.

Destruction of Vitamins

Many vitamins are destroyed by temperatures over 118 degrees Fahrenheit. Dog food processing temperatures are well above this level. If care is not taken to compensate for these losses, food that is deficient in vitamins is produced. Some companies use a micro-encapsulation process to avoid the destruction of vitamins and minerals in the manufacturing process. They also add extra vitamins and minerals to compensate for loss. In our research, we could not get a satisfactory answer to the question of how the manufacturer knows that the end product has sufficient vitamins. Perhaps there is no answer. Currently no guidelines exist that provide this information to the industry because the research has not been done.

Although dogs' needs for certain vitamins have been recorded, the National Research Council's findings tell us that *precise* quantities of these vitamins are not well established. The NRC found "reasonable" levels based on requirements of other species of animals as well as the dog. The needs of breeding and working dogs have not been calculated, but the NRC agrees that those animals need higher levels of some vitamins—how much more, no one seems to know for sure. No studies were presented to the NRC on the needs of the giant breeds or dogs over 75 pounds at maturity. The NRC states that some vitamins are unstable and may be destroyed by light, heat, oxidation and rancidity of other ingredients and that dog food should contain sufficient amounts in the manufacturing process to allow for the above considerations.

The conclusion can be drawn that the guidelines presented to the dog food companies, which form the basis of the recipes for making dog food, are incomplete. The industry has become aware of this and is in the process of updating the guidelines.

Minimum Daily Requirement (MDR)

When laboratory testing is done to determine how much of a certain substance a dog needs to live (minimum daily requirement) and how much of that substance would create toxic levels (hypervitaminosis), the dog is usually a young laboratory-bred beagle kept in a cage for the length of the experiment. Some of these puppies are fed a laboratory diet consisting of amino acids, soy protein and concentrated protein from milk. Other studies provide no information on the basic diet fed. It appears that no double-blind studies have been done, and those studies that have been done appear to be less than scientific. The information comes to the National Research Council from many laboratories, and to our knowledge, there is no one laboratory diet that is fed to all of these dogs. Further, no mention is made in most of the studies of the use of control dogs.

Dog foods are guaranteed to meet and not to exceed the *known* Minimum Daily Requirement of nutrients established to keep laboratory dogs alive for 24 hours. These requirements were changed in 1985 from the old requirements, printed in 1975, which stated that dog food should not only meet but *exceed* the known levels of nutrients. After 1985 the industry cut back on the levels of some of the nutrients put into dog food. We have noticed a decline in the overall health of dogs since these changes were made.

Dog foods are manufactured to meet the needs of the majority of dogs. There are many dogs whose needs are not met, and their diets will have to be supplemented in order for them to enjoy healthy lives.

How to Read the Charts

Each vitamin is listed by name, along with its purpose. Health states associated with each vitamin are included as well as digestibility and deficiency symptoms. Some of this information comes from studies done on dogs and other animals, but we have also included the latest, up-to-date information available from human research. If there are toxic symptoms associated with a vitamin, that too is listed. Toxic levels have been determined in a laboratory by feeding dogs 500 to 1500 times the level of the nutrient.

We have included a section on cravings. Our experience has been that dogs often crave certain foods such as vegetables, meats, fats, grasses and weeds. This usually signifies that their systems are out of balance. If your dog shows a craving for a particular food, pay attention.

Indicator Points

We have illustrated "indicator points" for most of the vitamins. These points can be used for diagnostic purposes. Biting, licking or scratching at these points may indicate a deficiency or excess of that particular nutrient. It may also indicate a genetic predisposition for a deficiency or an inability to digest that nutrient in the form being fed. Pimples, discolored skin and skin eruptions on these points will signify the same thing. Use kinesiology testing (chapter 13) to check your dog.

Vitamins

Supplement:	**Vitamin A.** Fat soluble.
Purpose:	Needed for the eyes, appetite, bone remodeling, nerve functions (especially the optic and cranial nerves), skin, hair, teeth and gums, as well as building resistance against respiratory disorders.
Credited with:	Healthy eyes, curing night blindness, laying down new bone during growth and promoting healthy teeth. After any kind of injury, vitamin A helps tissue repair and protects against infection. Gives healthy skin its structural integrity, as well as the mucous membranes (lining of the nose, eyes, intestinal tract, respiratory lining and the bladder). Acts as an antioxidant, protecting the body from rancid fat and air pollution. Promotes immune response. Works best if the diet contains adequate amounts of Vitamin D, zinc and high-quality protein.
Digestibility:	Available in oil form (fish oil), which is fat soluble, or beta carotene, which is water soluble. Vitamin A is stored by the liver, so avoid using high doses for long periods of time.

Deficiencies:	Eye diseases, deafness, inability to grow, skin lesions and susceptibility to infection and nerve damage.
Toxicity:	Lack of appetite and tenderness of joints, especially extremities, and an unwillingness to stand. Improper formation of long bones. Lesions in arteries and veins of the heart, gallbladder and urinary system as well as microhemorrhages. *Cleft palates in puppies.*
Cravings for:	Carrots, yellow fruit, green leafy vegetables, liver, eggs, milk products.

Supplement:	**Vitamin D.** Fat soluble.
Purpose:	Needed for proper absorption of calcium and phosphorus, which promote bone growth. As a hormone it helps to control the action of the parathyroid gland, which regulates calcium in the body.
Credited with:	Absorption of vitamin A, proper bone growth and strengthening of the teeth. Used in treatment of eye conditions.
Digestibility:	Now recognized as a hormone that can be synthesized from exposure to sunlight. Found in plant and animal tissue. Vitamin D_2 is the synthetic form and Vitamin D_3 is the natural form, which occurs in fish liver oils.

Needs to be taken with vitamin A, and is more effective with choline, vitamin C, essential fatty acids, calcium and phosphorus. It is stored by the body. |
| **Deficiencies:** | Rickets, imbalance in calcium and phosphorus levels, osteoporosis. |
| **Cravings:** | Fish, milk and dairy products. A small amount of vitamin D is found in mushrooms and dark green leafy vegetables. |

Supplement:	**Vitamin E.** Fat soluble.
Purpose:	An antioxidant, it prevents unsaturated fatty acids, sex hormones and fat-soluble vitamins from being destroyed in the body by free radicals. Gives the tissues oxygen and reduces the need for oxygen intake. Prevents rancidity when added to other substances. Dilates blood vessels and improves circulation. Prevents scar tissue from forming and aids in the healing of burns and sores. Helps to prevent blood clots.

Protects lungs and other tissues from air pollution. Retards the aging process. Essential for healthy function of reproductive organs. Used successfully in the treatment of sterility, heart disease, arthritis in old dogs (together with selium, which enjoys a symbiotic relationship with vitamin E), leg ulcers and hypoglycemia. Promotes testicle growth and production of sperm. Prevents weak and dead puppies, and weakness of the skeletal muscles. Vitamin E is stored in fatty tissues. It is essential for nuclei of cells and utilization of sex hormones, cholesterol and vitamin D. Destroyed by rancid fats or ultraviolet light (sunlight).

Digestibility: Comes in the following forms: Alpha, beta, gamma and delta tocopherols. D-Alpha is natural and is the most potent form of vitamin E. The synthetic version is called dl-Alpha and is the one used in most dog foods. Available as mixed tocopherols. Found in some dairy products and liver, the best source is cold pressed vegetable oils, safflower oil containing the largest amount. Wheat germ oil also contains vitamin E. Available in oil, capsules or tablet form.

Deficiencies: Destruction of red blood cells, muscle degeneration, reproductive disorders, poor sperm count, inability to breed or carry puppies full term through gestation period, prolonged deliveries, heart and circulation problems, plus some anemias. Elevated plasma creatinine phosphokinase values. Retinal degeneration. A combined vitamin E and selenium deficiency could show up as muscle weakness(especially in old dogs), edema, lack of appetite, depression, heart and renal disease.

Cravings: Lettuce, celery, green leafy vegetables, broccoli, Brussels sprouts, whole wheat bread, alfalfa, salad dressings made with safflower oil.

Supplement: **Vitamin K.** Fat soluble.

Purpose: Essential in the formation of the blood-clotting factor, prothrombin. Can be destroyed by rat poisons (Warfarin).

Credited with: Although no studies were presented to the NRC to prove vitamin K was necessary to dogs if fed an

Digestibility: adequate diet, the NRC guidelines suggest it would be prudent to add it to the diet for its blood-clotting abilities. Most foods contain vitamin K.
Vitamin K_1 and K_2 are made by the body from naturally occurring bacteria in the intestines. Vitamin K_3 is the synthetic kind found in dog food, listed as menadione sodium bisulfite complex. It is a fat-soluble vitamin.

Deficiencies: Diarrhea and colitis can be symptomatic. It helps prevent massive hemorrhages, internal bleeding and nosebleeds.

Toxicity: Too much Vitamin K_3 can cause hemolytic anemia.

Cravings: Yogurt, alfalfa, egg yolk, safflower and soybean oils, kelp, green leafy vegetables, fish and fish liver oils, cabbage, kale and cauliflower.

Supplement: **Vitamin C.** Water soluble.

Purpose: Needed for healthy teeth, gums and bones. Strengthens all connective tissue. Speeds wound healing and promotes capillary integrity. Helps provide immunity to disease. Used in growing dogs to promote collagen production. Females in season, in whelp, and nursing mothers, as well as geriatric dogs that are getting a bit stiff in the joints, all benefit from vitamin C supplementation. Helps to bring down temperatures. Should always be used in conjunction with steroid therapy. Use when any drugs are being used—e.g., antibiotics, wormers, etc.

Credited with: Helping to maintain the correct pH balance for the urinary tract, thus reducing symptoms of cystitis and other bladder infections. Invaluable for keeping the whole digestive system acidic. Essential to the function of several amino acids. Important in the formation of collagen. Necessary for the growth and repair of tissue cells, gums, blood vessels, bones and teeth. Helps the body absorb iron. Accelerates healing after surgery. Used as a preventative, claims have been made that it prevents hip displaysia, distemper, bronchitis, fever, loss of appetite, coughing, allergies, cystitis, spinal degeneration and stress if fed to young, growing puppies. Anti-fatigue vitamin, increases endurance. Used in cancer therapy.

Vitamin C is a detoxifier and diuretic. Promotes production of interferon, an antiviral agent, and transportation of material through cell structures. As an antioxidant it is used to prevent aging and to counteract effects of preservatives used in dog food.

Digestibility: Ascorbic acid, sodium ascorbate, calcium ascorbate. Comes in powder, tablet or crystal form. A water-soluble vitamin that passes through the body in 4 to 8 hours. Vitamin C overdosing can be judged by bowel tolerance. Too much creates a runny stool. Helps absorption of other vitamins, especially B-complex vitamins and amino acids. Young and old dogs, as well as pregnant or lactating females, seem to do best on calcium ascorbate. We use vitamin C in the form of calcium ascorbate as it is the buffered and most gentle form of vitamin C and produces the least incidence of allergic reactions. Ascorbic acid and sodium ascorbate are tolerated well by most dogs in small doses. Most effective when doses are given every 4 hours to keep levels constant in the body. Necessary when traveling, showing, visiting the veterinarian or any other occasion when your dog becomes stressed.

Ester-C is a new form of vitamin C that acts more like a time-released product, staying in the body longer than other types of vitamin C. More expensive than other varieties, only half the amount is given. Used in some of the natural dog foods. All vitamin C should be stored in a cool, dry place out of the light to stop the oxidization process, which renders it useless. Too much vitamin C depletes the body of sulphur. The dog's body manufactures vitamin C, the levels of which are quickly depleted when small amounts of stress are experienced.

Deficiencies: Urinary tract and skin infections, bladder stones, poor immune system. Vitamin C can only do its work when the essential amino acids are present in every meal the dog eats.

Cravings: Tomatoes, citrus fruits, green peppers, cabbage, parsley, watercress, cantaloupe, watermelon, raspberries and certain grasses and weeds, especially goldenrod.

Supplement:	**Vitamin B-complex.** Water soluble.
Purpose:	As coenzymes, they promote biochemical reactions acting with enzymes to change carbohydrates into glucose, which provides energy. Necessary for fat and protein assimilation.
Credited with:	Promoting growth, helping to fight motion sickness. Helps the body deal with stress. Promotes healing after surgery. B-complex vitamins are important to the proper functioning of the nervous system and help energize and relax the system if suffering from fatigue. The liver, skin, hair, eyes, mucousal linings of the body, especially those around the mouth, are affected by the B vitamins. The whole gastrointestinal tract works better with correct levels of vitamin B in the system. Promotes proper bowel function. Used in cases of hyperactivity, many skin conditions, rashes, dermatitis, cracks around the mouth, as well as burning or sore tongue.

Comes as a complex containing all the B vitamins. Using a complex tablet is more effective than using an isolated part of the B-complex as the action of each vitamin depends on the amount of the others in the body. In nature, the B vitamins come together in the same food, and there is no case reported of a B vitamin found by itself. *Many B-complex vitamins are destroyed by cooking and food processing.*

| Digestibility: | Water soluble, flushes through the body in 4 to 8 hours. Must be replaced daily. No known cases of toxicity, but it would be inadvisable to overdose on one single part of the complex. Works in conjunction with other vitamins and is more effective when diet contains phosphorus. B-complex is made up of the following vitamins: |

B_1	Thiamine
B_2	Riboflavin
B_3	Niacin
B_5	Pantothenic Acid
B_6	Pyridoxine
B_9	Folic Acid
B_{12}	Cyanocobalamin

B_{13}	Orotic Acid
B_{15}	Pangamic Acid
B_{17}	Laetrile
	Biotin
	Choline
	Inositol
	PABA (Para Aminobenzoic Acid)

Deficiencies: Constipation, skin conditions, neuritis, hair loss and early graying, increased cholesterol levels, weakness of back legs, loss of appetite, stool eating, poor immune system, attracting fleas and other parasites, stress, fatigue, anxiety, nervousness, edema, heart disease and poor reaction to vaccines; see individual vitamins for other symptoms.

Cravings: Liver, milk, eggs, brewers yeast, wheat bran, wheat germ, kelp, molasses, kidney, heart.

Supplement: **Vitamin B$_1$ (thiamine)**
Purpose: Helps in protein and carbohydrate digestion, helps to produce hydrochloric acid in the stomach, improves the movement of food through the digestive tract (peristalsis), keeps the nervous system functioning normally. Needed more by dogs with *hypothyroidism*, females during lactation and growing puppies. Needs are affected by levels of protein, fat, vitamin C, lactose, sorbitol and penicillin in the diet. Dogs that eat their stools (*copraphagy*) show an increased need for thiamine. Losses of 74% have been noticed in cooked dog food. No known data has been presented to NRC regarding pregnancy or lactation.

Credited with: Promoting growth, improving mental attitude, fighting nausea from travel sickness. Used in treatment of herpes virus (suspected in fading puppy syndrome).

Deficiencies: Malnutrition where diets are high in processed rice and carbohydrates and low in protein and fat, as seen in many weight-loss diets for dogs. Stool eating, lack of appetite, depression of the central nervous system, going around in circles, convulsions, stiff and twisted neck, spasmodic contractions of the

31

neck muscles, partial paralysis of the back legs, muscular incoordination, overall muscular weakness, diseases of the brain and nervous system, and enlargement of the heart. Diseases expressed on the right side of the heart. Disintegration of the substance surrounding the nerves (myelin sheath).

Supplement:	**Vitamin B$_2$ (riboflavin)**
Purpose:	Acts as a precursor to two coenzymes that are important in energy production. Necessary for carbohydrate and fat digestion. Helps cells utilize oxygen and is necessary for proper cell growth. Counteracts **stress** during growth, reproduction, lactation and old age.
Credited with:	Promoting growth and reproduction. Promotes healthy skin, hair and nails, helps to eliminate lesions and cracks of mouth, lips and tongue. Useful in treatment of bloodshot eyes, itching and burning eyes and cataracts. Counteracts oily skin and hair, and splitting nails. Prevents stool eating.
Digestibility:	Good. Destroyed by sulphur drugs and hormone therapy. Should be used when dieting your dog. More effective when used with B-complex.
Deficiencies:	Lesions of mouth, skin, genitalia, cracked nails and poor, oily coat. Loss of weight, muscles in hindquarters weak. Dry, flaky skin, plus red patches on hind legs, chest and abdomen. Excessive shedding (dogs that shed year round), greasy feeling to coat (residue left on your hand after petting dog). Extreme "doggy" smell. Lesions, followed by discharge from the eyes. Stool eating. Redness, itchiness in the eyes and excessive tearing. Digestive upsets and skin ulcers. Leg cramps.

Supplement:	**Vitamin B$_3$ (niacin, niacinamide, nicotinic acid)**
Purpose:	Acts as part of two coenzymes that influence more than 50 different metabolic reactions. It plays an important role in glycosis (extracting energy from carbohydrates and glucose), in the processing of waste from amino acids (protein) and in the utilization of fatty acids. Helps certain drugs work better. One of the most stable of the B vitamins, being less susceptible to heat, light and oxygen than other

32

members of this family. Can be manufactured from the essential amino acid tryptophan, so if there is sufficient protein from a quality animal source, extra niacin is not necessary. When the diet is low in protein, extra niacin is needed. Mellows the personality. Prevents "black tongue" disease. How much niacin is needed depends on the dog's diet. **Diets high in corn require more niacin** than those where there is adequate animal protein provided. Cereal grains contain niacin, but they are bound up and the dog cannot digest them as easily. Niacin is added to most dog foods.

Credited with: Relieving irritability as well as allergic reactions to some fruits and vegetables. Stimulates circulation, reduces cholesterol level and is important to the normal function of the nervous system and the brain. It is needed for the proper synthesis of sex hormones such as estrogen, progesterone and testosterone and corticosteroids. Improves food utilization and has been used successfully in cases of digestive disorders such as diarrhea, constipation and indigestion. Helps in production of hydrochloric acid in the stomach, and aids in the regulation of blood sugar. Useful in the treatment of skin, teeth and gum diseases.

Digestibility: Good. Caution must be used when isolating this vitamin. Too much niacin causes "flushing" and increased blood pressure. If your dog is being treated for diabetes or liver or uric acid problems, use only small amounts. Dependent on the amount of tryptophan in the diet.

Deficiency: Four Ds: dermatitis, diarrhea and dementia (madness) followed by death. A deficiency of niacin was the cause of many human deaths in the American Civil War. It was caused by a diet high in corn, which contains niacin but in a form that is not digested well by the body. The term *redneck* was coined in the South to describe workers in the fields at the turn of the century. Workers whose necks were exposed to too much sunlight became extremely sensitive. They developed skin that was rough, thick, dry and darkly pigmented. This niacin deficiency caused death.

Symptoms include irritability and aggression, inability to eat, inflammation and ulceration of the inside of the mouth and pharynx, profuse salivation, bloody saliva hanging in ropes from the mouth, tender gums, foul breath. Bloody diarrhea, inflammation of the small intestine and degeneration of the large intestine. Absorption of food greatly disturbed; poor conditioned reflexes and degeneration of the spinal cord.

Supplement:	**Vitamin B$_5$ (pantothenic acid)** Also known as calcium pantothenate.
Purpose:	Stimulates adrenal glands to produce natural cortisone and hormones and as such is known as the ***"anti-stress"*** vitamin. It is thought to help prevent aging and is important to healthy skin and nerves. Through support of the adrenal gland, B$_5$ may reduce toxic effects of antibiotics and radiation. Necessary for proper utilization of fats and carbohydrates and supports many neurotransmitter (brain) functions. Essential for the synthesis of fatty acids, cholesterol and steroids. Used after surgery for paralysis of the gastrointestinal tract to stimulate peristalsis.
Credited with:	Helping to prevent hair loss, turning graying hair back to natural color, anti-stress vitamin, anti-aging, involved in all functions of the body; helpful in treating hypoglycemia; painful, burning feet; adrenal and emotional exhaustion. Used in dogs that grind their teeth at night or who have epilepsy, neuritis and multiple sclerosis; used as treatment for mental diseases in humans. As calcium pantothenate it has been helpful in reducing joint pain, stiffness and reducing arthritis symptoms.
Digestibility:	Produced by intestinal bacteria. Available in many foods, although a great percentage is lost in food processing, half in the milling process of grains and one third in cooking meat. Water soluble.
Deficiencies:	Emotionally oversensitive, premature graying of hair, low blood sugar, Addison's disease. Erratic appetite, ***lowered antibody response***. Spastic movements of the hind end. Reduced blood cholesterol. Studies in rats deficient in B$_5$ showed graying of fur, decreased growth, destruction of adrenal glands and

hemorrhage. Deficiency causes a decrease in hydrochloric acid production in the stomach (necessary as the first step in the digestive process) and problems in blood sugar metabolism. Reduces immunity and worsens all allergy symptoms.

Note: Pantothenic acid taken alone for longer than 6 months without being balanced with other B-complex vitamins displaces sulphur in the body.

Supplement: B_6 (pyridoxine, pyridoxal and pyridoxamine)

Purpose: Aids in absorption and conversion of many amino acids. As such, it is one of the most important nutrients needed in the diet. Needed by the pituitary gland to balance electrolytes (sodium and potassium) in the body. Must be present for the production of antibodies and red blood cells. Increased requirement in high- or very low-protein diets. Required for the body to be able to absorb vitamin B_{12}. Necessary for the formation of hydrochloric acid and magnesium. Needed for proper conversion of essential amino acid (tryptophan) to nonessential amino acid. Cortisone drugs deplete the body of B_6.

Credited with: Essential for females in retaining correct fluid balances. Needed for correct assimilation of protein and fat. Helps to prevent skin disorders and nervousness. Alleviates nausea in pregnancy, helps with the whelping process, reduces edema, muscle spasms, leg cramps, numbness in extremities experienced at night. Acts as a natural diuretic. Helps fight mental depression, skin disorders, sore mouth and lips, bad breath, kidney stones, loss of muscular control and senility. Controls dandruff. Used in treatment of epilepsy.

Deficiencies: Destroyed by cooking, food processing and improper storage and when exposed to sunlight. Some B_6 is stored in the muscles and some is produced by intestinal bacteria. Almost all the subtle things that go wrong with our dogs can in some way be related to a vitamin B_6 deficiency. Since it is necessary for the proper assimilation of protein in the diet, all the deficiency symptoms applying to protein would apply here.

B_6 may be **the most significant ingredient in our dogs' food,** because it is necessary for the proper function of other vitamins and minerals that in turn affect the ability of the body to assimilate fats and carbohydrates as well as other vitamins and minerals.

When the body is stressed for any reason—a visit to the veterinarian, the use of vaccines, wormers, drugs, dips, flea powders, surgery, etc.—the need for B_6 is greater. Leaving your dogs in a kennel or taking them on vacation, to an obedience class or even the shopping center will have an effect on vitamin B_6 levels.

Growing puppies are especially vulnerable to depletion of B vitamins. **The levels of B_6 in their systems will determine their reaction to vaccines.** B_6 is needed to build antibodies.

Deficiencies also cause anemia, decrease in the number of white blood cells, inflammation of the tongue, dermatitis and problems in pregnancy, whelping and proper growth of puppies in utero. Research conducted on B_6 shows a direct correlation between the intake of this vitamin and heart disease. The increase in **dental decay** in dogs is thought to be due to a B_6 deficiency. Drugs that influence the metabolism of B_6 are hormones, drugs for high blood pressure and some antibiotics. Magnesium is needed for B_6 to function well. Overdosing on B_6 causes vivid dreaming.

Supplement:	**Vitamin B_{12} (cobalamin)** Named the "red" vitamin, it is unusual as it is the only vitamin that contains an essential mineral cobalt. It is also unique because it is required in such tiny amounts in comparison to other B vitamins.
Purpose:	Forms and regenerates red blood cells, prevents pernicious anemia, promotes growth and increases appetite in puppies. Increases energy, helps the body assimilate fats, carbohydrates and protein. Involved in metabolic and enzymatic processes of protein breakdown and assimilation. Helpful for females going into season and coming out of season. Dogs

fed high cereal-based (soy) diets will need more than dogs fed a diet with animal source proteins, where B_{12} is abundant. It is sensitive to light but is less affected by heat than some of the other B vitamins.

Credited with: Longevity, healthy digestive function, preventing fatigue, allergies, eczema, bursitis, hepatitis, asthma, memory loss and poor balance. Stimulates growth in malnourished animals. Relieves irritability and improves concentration. Helps to prevent cataracts and excessive watering of the eyes.

Digestibility: Hydrochloric acid in the stomach is needed for absorption, as are calcium and thyroid hormones. Needs calcium to be properly absorbed. Can be used in injectable form. **Thyroid gland needs to be functioning properly for proper absorption.**

Absorbed by small intestine, highest concentrations in the body are found in the liver, heart, kidney, pancreas, brain, testes, blood and bone marrow. Present only in animal-protein foods.

Deficiencies: Vegetarian diets are often deficient in this vitamin. Brain damage, anemia, extreme fatigue, defective bone marrow, poor red blood cell production are signs of a deficiency. Fluid on the brain (hydrocephaly) has been seen in rat pups deficient in B_{12}.

Supplement: **Biotin**

Purpose: Essential for normal metabolism of fat and protein. Vitamin C needs biotin to be effective. Very stable and not affected by heat.

Credited with: Helps to keep hair from turning gray; prevents some forms of baldness; restores healthy hair growth; alleviates eczema, dermatitis, dandruff, skin disorders, lung infections, loss of appetite and lethargy.

Digestibility: Egg yolk is a rich source of biotin. Raw egg white, which contains avidin, inhibits the absorption of biotin. When eggs are fed, they should be fed whole and cooked. Affected by sulphur drugs and antibiotics. Naturally produced by the intestines.

Deficiencies: Skin eruptions, sensitivity to touch, inflamed eyes, hair loss, muscle weakness, bald spots, elevated cholesterol, anemia, and heart conditions.

Cravings: Egg yolks, liver, brewers yeast and milk products.

Supplement:	Choline
Purpose:	Fat emulsifier. Works with inositol to utilize fat and cholesterol. Penetrates the blood-brain barrier to produce a chemical that aids memory. Choline is heat sensitive and is lost in food processing and through improper food storage.
Credited with:	Helps memory function in older dogs. Keeps the thymus healthy, as well as the liver and gallbladder. Used for nerve conditions such as muscle twitching, especially in the face. Aids in detoxifying the liver and reduces stones in the gallbladder. Is used in the treatment of many kidney conditions. Choline reduces fat around the liver and maintains the integrity of the myelin sheath (the covering around nerve cells).
Digestibility:	Can be made by the body from the amino acid glycine. Choline combines with glycerol and phosphate in the body to make lecithin. It is part of the neurotransmitter acetylcholine and helps to keep the "electricity" flowing between the nerves. *Choline is dependent on the level of the amino acid methionine* in the diet to work properly.
Deficiencies:	Fatty degeneration of the liver. Hardening of the arteries. Improper nerve function. Disruption of protein metabolism. Thymus gland (producer of immune fighting cells) degeneration.
Cravings:	Egg yolk, brewers yeast, wheat germ, fish and liver.

Supplement:	Folic Acid (Folacin)
Purpose:	Made up of paraminobenzoic acid (PABA) and glutamic acid, this vitamin is found inside another vitamin. Very fragile and is destoyed by heat, light, food processing and when left at room temperature for any length of time. Needed to form red blood cells. Aids in protein metabolism. Necessary for the growth and division of all body cells so is needed more in pregnancy and during puppy growth. Helps to build antibodies. Helps to heal and prevent infections.
Credited with:	Correcting pigmentation problems. Stops spontaneous abortion, difficult labor, dead puppies. Improves lactation. Essential in the utilization of

amino acids and glucose. Useful when adrenal gland is not functioning well. Needed by **epileptics** taking drugs to control seizures, old dogs and when weight-reducing diets are used. Extra folic acid is needed when hormone treatment is being used or large doses of vitamin C are added to the diet. Lactating females have a greater need for folic acid. Has been used successfully for chronic diarrhea, malabsorption problems and to stimulate the appetite. ***Counteracts birth defects***.

Digestibility: Good. Look to see that this is added to the dog food you feed. *When B-complex is used as a supplement make sure it has folic acid in it.*

Deficiencies: Dogs fed a folic acid–deficient diet take twice as long to **build antibodies to hepatitis and distemper vaccines**. *Vitamin B$_{12}$ deficiency and a folic acid defi*ciency often are confused. One can cover up the other. Feed these vitamins *together*. Needs are higher after surgery, during long-term drug use or if the diet fed is cereal based. Folic acid is crucial during pregnancy to prevent birth defects of the nervous system and the spine. Deficiency of this vitamin causes inflamed tongue, watery discharge from the eyes, anemia, erratic appetite and poor tolerance to vaccines.

Cravings: Raw green leafy vegetables, raw liver, raw kidney, brewers yeast and some raw fruits.

Supplement: Inositol

Purpose: Maintains cell membrane integrity. Crucial for cells in bone marrow, eye tissue and intestines. Helps to lower cholesterol levels. Helps hair growth and prevents skin problems. Burns up fat. Combines with choline to form lecithin.

Credited with: Helping to reverse symptoms of myelin sheath degeneration, which can cause paralysis of lungs, front feet and limbs. Aids in weight loss. Used in treatment of diabetes.

Deficiencies: Bald spots, skin problems, eye abnormalities, high blood cholesterol and constipation.

Cravings: Brewers yeast, blackstrap molasses, liver and cantaloupe.

Supplement:	**PABA**
Purpose:	Keeps skin healthy and supple. In combination with other B-complex vitamins and vitamin E, helps restore color of coat.
Credited with:	Has been used in skin lesions from lupus. Used for short-coated dogs in hot climates to protect against sunburn. Reduces pain from burns. Used in the treatment of hypopigmentation (snow noses, eye rims and mouths) together with other B vitamins, hydrochloric acid, vitamin C and amino acids.
Deficiencies:	Eczema, extreme fatigue, premature gray hair, reproductive disorders, infertility, lack of libido in breeding animals, anemia and loss of pigmentation.
Note:	Penicillin or sulfur drugs destroy PABA. Use more B-complex containing PABA when using these drugs.
Supplement:	**Vitamin B_{13} (orotic acid),** which helps to metabolize folic acid and B_{12}, is not mentioned in the guidelines. Found naturally in carrots, beets and artichokes and has been used in the treatment of liver disease.
Supplement:	**Vitamin B_{15} (pangamic acid),** which extends cell life, is not mentioned in the NRC guidelines. B_{15} aids in protein assimilation, regulates fat metabolism and stimulates the immune response. Used to treat the buildup of lactic acid in the muscles of athletes. Naturally found in beef blood, brown rice and brewers yeast. Deficiencies are responsible for glandular and nerve disorders, heart disease and poor oxygenation of tissues.
Supplement:	**Vitamin B_{17} (laetrile)** Not mentioned by the NRC, it is a controversial vitamin used in countries outside the United States for cancer treatment. Part of one molecule in laetrile releases cyanide, which poisons cancer cells. It is found naturally in the seeds of apricots, plums, cherries, peaches, nectarines and apples.

Supplement:	**Vitamin F (unsaturated fatty acids—linoleic, linolenic and arachidonic)**
	Mentioned under "Fat" in NRC guidelines.
Purpose:	Promotes healthy skin and hair.
Credited with:	Preventing cholesterol buildup, influencing glandular activity and making calcium available to cells. Combats heart disease. Burns saturated fats. Gives some protection against the harmful effects of X-rays. Has been credited with preventing allergic reactions to corn and wheat.
Digestibility:	Good. More effective if taken with vitamins E, A, C and D, as well as phosphorus. Needed more in heavy cereal grain diets. Vegetable oils need to be kept refrigerated when opened to avoid rancidity.
Deficiencies:	Skin conditions from eruptions to flaky dandruff. Skin lesions on the abdomen, thighs and between the shoulder blades. Poor hair coat. Stiff joints in older dogs. Itching. Allergies to corn and wheat. Being in the sun too long depletes the body of vitamin F. Right ear inflammations (swimmers' ear).
Cravings:	Vegetable oils—safflower, sunflower, wheat germ and linseed oils. Some vitamin F found in corn oil.
Supplement:	**Vitamin P (bioflavanoids)** Water soluble
Purpose:	Not mentioned by NRC. Found in citrin, hesperidin, quercitin, rutin. Considered as part of the vitamin C complex. Increases capillary strength and prevents the appearance of blue/purplish spots on the skin. Prevents vitamin C being destroyed by oxidation and helps build resistance to infection.
Credited with:	Alleviating respiratory infections, bleeding gums, skin problems, hemorrhages in the eyes, radiation sickness and diseases of the inner ear.
Digestibility:	Water soluble. Works together with vitamin C.
Deficiencies:	Capillaries breaking at the surface of the skin; bruising easily.
Cravings:	Citrus fruit, strawberries, prunes, apricots, blackberries.

Summary

1. **SOME VITAMINS ARE WATER SOLUBLE,** PASSING THROUGH THE BODY WITHIN 4 TO 8 HOURS AFTER INGESTION. Water soluble vitamins need to be fed twice a day to keep the balance steady in the body. Dogs that work long hours, dogs that are shown, old dogs and those used for breeding have a greater need for vitamins than do pet dogs not exposed to stressful situations. Dogs that live outside and those that get little human attention require more B and C vitamins.

2. **USE FAT SOLUBLE VITAMINS** (A, D, E AND K, WHICH ARE STORED BY THE BODY) **ONLY IN MODERATION.** They could cause toxic symptoms if used in large doses for long periods of time.

3. **MANY VITAMINS ARE AFFECTED BY OXYGEN, HEAT AND LIGHT** AND SOME ARE DESTROYED IN THE PROCESSING OF DOG FOOD. Supplementing with a high-quality vitamin/mineral supplement is crucial to good health.

4. STUDIES DONE AT CORNELL UNIVERSITY IN THE 1960s SHOWED THAT **PUPPIES WITH LOW VITAMIN B-COMPLEX** IN THEIR BODIES **RESPONDED LESS WELL TO VACCINES** AND TOOK LONGER TO BUILD ANTIBODIES THAN DID THOSE ADEQUATELY PROVIDED WITH B-COMPLEX VITAMINS.

5. **EXTRA VITAMINS ARE NEEDED WHEN ANTIBIOTICS,** STEROIDS AND SULFUR DRUGS ARE BEING USED.

6. THE NRC GUIDELINES HAVE LITTLE DATA ON WHAT VITAMINS ARE NECESSARY FOR GROWING OR ADULT DOGS. There is no data on the needs of giant breeds, older dogs, pregnant or lactating females. Supplementation is recommended.

7. DO NOT USE ISOLATED VITAMINS FROM THE B-COMPLEX FAMILY FOR PROLONGED PERIODS. ALWAYS USE *WITH* A B-COMPLEX TABLET.

8. **VITAMIN DEFICIENCIES SHOW UP IN CASES OF POOR GROWTH;** ANY FORM OF DIGESTIVE DISORDER; ELIMINATION PROBLEMS; POOR RESISTANCE TO DISEASE; STOOL EATING; GREASY, SMELLY COATS; WARTS; SEIZURES; ADDISON'S DISEASE; THYROID MALFUNCTIONS; AGGRESSION; TIMIDITY; INABILITY TO COPE WITH STRESS; POOR ASSIMILATION OF FOOD; STERILITY; AND IN ALMOST ALL DISEASE STATES.

9. CORN AND WHITE RICE DIETS REQUIRE SUPPLEMENTATION OF VITAMIN B-COMPLEX.

Chapter 6

Minerals

What Do They Do?

Minerals, together with vitamins, make up less than 2 percent of any formulated diet for dogs. They are the most critical nutrients. Minerals do not contain any calories or energy themselves, but they assist the body in energy production. Although the dog's body can make some vitamins, it cannot make minerals. Natural minerals come from the food dogs eat, but the availability of the minerals is complex.

Like vitamins, minerals function as coenzymes, enabling the body to perform its activities quickly and accurately. They are needed for the proper composition of body fluids, the formation of blood and bone and the maintenance of a healthy nervous system. Minerals are stored primarily in the body's bone and muscle tissue. In extremely large doses, minerals can be toxic.

Destruction of Minerals

Between 50 and 88 percent of minerals are lost during food processing and can cause mineral deficiencies. While some minerals are not destroyed by heat, many of them are water soluble and are lost during the cooking process.

Minimum Daily Requirement

The National Research Council provides dog food manufacturers with the Minimum Daily Requirement of known nutrient figures to use in the recipes for dog food. The NRC tells us that the research data presented to them has been limited, is not complete in many nutrients and life stages, and that much of the data is over three decades old.

The sum total of minerals, together with the cereal grains contained in all of a food's ingredients, determine the acid/alkaline balance of the body.

Most minerals are only moderately well absorbed even when the digestive system is functioning well.

How Much Does Your Dog Need?

The way dog food is made, the source of ingredients, the breed and age of the dog and the climate in which the dog lives all will have an effect on mineral needs. The need for minerals for differing life stages has not been calculated, but the assumption of the NRC is that more are needed during growth, gestation, lactation, old age and when a dog is working. The theoretical estimates in the guidelines are based on these beliefs.

Types of Minerals

Minerals are either **elemental or chelated**. Elemental means they come from the earth and are composed of chemical molecules that cannot be reduced to simpler substances. They are basic constituents of all living matter and they exist in an inorganic form in the earth. Chelated minerals are suspended in an amino acid or other organic substance (such as orotates or arginates), which makes them easier for the body to absorb. Minerals are also available in water— "hard" water containing more minerals than "soft" or treated water.

There are approximately 17 essential minerals, which are divided into macrominerals and trace minerals. The eight macrominerals are calcium, phosphorus, sodium, potassium, chloride, sulfur, magnesium and silicon. The nine trace minerals are iron, zinc, copper, cobalt, iodine, manganese, chromium, molybdenum and selenium.

Minerals are absorbed by the gastrointestinal tract. They fine-tune levels of other nutrients to obtain maximum body function. They are eliminated through the kidneys into urine, or through the liver, bile or other digestive secretions. Minerals can be stored by the body and are found primarily in bone and muscle tissue.

Supplementation

Some minerals can be toxic if fed in large amounts. It is unwise to separate or supplement with one mineral alone for any length of time because of the chain reaction produced in the body with other nutrients. If supplementation is necessary, look for a mixture of vitamins and minerals from a natural source—for example, herbs—rather than a chemical source that contains minerals not easily broken down and absorbed.

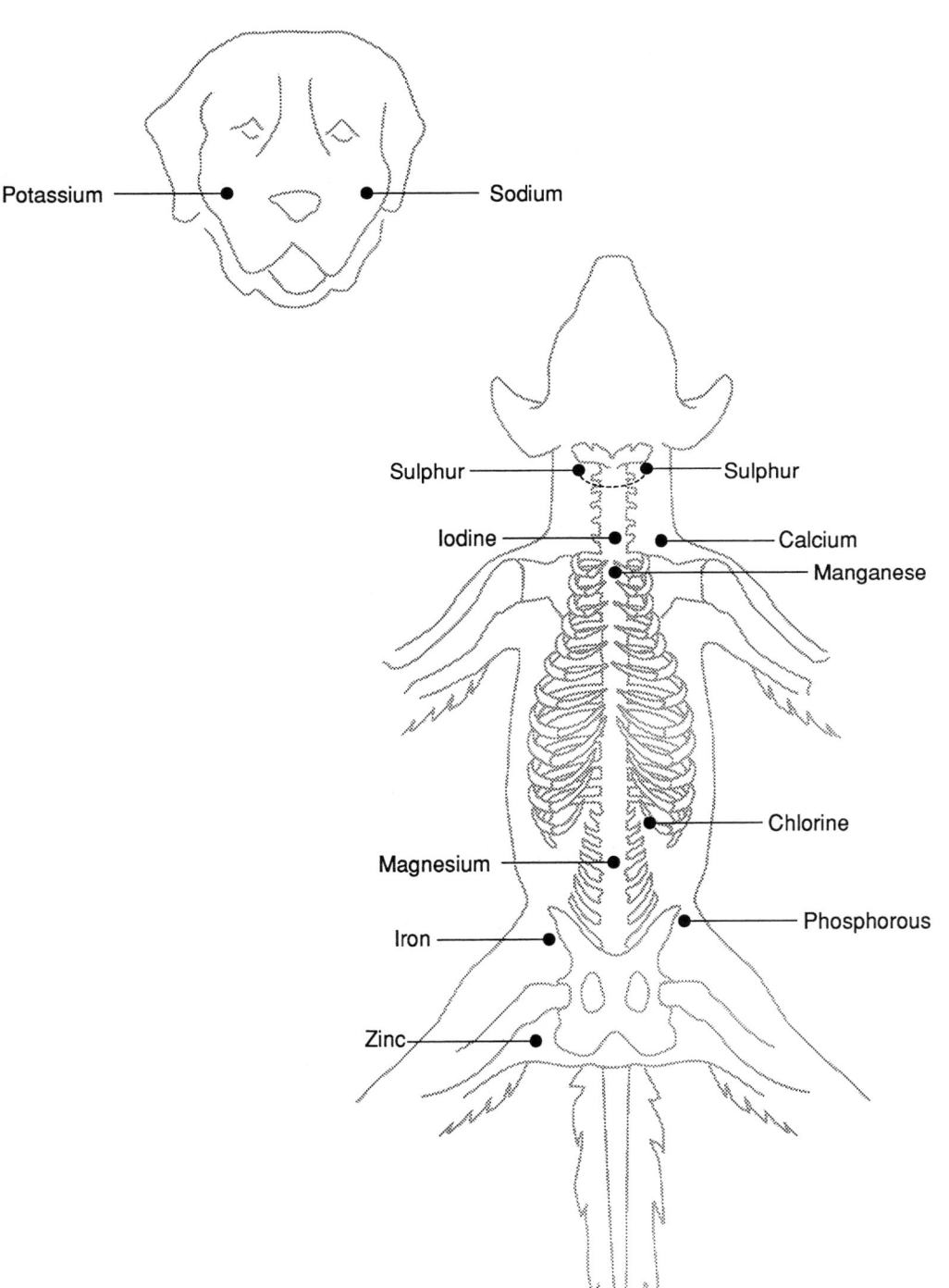

6–1: The Mineral Dog

Minerals are in the ingredient list for all dog foods. Minerals listed in a chelated form will provide a source of nutrients that are more readily available to your dog. Higher-quality foods generally will list the same mineral coming from different sources.

The following list of minerals does not contain all of the essential and trace minerals that are known. Rather it is a compilation of those mentioned in the NRC guidelines that are considered essential for the dog plus information of those trace minerals we feel are worthy of mention.

Supplement:	**Calcium.** Comes in the form of oyster shell, dolomite, bone meal, calcium chelated with amino acids, calcium gluconate, calcium carbonate, calcium iodate, dicalcium phosphate, calcium orotate and calcium lactate.
Purpose:	Needed for proper bone and teeth formation, proper heart function and normal clotting of blood. Needed in pregnancy and lactation. Helps to maintain correct balances of sodium, potassium and magnesium. Needed for the utilization of phosphorus and vitamins A, C and D. Affected by the functioning of the parathyroid gland. Competes with phosphorous in the intestines for absorption.
Credited with:	Preventing porous bones, rickets and muscle cramping. Needed for proper growth of the skeleton, teeth and jaws; regulating the heartbeat; and proper functioning of the nervous system. Influences the release of the neurotransmitters *norepinephrine* and *serotonin*, which act in the brain to excite or calm; crucial for the developing puppy. Necessary for the release of prothrombin, which is essential to blood clotting.
Digestibility:	Calcium is most critical during the third and fourth month of growth, when the dog's body retains higher levels than at any other time. Affected by the amount of phosphorus, magnesium and vitamin D in the diet as well as stress and exercise levels. Between 3 and 5 months, puppies develop their teeth, and general growth is optimum.
	Calcium levels must be monitored, as too much will create the same symptoms as too little. The correct amount of calcium in the diet makes the difference between good and poor bone growth, and is necessary for correct tooth and jaw formation.

Mistakes made during this time are generally not able to be fixed at a later date.

Most forms of calcium are well absorbed, but bonemeal is probably best for the dog because it contains phosphorus and magnesium in the correct ratio to calcium. Calcium amino acid chelates, calcium carbonate and lactate are also well absorbed. If calcium supplementation is considered, add a small amount of cod liver oil (vitamins A and D), so that it can be correctly utilized. Calcium lactate should be avoided if there is a milk allergy. NRC suggests that a diet containing a ratio of calcium to phosphorus of 1.2 to 1.0 is adequate. Magnesium should be in the ratio of .6.

Deficiencies: Muscle cramps, porous or fragile bones, rickets, hip problems, lameness, brittle nails, joint pains, tooth decay, gingivitis, loss of teeth, nervousness, mental depression, irritability or aggression, kidney stone formation, calcification of soft tissues, toxemia in pregnancy, anxiety, muscle twitching, palpitations, insomnia and confusion.

Toxicity: Too much as well as too little calcium and phosphorus in the diet results in lameness, pain in joints, too much extension in the carpus (wrist) joints, going down in the pasterns (wrists), and improper growth of the long bones.

Many breeders of giant breeds experience difficulty in growing puppies properly. They have successfully put pups of 4–6 months on adult food to avoid bone growth problems. Because the ratio of protein and fat in the diet affects the need for calcium and phosphorus, some puppy foods **may be** improperly balanced for proper growth of these breeds. There was no research data presented to the NRC on the needs of dogs maturing over 75 pounds.

Cravings: Milk (goats' milk is excellent for raising puppies), cheese, eggshells and most raw vegetables, especially dark green, leafy vegetables, such as romaine lettuce, watercress and broccoli. Other cravings include dandelions, Brussels sprouts, sesame seeds, almonds, walnuts, millet, comfrey, yogurt, sardines, blackstrap molasses, dried fruit, parsley and kelp.

Supplement:	**Phosphorus**
Purpose:	It is the second most abundant mineral in the body next to calcium and *is involved in most biochemical reactions* in the body. It is essential to calcium metabolism and is mostly controlled by the parathyroid gland. It is necessary for proper bone and teeth construction and *is contained in every cell in the body.*
	It is a component part of fat molecules, which are essential to cell membranes and which in turn allows nutrients to pass in and out of the cells. It is used by the body in the digestion of protein, and in production of RNA and DNA, the substances that carry genetic information. It helps kidney function and acts as a buffer for acid in the body. Phosphorus helps regulate muscle contractions, including the heartbeat, and it supports the function of the nerves. It helps some of the B vitamins (niacin and riboflavin) convert to enzymes. Cancer research has revealed that cancer cells lose phosphorus more quickly than healthy cells, so phosphorus is being studied as a possible support of cancer patients.
Credited with:	Normal brain function, stimulating hair growth, controlling acid levels in the body, maintaining bone mass and helping to control arthritis. Keeps teeth enamel strong.
Digestibility:	Good. Needs to be taken in a balance with correct amounts of calcium and magnesium as well as vitamins A and D. Many foods are high in phosphorus, and it is unlikely that a dog would be deficient in this alone.
Deficiencies:	Rickets, weight loss, stiff joints, bone pain and bone fragility. Poor tooth or jaw development. Some skin disease, arthritis, tooth decay, loss of memory, failing eyesight, cataracts and excessive shedding.
Cravings:	Milk products, cheeses and eggs; meat, chicken, fish, turkey, dairy products, whole grains, brewers yeast, wheat germ and bran. Care must be taken in supplementing with cottage cheese, which has an incorrect calcium/phosphorus ratio.

Supplement:	**Magnesium**
Purpose:	Needed for the transport of sodium and potassium. Half of the magnesium in the body is combined with

calcium and phosphorus to assure strength of bones and teeth. The rest is found in body tissues, muscles and red blood cells. *Magnesium is an important catalyst in enzyme reactions.* It helps with the utilization of vitamins B and E, fats and other minerals. It is helpful in reducing cholesterol levels, and in the treatment of nervousness, neuromuscular problems and depression.

Authors' note: We have been successful in some cases of "rage syndrome" supplementing with small amounts of magnesium oxide in those cases where the individual dog has been unable to assimilate magnesium as provided in dog food. This inability was determined by blood testing. There appears to be a genetic factor here. This research was done before magnesium amino acid chelates were available and bears further investigation.

If extra calcium is supplemented in a diet, magnesium needs to make up half the amount of calcium. Should be used in conjunction with calcium/ phosphorus supplements. Calcium and magnesium are both alkaline-forming minerals and not well absorbed when taken with food. Better taken between meals or on an empty stomach, which will be a more acidic environment. Some supplements supply hydrochloric acid and vitamin C as well as calcium and magnesium, which is the best combination for absorption.

For a dog the proportions should be calcium 1.2, phosphorus 1.0 and magnesium .6.

Credited with: Helping in the treatment of arrhythmias, angina pectoris, hypertension, bronchial asthma, epilepsy, hyperactivity, false pregnancies (together with calcium), kidney stones, fatigue, anxiety, insomnia and muscle cramps.

Digestibility: Magnesium chelated with amino acids or in the form of orotate seems to be the easiest to absorb, followed by less digestible forms such as magnesium oxide, bicarbonate, and carbonate. More magnesium is needed if cholesterol levels are high. More effective when taken with vitamin B_6, vitamin C, vitamin D, calcium, phosphorus and protein.

Deficiencies:	Loss of appetite in puppies, overextension of front legs, aggression, irregular muscle movements of hind legs, muscle twitching, restless sleep, convulsive seizures and changes in potassium levels in body. Kidney stones, gallbladder stones, epilepsy, impaired protein assimilation and calcification of the joints.
	Found where soft water is consumed. Deficiencies often occur after trauma from injury, surgery, burns or when there are other diseases present such as diabetes and liver disease. Rapid heartbeat, learning difficulties, poor memory and tetanus also are indicators of deficiency. Twenty percent of laboratory animals that were deprived of magnesium developed cancer.
Cravings:	Kelp, almonds, apples, raw and cooked green leafy vegetables, figs and safflower oil.
Supplement:	**Potassium.** Comes in the form of sulfate, chloride, oxide or carbonate. An alkaline-based forming mineral, it is an electrolyte that carries electrical energy to the body.
Purpose:	Together with sodium it is responsible for maintaining the proper fluid balance in the body's cells. Regulates heart muscle action and blood pressure. Helps in enzyme action and regulates blood pH level. Helps in the formation of glycogen in the liver muscles and cartilage and is found in concentration on the right side of the brain. Facial paralysis of the right side may respond to potassium. It helps the body in eliminating waste through the kidneys and helps purify the blood.
Credited with:	Proper functioning of the heart and nervous system, metabolism of protein and carbohydrate and helping in the elimination of wastes from the body. It is an aid in the treatment of certain milk and cheese allergies. If properly balanced with sodium, edema can be prevented. Mental and physical stress can lead to potassium deficiencies, as can hypoglycemia and diarrhea and vomiting.
Digestibility:	Well absorbed by the body in most of its forms.
Deficiencies:	Fatigue, edema (swelling), water retention, low blood sugar, poor growth, restlessness, paralysis of the neck and the forepart of the body, muscular

paralysis, a tendency to dehydration and lesions to the heart and kidneys. Depletion occurs during stress. Caution should be observed to provide enough potassium when prolonged vomiting or diarrhea have been observed. Potassium is lost when dogs excessively pant in hot weather. Dieting incorrectly causes potassium losses.

Some studies state that the content of sodium and potassium in the diet determines the ability to adapt to different climates. Lack of potassium can produce sciatica on the right side of the body. Deficiencies common in older dogs and those that experience chronic disease.

Use of Prednisone, ACTH, Digitalis or Lasix (diuretics) will deplete potassium levels in the body.

Cravings: Bananas, potatoes, green leafy vegetables, citrus fruits, mint leaves, bee pollen, alfalfa, tomatoes, parsley, rice bran, dried apricots and dates.

Supplement: Sodium

Purpose: "Where sodium goes, so goes water." Acts as an electrolyte together with potassium and chloride. Comes in the form of salt or sodium chloride. Found in the fluids surrounding cells as well as inside cells and bones. Sodium is closely connected with water inside the body. Without sodium the blood clots, causing a stroke on the left side of the body. Found in abundance in natural foods, processed foods have too much salt added. It is used as a preservative in some instances.

Credited with: Helping in the proper function of muscles and nerves and preventing heat prostration. Keeps water levels in the body constant and prevents dry skin and loss of hair coat; prevents exhaustion and fatigue. Contributes to the formation of saliva and digestive enzymes. Helps in contracting mammary gland muscles. Helps prevent water retention. Has been credited with retarding aging by neutralizing waste products and eliminating them through the lymph system. Eliminates fermentation of foods in the gastrointestinal tract.

Digestibility: Better when obtained from natural foods, which are easily digested. Sodium chloride and salt are harder for the body to use. More efficient if fed with vitamin D and potassium. Low-sodium diets can lead to a depletion of potassium, causing a stroke or paralysis on the left side of the body. Best supplemented in the form of easily digested vegetables rather than hard to digest salt.

Deficiencies: Allergies, especially in hot weather when the appetite is depressed. Watery discharge from the eyes (tears). Diarrhea, increased gas and arthritis of the left knee and sciatica on the left side. Nausea, muscular weakness, heat exhaustion, mental apathy and respiratory failure.

Too much sodium creates high blood pressure, problems with females before going into season and toxemia in pregnancy.

Cravings: Kelp, celery, carrots, spinach, okra, strawberries, apples, asparagus, beets, cucumbers, plums, radishes, Swiss chard and turnips.

Supplement: **Chlorine.** An essential mineral, together with sodium and potassium. Chlorine compounds are found mainly inside cells. It is a cleanser, expelling waste materials and helping to clean the blood with a tendency to reduce excessive fat. It unites with hydrogen and other elements to form hydrochloric acid which is needed for the digestion of protein and minerals. It aids the liver in detoxifying the body.

Purpose: Helps to replace sodium in the body when used in the form of sodium chloride. Necessary to replace minerals that can be depleted through heavy exercise. Helps to kill bacteria and other micro-organisms.

Credited with: Helping with proper digestion.

Digestibility: Good. Listed as sodium chloride in most dog foods.

Deficiencies: Impaired digestion, obesity, goiter, overactive adrenal glands (Cushing's syndrome), loss of hair and teeth. Can affect acid/alkaline base, turning body too alkaline, especially when there is prolonged diarrhea or vomiting.

Toxicity: Excessive drinking of water that has been chlorinated will deplete the body of potassium and sodium and may cause adrenal gland exhaustion (Addison's disease).

Cravings for:	Tomatoes, celery, iceburg lettuce, kelp, spinach, cabbage, parsnips and radishes.
Supplement:	**Iron.** Comes in the form of ferrous sulfate or ferrous carbonate and iron amino acid chelate.
Purpose:	Essential for life; necessary to produce hemoglobin (red blood cells) and myoglobin (red pigment in muscles) and certain enzymes. *Lost easily* in the body and *must be replaced.* Needed to prevent anemia.
	Works with copper in the body as well as chlorophyll, the green coloring in plants and vegetables. Hemoglobin transports oxygen in the blood from the lungs to tissues that need oxygen for energy. Found in every cell in the body, combined with protein. Needed for proper protein metabolism.
Credited with:	Aiding growth and resistance to disease, preventing fatigue and anemias, aiding in good skin tone.
Digestibility:	Soy protein adversely affects absorption of iron. More effective taken with vitamin B_{12} and folic acid. Easily digested from meat sources and is found in abundance in beef, liver and other organ meats, pork, lamb, chicken, shellfish, egg yolks and salmon. Less available from grains—75 percent of the iron is found in the outer brans and germs. Enriched grain foods contain iron in the ferrous state and are poorly digested.
Deficiencies:	Anemia, pale skin, fatigue, brittle nails, shortness of breath, depression, red and inflamed tongue, low blood pressure, rheumatism of the back legs, dizziness and infertility. Rubbing the head on the right side near the eyes.
Toxicity:	Too much iron can cause gastrointestinal lesions.
Cravings:	Liver, molasses, kelp, yellow dock, beets, green vegetables, brewers yeast, wheat bran, wheat germ, parsley, millet, prunes, raisins, eggs, lamb, pork, lentils, peanuts, brown rice, ripe olives, chicken, artichokes, broccoli, whole wheat bread and cauliflower.
Supplement:	Copper
Purpose:	Required to convert iron into hemoglobin. Necessary for the function of the amino acid tyrosine, which is needed for the production of the

pigmentation factor for hair and skin. Essential to the utilization of vitamin C but interferes with the absorption of zinc. Copper and zinc need to be taken together. Can be found in the form of amino acid chelate or copper sulfate.

Necessary for the central nervous system. Contributes to the hair and skin color and also stimulates the brain. Copper promotes red blood cell production in bone marrow and increases respiration of tissue and is part of the substance called elastin, which is contained in muscle fibers.

Credited with: Preventing anemia. Copper in red blood cells is bound to erythrocuprein, which enhances energy. It is part of the system for cell respiration, an energy-releasing process. It helps to oxidize vitamin C and works with this vitamin to form collagen (supportive substance for muscles and connective tissues).

It is found in many enzymes that play a role in oxygen-free radical metabolism and in this way has a mild anti-inflammatory effect. It is necessary for certain amino acids to function, especially tyrosine, which converts into melanin, the substance which gives hair and skin their pigmentation and color.

Copper together with zinc is important in converting the thyroid hormones T3 to T4. Low copper may reduce thyroid functions. It controls histamine, which limits allergic inflammatory reactions.

Digestibility: Since the line between therapeutic and toxic levels is so narrow, it is better not to give a copper supplement. It is found in whole wheat, some other grains, beans, peas, liver and seafood.

Digestibility depends on zinc levels in the body as well as iron and cobalt. Copper toxicosis found in Bedlington Terriers and West Highland White Terriers has been well studied. These dogs have a genetic abnormality that affects their ability to metabolize and eliminate copper from their systems.

Deficiencies: Anemia, loss of hair, poor respiration, premature graying, lack of pigmentation, low blood pressure, reduced thyroid function, reduced immune response, reduced activity of white blood cells and reduced thymus production.

Toxicity:	Copper can leak into the water supply from copper pipes. Swimming pools can create copper contamination where fungicides and algaecides are used. High copper levels are found when zinc levels are low. This can create stress, anxiety, joint and muscle pain, depression, poor memory, lack of concentration, senility, epilepsy, hyperactivity, eclampsia in pregnancy, nausea, vomiting, diarrhea, liver damage, gingivitis, dermatitis, and discoloration of hair and skin.
Note:	If your dog is suffering from thyroid problems (hypothyroidism), test the copper levels in his blood to see if the food you are feeding contains enough or too much copper. Check whether the copper can be eliminated from your dog's system.
Cravings:	Green leafy vegetables, liver, whole wheat products, prunes, raisins, almonds and beans.

Supplement:	**Manganese.** Comes in the form of manganese amino acid chelate, or manganous oxide.
Purpose:	There is no published data on what is needed for dogs. The NRC guidelines contain information taken from other species. Manganese helps activate enzymes necessary for the body's proper use of biotin, vitamin B_1 and vitamin C.
	Needed for normal bone structure. Important for the formation of thyroxin, the principal hormone of the thyroid gland. Also needed for the reproductive and nervous systems. Used to treat deafness (tinnitus) and to control allergic reactions to rice. Used in the treatment of arthritis. Necessary for synthesis of dopamine, cholesterol and mucopolysaccharides.
	It is present in the body cells, particularly those containing an antioxidant enzyme, superoxide dismutase (SOD). Large amounts of calcium and phosphorus will interfere with the absorption of manganese. It activates arginase, an enzyme that helps to form urea in the body.
Credited with:	In its interaction with cells containing SOD, manganese acts as an anti-inflammatory. Has been used to counteract fatigue, poor memory, nervousness, irritability and dizziness. Used along with zinc it

helps to decrease copper levels in the body. Helps to alleviate muscle twitching and muscle rigidity. May help in the treatment of epilepsy. Tumors and cancer cells are low in manganese and it may have a role in preventing cancer cell production.

Digestibility: Best taken in a multimineral preparation than by itself.

Deficiencies: Decreased glucose tolerance, poor pancreatic funtion, sterility, poor growth during pregnancy, decreased brain function and poor production of milk in a lactating bitch. Lack of thyroid hormone production. Associated with poor bone and cartilage growth as well as spinal disc degeneration. Low or deficient manganese has produced slipped patellas in chickens. Seizures, irritability, aggression, deafness and allergies have been observed. Together with amino acid and zinc deficiencies, has been associated with "spinning" in Bull Terriers.

Cravings: Eggs, whole grain cereals, green leafy vegetables, peas and beets.

Supplement: **Iodine**

Purpose: Prevents goiter and is necessary for a healthy, functioning thyroid gland.

Credited with: The thyroid hormones are responsible for the rate at which the body burns energy. Needed for proper growth and development, protein digestion and energy metabolism.

Regulates all body functions. Bone and nerve formation, reproduction, condition of skin, hair, nails and teeth and mental state are all governed by the thyroid.

Affects how vitamins are broken down as well as protein, cholesterol and carbohydrates and how they are used by the body. Combines with the amino acid tyrosine to make the thyroid hormones T3 and T4. Used for excessive weight gain when thyroid is not functioning well.

Digestibility: Best absorbed from natural sources rather than salt. Found in iodized salt and kelp.

Deficiencies: All of those common to hypo- or hyperthyroidism: weight gain, blackened skin, fatigue, sluggishness, patches of dry fur, thickening skin, decreased resistance to infection, feeling cold, inability to regulate body temperature, mammary tumors. Deformities such as thick tongue, short broad head, wide nose, short bodies, heavy extremities, delayed shedding of puppy teeth, hairlessness, dullness and timidity.

Cravings: Kelp, Swiss chard, turnip greens, watercress, pears, pineapples, artichokes, citrus fruit and egg yolks.

Supplement: **Fluorine.** Sodium and calcium fluoride.

Purpose: To prevent mottling of the enamel of young adult teeth and tooth decay. Helps to reduce bone loss.

Credited with: NRC has not established requirements for this mineral. Fluorine is added to most city and town drinking water.

Deficiencies: Pitted adult teeth, which happens when the enamel is being formed. Tooth decay. Possible bone fractures in older animals.

Toxicity: Toxic levels are of more concern than are deficiencies with this mineral. Arthritis, decreased growth and cellular changes in liver, kidney and adrenal glands has resulted. Fat and carbohydrate metabolism have been changed from the use of excess fluoride. Bone malformations and cancer have been linked to toxic levels. Dogs that drink too much fluorinated water could become toxic.

Cravings: Oats, milk, cheese, carrots, garlic, beet tops, green vegetables, cabbage and watercress. Abundant in sea water and naturally hard (mineralized) water.

Supplement: **Selenium (sodium selenite)**

Purpose: Vitamin E and selenium are more effective together than each is alone. Antioxidants, they are needed by males for correct functioning of reproductive organs. Needs to be replaced when using dog for breeding, as selenium is stored in testes and lost in the semen.

Credited with: Elasticity in the tissues. Effective with vitamin E in treating lameness in older dogs. Helps to neutralize certain carcinogens and provide protection against cancer of the gastrointestinal tract. Used in treatment of dandruff. Essential for correct enzyme activity. Together with iodine, necessary for correct thyroid function.

Digestibility:	Could cause allergy for dogs with allergies to yeast because that is where most forms of selenium come from. Can be used with vitamin E. *Selenium can be toxic in large doses.* Use sparingly.
Deficiencies:	Liver problems, muscle degeneration, premature aging, heart disease, muscular dystrophy. Long-term deprivation has led to cancer of the gastrointestinal tract, muscular weakness of newborn pups, persistent diarrhea, dead and weak offspring. (Look for low levels of CPK and SGOT on blood work.) Research has shown that vitamin E and selenium deficiencies are more widespread in animals than had been realized.
	Found mostly in grains, theoretically there should be enough selenium in our food supplies. North America and southern Canada, where most of the grains used in dog food are grown, have been found to be deficient in selenium. It is added to most dog foods in the form of sodium selenite.
Cravings for:	Bran, tuna, tomatoes, broccoli and brewers yeast.

Supplement:	**Sulfur**
Purpose:	Not mentioned in NRC guidelines separately as it is contained in many food substances, especially protein. It is present in four amino acids and in some B vitamins, and is abundant in meat, fish, dairy products, eggs and molasses plus some vegetables. It is absorbed by the small intestine and stored in all body cells, especially in the skin, hair and nails. Dogs fed vegetarian diets may be deficient in sulfur.
Credited with:	Preventing skin disorders, eczema and dermatitis. Used topically in many preparations for wound healing and skin problems. Painful joints are helped by bathing in water high in sulfur.
	Taurine, one of the sulfur amino acids, is used in the treatment of epilepsy along with zinc. Another form of sulfur called MSM (methylsufonyl methane) has just become available for use in treating allergies.
Digestibility:	Good.
Deficiencies:	Any skin condition or coat discoloration. Sulfur deficiencies are seen when grains are grown on sulfur deficient soils, or when the diet is deficient in

animal protein and when the intestinal bacteria is depleted, evident after prolonged use of antibiotics.

Supplement:	**Zinc.** Zinc amino acid chelate, zinc oxide
Purpose:	Needed for proper growth. Involved in many enzyme systems. Helps the liver to detoxify poisons. Helps to maintain vitamin A levels in the body. Needed for healthy skin, hair and nails. Helps in the formation of collagen and improves wound healing.

It is a cofactor in the enzyme alkaline phosphatase, which helps contribute phosphates to bones. Important in producing reproductive fluids. Helps in protein digestion and has some antioxidant function. It is part of SOD and acts as an anti-inflammatory as well as an antioxidant.

It supports the immune system, improves antibody response to vaccines and regulates white blood cells. Important in insulin activity and aids in the acid-alkaline balance of the body. Helps to detoxify the body from environmental pollutants.

Credited with:	Proper growth and wound healing. Zinc uptake is affected by the kind of diet fed, and greater amounts than are currently used may be necessary.

Zinc used topically has been successful in cases of bedsores, boils, general dermatitis and acne. Ulcers on the legs respond well as do gastric ulcers. Cataracts also have been helped by using zinc, and many eye medications now contain zinc. Zinc has been used successfully in treating colds, herpes and allergies. Studies continue on the influence of zinc and leukemia.

Digestibility:	Zinc affects levels of copper in the body, which in turn affects iron. Zinc is more effective if used along with copper, B-complex, vitamin A, calcium and phosphorous.
Deficiencies:	Skin lesions on the abdomen and extremities. Eye diseases, including dry eye. Fatty changes in the liver and gallbladder. Kidney damage and inflammation of skin. White tipping, browning out or red tinges on the fur of solid-colored dogs.

"Spinning" in Bull Terriers is partially associated with a zinc deficiency plus deficiencies in manganese and amino acids. Parasites cause zinc depletion, which in turn affects the ability to absorb food.

Premature aging, dwarfism, cataracts, epilepsy, Crohn's disease, ulcerative colitis, lack of appetite, diabetes, immune suppression, infections, male infertility, learning disabilities, toxemia in pregnancy, environmental sensitivities and allergies are all related to zinc deficiencies.

Cravings for: Beef, liver, seeds of sunflowers or pumpkins, tuna fish, peanuts, whole grains. Small amounts are found in peas, carrots, beets and cabbage.

Supplement: **Trace minerals.** While the NRC acknowledges the need for some of these minerals, no levels have been established. Cobalt, molybdenum, tin, silicon, nickel, vanadium, chromium, lead and arsenic are all mentioned, but they feel that since dog food comes from natural ingredients, there is enough of these minerals in the food itself to satisfy known requirements.

Chromium works as a co-factor with insulin to move glucose from the blood into the cells and is responsible for sugar metabolism in the body. It improves carbohydrate digestion. When dogs are fed semi-moist foods, or a large amount of dog treats preserved with sugar, their bodies will be depleted of chromium which may cause heart problems. Found in liver, brewers yeast, brown rice, chicken and corn.

Molybdenum takes part in the metabolism of waste from protein (purines) and converts it to uric acid. It is antagonistic to copper and may have a protective action in copper poisoning. It is involved with carbohydrate metabolism. Deficiencies in people relate to esophageal cancer. It is found in liver, brewers yeast and cereal grains.

Silicon is sand found in stems of certain grasses. It is found in the bones, hair, nails and teeth and is used in the treatment of poor hair coat, brittle nails, crooked and poorly formed teeth. Beneficial to the healing of wounds and protects against skin disorders. Throws off pus in the body from boils, abscesses, carbuncles and postules. Lack of silicon can create epilepsy in people. If your dog eats dirt or the stems of plants, he probably needs silicon. Silicon pushes foreign objects out of the body and dogs that need to be wormed eat dirt in an attempt to push the worms out of their systems.

Summary

1. DEFICIENCIES OF MINERALS ARE MORE COMMON THAN DEFICIENCIES OF VITAMINS.

2. MINERALS ARE ESSENTIAL TO PHYSICAL AND MENTAL HEALTH AND ARE A BASIC PART OF ALL CELLS.

3. MINERALS ARE NECESSARY FOR PROPER FUNCTIONING OF BLOOD, NERVE AND MUSCLE CELLS, BONE, TEETH AND ALL SOFT TISSUE.

4. SOME MINERALS HELP TO REGULATE THE ACID-ALKALINE BALANCES IN THE BODY. Others are a part of enzymes, which aid in the production of energy.

5. MINERALS ARE STORED BY THE BODY AND CARE MUST BE TAKEN WHEN SUPPLEMENTING WITH INDIVIDUAL MINERALS. This may cause a chain reaction that affects the absorption of other nutrients.

6. SUPPLEMENTING YOUNG PUPPIES UNDER 6 MONTHS OF AGE WITH *CALCIUM* SUPPLEMENTS *ALONE CAN CREATE AN IMBALANCE* IN MANY OTHER MINERALS AND VITAMINS, THEREFORE CAUSING BONE GROWTH ABNORMALITIES.

7. PUPPIES EATING PUPPY FOOD NEED *SUPPLEMENTATION*. Use *vitamins C and B-complex,* together with *digestive enzymes,* so that the minerals in the food can be better assimilated.

8. REMEMBER THAT MOST PROCESSED DOG FOODS LOSE A NUMBER OF THEIR MINERALS IN THE COOKING PROCESS. Some are lost along the chain of distribution.

9. WHEN A DOG IS EXPOSED TO STRESS OF ANY KIND, IT USES ITS VITAMINS AND MINERALS UP AT A FASTER RATE THAN NORMAL. Correct supplementation is beneficial at these times.

10. THERE IS AN OLD ADAGE THAT SEEMS TO PREVAIL AMONG CARETAKERS OF DOGS THAT IF A LITTLE OF SOMETHING IS GOOD, THEN A LOT MUST BE BETTER. **This is wrong when using mineral supplementation.** Too much of something creates as many problems as too little.

11. SOY PROTEIN ADVERSELY AFFECTS THE ABSORPTION OF IRON.

12. CUSHING'S DISEASE—HYPERACTIVE ADRENAL GLANDS—CAN BE CAUSED BY DRINKING TOO MUCH CHLORINATED WATER.

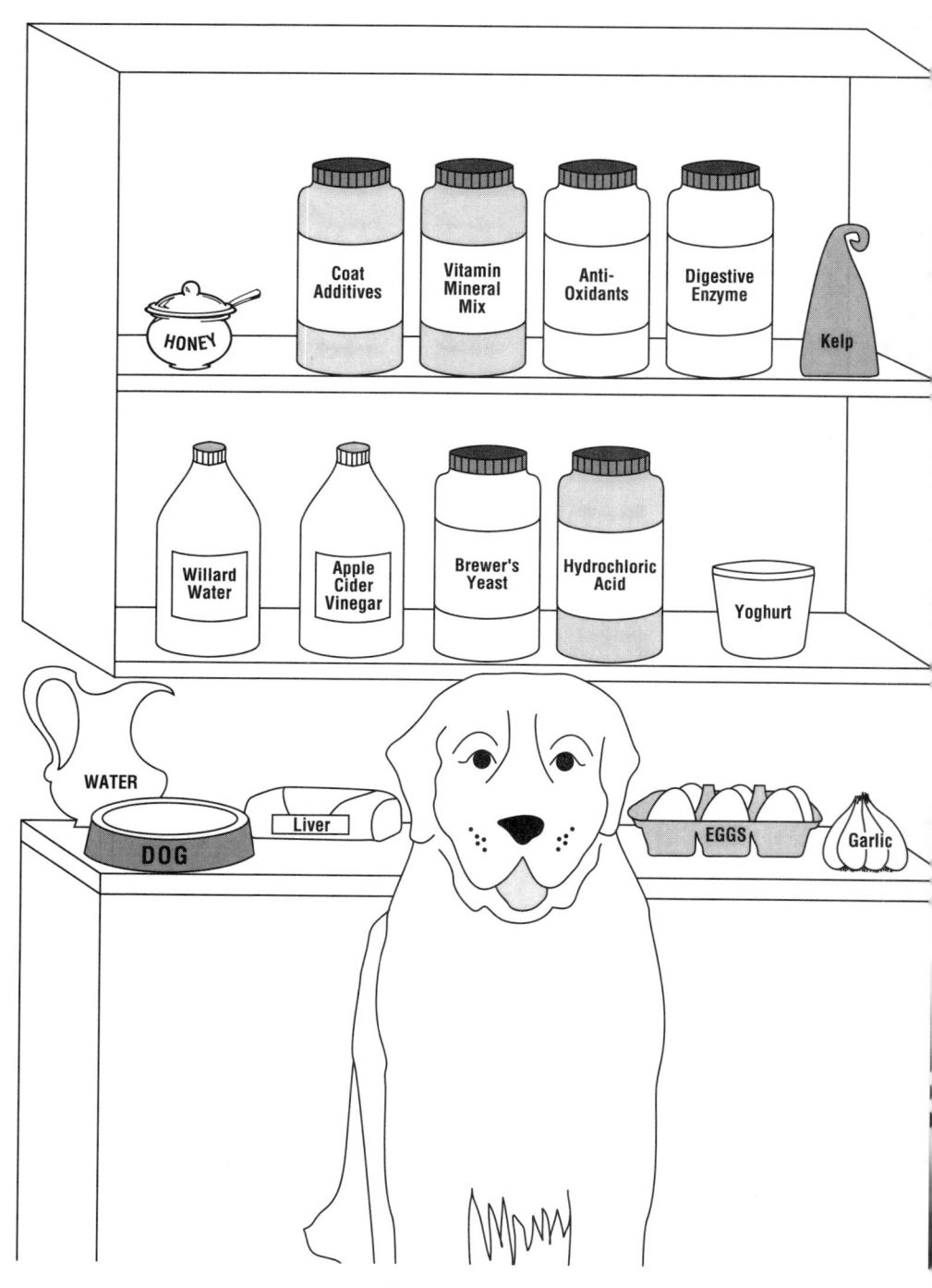

7–1: The Supplement Dog

—Chapter 7—

Water, Enzymes and Other Essential Nutrients

Water: Where Does It Come From?

Water, Water Everywhere, and Not a Drop to Drink!

If you or your dog is drinking water from the faucet in your house or apartment, you both may be ingesting bacteria, viruses, lead, gasoline, radioactive gases and carcinogenic industrial compounds. So says an article in the November 15, 1993 issue of *Time* magazine.

> By-products of chlorine, which is used to kill water borne pathogens at the water plants, is also found in water supplies, and kills more than 10,000 people of rectal and bladder cancer. Neurological problems and high blood pressure in over a million cases can be traced to lead in the water and lung and rectal cancer to radioactive contamination found in the water supplies of 50 million Americans.

Have you experienced inexplicable problems with your own health or that of your dog? Your water supply could be the cause.

Why Water Is Necessary

Water is the most necessary ingredient dogs need. Without water your dog will die. If they have adequate water, dogs can live about 3 weeks without food, but they will die in a few days without water.

Water is used by dogs for all digestive purposes, both the breaking down and absorption of nutrients, as well as maintenance of body temperature. It helps to detoxify the body and transport toxic substances out of the body through the eliminative organs. It is used to keep the acid levels of the blood constant.

The kind of food you feed will determine how much water your dog needs. Dry food contains little moisture—about 10 percent—and it is calculated that your dog needs about a quart of water for every pound of dry food eaten. A dog fed only canned food, which contains up to 78 percent moisture, will drink much less. If fed raw natural foods, a dog may drink up to 1 cup of water a day, as these foods contain large quantities of water.

The city water supply is freed from parasites and bacteria by using various chemicals such as chlorine, aluminum salts, soda, ash, phosphates, calcium hydroxides and activated carbon. According to a study done by *Consumer Reports* in 1990, the main contaminants remaining are lead, radon and nitrates. Lead will come from the pipes through which water passes. Radon is a byproduct of uranium found in the earth's crust and is more prevalent in water from wells and ground water in the Northeast, North Carolina and Arizona. Water from lakes and rivers will be less contaminated with radon. Nitrates come from ground water sources that contain agricultural contaminants.

Testing the Water

We found a simple way to test our water. Wal-Mart department store carries a small water-testing kit that you can buy for about $4, which tests chlorine, hardness (mineralization), pH (acidic) level, nitrate/nitrite and iron levels. This is not a complete test. If you are in doubt, take a sample of your water to your local cooperative extension office, which offers a water screening service. Independent laboratories also will check out the water supply for you. If you or your dogs are experiencing chronic health problems, having your water supply checked is well worth the investment. Dogs should have clean, cool drinking water at all times. There is considerable controversy about having water available directly after eating. We think if your dog is fed a high-quality diet with a small amount of dry food (up to 2 cups per meal) and the addition of fresh raw foods, and you allow a couple of hours quiet time after eating, the dog will be fine with water available all the time. Digestive troubles occur when dogs are fed diets that require an enormous amount of food (over 5 cups per sitting), drink large quantities of water, and then are allowed free exercise.

The Acid-Alkaline Balance

The more alkaline the food, the more your dog will drink to maintain the acid-alkaline balance required. Try putting a pH strip into your dog food to test the acidity. It needs to be between 6.2 and 6.5. Check the dog's urine (first thing in the morning is best) to see how your particular dog's body deals with the food. A very general rule of thumb is that primarily cereal-based foods produce a more alkaline urine, and foods high in animal proteins produce a more acid urine. Look for a food that satisfies your dog with the least amount of bulk so that the smallest amount of water is needed.

If you notice that your dog is suddenly drinking more water than usual, it could be a sign of kidney or bladder infection. Go to your veterinarian. Generally, a healthy dog drinks only what is needed. An older dog with weakened kidneys will drink more than a younger dog.

All dogs should have fresh, clean, cool water available to them at all times.

Willard Water

Any discussion of water would be remiss without mentioning Willard Water. It is still something of a mystery. In November 1980, Harry Reasoner of CBS's *60 Minutes* visited Dr. John Willard to find out if in fact the claims made by those who use it were valid. Reasoner and his crew were primed to be "alert to the first whiff of snake oil."

They saw Dr. John Willard, a professor emeritus of chemistry at the South Dakota School of Mines and Technology, drink this water for his emphysema. They talked to farmers who used it on their crops and cattle ranchers who used it for their cattle. On camera a young man sprayed Willard Water on his second- and third-degree burns suffered during a welding accident. *Sixty Minutes* returned a few weeks later to find the burns healed, with healthy, pink, unscarred skin on those areas. Harry Reasoner spoke with doctors, health officials and a biochemist and was unable to find anyone who could find evidence that Willard Water was *not* responsible for these miraculous results. Mr. Reasoner had the water analyzed by a laboratory, which was unable to find anything harmful in the water. In the conclusion of his report, Mr. Reasoner states "We haven't proved anything, and we didn't expect to. But we've met a lot of nice people, and we've found a product that everyone agrees can't hurt you. Maybe that's enough."

In the book *Aqua Vitae* by Roy Jacobsen many interesting uses of Willard Water are described:

- Ranchers who add it to their cattle's drinking water find that they are much less stressed, are healthier and utilize their food better.
- Many farmers soak seeds in Willard Water before planting and find that their crops survive even during droughts, and growth is much better than seeds not soaked in it.

- Using it on house plants makes them grow better.
- A kennel that specialized in racing greyhounds reported that they were able to get rid of a stubborn virus.
- Dog owners describe aggressive dogs becoming mellow after using Willard Water in their drinking water.

It works topically as a treatment for many skin disorders, especially hot spots. It acts as an eye wash, and you can clean out your dog's ears with it. When you are traveling with your dog, add it to the drinking water. It helps keep stress levels under control. You can soak your dog food in Willard Water.

What Is Willard Water?

Dr. Willard discovered a unique catalyst that alters the molecular structure of ordinary water. In his product Willard Water XXX one of the ingredients is fossilized organics from refined lignite. The lignite, which is rich in carbon, is added to "re-activate" the CAW (catalyst-altered water). Lignite is a source of trace minerals, nutrients and amino acids, humic acids and carbon, natural ingredients that act as growth accelerators in plants. Researchers have also found traces of antibiotics that occur naturally in lignite. We recommend *Aqua Vitae* as an excellent source for anyone interested in learning more about Willard Water.

How to Use Willard Water

We have used Willard Water in our kennel for the last several years. We use it for everything. If a dog gets a hot spot, we spray on Willard Water, which dries up the inflamed area over night. If a dog has a cut pad, we spray on Willard Water, which not only stops the bleeding but seems to relieve pain. If a dog is stung by an insect, we spray Willard Water on the site of the sting, reducing the swelling and irritation. When we travel, we use it in the dogs' water and in their food.

You buy this product in a concentrated form and add one ounce to a gallon of distilled water. It can be used topically on your dog in this dilution or you can dilute it down again when you add it to a bowl of water. Because it is successful in reducing stress, we use it at our training camps to relieve dogs of diarrhea often experienced when they have traveled a long way. It can be used for cleansing any wound, as well as after surgery to keep the surgical site clean. It promotes healing and, if used when sutures are still in, Willard Water can reduce scarring.

The easiest way to use Willard Water is to keep some in a spray bottle. In treating hot spots, the dog's hair can be parted and the water sprayed in. If you catch the hot spot and spray it before it becomes too hot, there is no need to shave the dog. We also use it to spray on the coats of long-haired dogs when grooming, and it works as a coat conditioner.

This product is as much a part of our daily routine as feeding the dogs. We use it for everything. See the Source List (Chapter 19) for where to obtain Willard Water.

Liver—the Wonder Food!

In 1972 Donald Collins, DVM, wrote *The Collins Guide to Dog Nutrition*. It has been the bible of dog feeders since that time. On page 71 he talks about the miracle of adding liver to a dog's diet. He gives anecdotal information on failing puppies being revived overnight by adding a teaspoon of chopped liver to their mother's food, of listless stud dogs and dogs not recovering as they should from surgery all being much improved by the addition of liver to the diet. He says that "if there is one single food that every dog should have in its diet, that food would have to be liver."

Liver and Toxins

Liver has fallen out of favor in the last decade or so. More informed dog feeders now know that the liver is one of the filtering organs of the body and many toxins end up there, and thus they are afraid to feed it. They are aware of all the additives put into cattle feed, from hormones to antibiotics and residues of pesticides and herbicides and fumigants used in grains, much of which would presumably end up in the cow's liver.

Let's look at this argument a little more closely. If you feed commercial dog food, you may already be feeding liver in small quantities to your dog. Look at the package. By choosing the convenience of using a commercially prepared diet, you are already feeding a product containing all of the above. Unless they are raised on organic grains, most chickens, beef cattle, sheep and turkeys are given feeds that contain all of the above ingredients. Animals fed organic grains do not end up in dog food. So not feeding liver doesn't make sense.

Buying liver at the grocery store is a good idea. It has had to pass government veterinary inspection, is free from disease, and is prepared in a clean environment. It's the best you can do.

Beef liver is full of wonderful vitamins and minerals. Certainly, those of us who raise our dogs naturally wouldn't be without it. Like anything else, it should be fed in moderation—less than an ounce a day for a 10-pound dog and up to $4^1/_2$ ounces for a 100-pound dog, no more than five times a week. Too much liver can cause dark, runny stools. We use raw beef liver in our food, but many dogs do not like the texture. If you have to cook it, put it in a pot with sufficient water to cover the liver and bring it to a boil. Immediately turn off the heat. Pork liver should be cooked a few minutes longer. Remember that B vitamins and enzymes are killed in the cooking process.

Following is a chart reprinted from *The Collins Guide to Dog Nutrition* giving the breakdown of nutrients in raw beef and pork liver.

The Nutrient Content of Beef and Pork Livers in 100 Grams or 3.53 Ounces

Nutrient	Beef	Pork	Comments
Water (%)	69.7	72.3	Similar to canned food
Protein (%)	19.7	19.7	Better bioavailabiity than canned meat
Fat (%)	3.2	4.8	
Carbohydrate (%)	6.0	1.7	
Crude fiber (%)	0	0	
Total ash (%)	1.4	1.5	
Calcium (mg)	7	10	
Phosphorus (mg)	358	362	
Iron (mg)	6.6	18.0	
Sodium (mg)	110	77	
Potassium (mg)	380	350	
Copper (mcg)	2,450	—	About 5× more than most sources
Vitamin A (IU)	43,900	14,200	
Vitamin D (IU)	34	44	Same as milk, more than plants, less than fish liver oils
Vitamin K		115–230	
Vitamin B_1 (mg)	0.26	0.40	
Vitamin B_2 (mg)	3.33	2.98	
Niacin (mg)	13.7	16.7	
Folic acid (mcg)	294	221	10× more than most foods
Pantothenic acid (mcg)	5660–8180	5880–7300	5× more than most natural sources
Biotin (mcg)	100	—	10× more than most natural sources

Nutrient	Beef	Pork	Comments
Vitamin B$_6$ (mcg)	600–710	290–590	About equal to most natural sources
Choline (mg)	480–700	470–620	5× more than most natural sources
Vitamin C (mg)	31	23	

Eggs

Eggs are misunderstood. They are a great food for dogs, if you don't go overboard and feed too many. They are complete in protein and contain lecithin as well as choline, many of the B vitamins, vitamin E, magnesium, phosphorus and selenium. Egg yolk is high in vitamin A. Lecithin and choline help to break up the Low Density Lipoproteins (LDL)—the "bad" cholesterol—and help clean out the arteries. Eggs contain the sulfur amino acids cysteine, cystine and methionine, needed for cell and tissue regeneration. We have noticed that German Shepherd Dogs, Labrador Retrievers, Boxers, Newfoundlands, Rottweilers and Pembroke Welsh Corgis seem to need more sulfur amino acids than other breeds.

We like to use eggs whole, *including* the shell. The shell is a pure form of calcium, and a dog going through a growth spurt may need extra. If needed, the eggshell is utilized; if not, it passes right through and you see it in the dog's stool. We cook the eggs 4 to 5 minutes in boiling water to kill any bacteria or other contaminants. Cooking them longer reduces the protein level. The green ring you see around the yolk is the dead protein. Brown eggs are better than white. Brown eggshells seem to absorb less bacteria than white. Organic eggs are best, if you can find them. If the eggs are cracked, throw them away, as the risk of contamination is too great.

Do not feed eggs more than three times a week. A dog over 50 pounds can have a whole small egg. A 100-pound dog can have a large egg three times a week, and a small dog (around 25 pounds) can have $^1/_2$ of a cooked egg three times a week.

Garlic

Nature's antibiotic, garlic contains a wealth of vitamins, minerals and oils, as well as protein and fat.

Garlic used in your dog's food helps to kill internal parasites. The smell of garlic excreted through the skin often makes your dog unpalatable to fleas. The oil of garlic has been used to clear up cases of ringworm, skin parasites, some warts and tumors of the skin. Used in diluted form as an enema, it can alleviate bowel infections and parasites. Used as a douche, it can correct yeast infections. You can use it with olive oil to make a mild ear medication. Peel the garlic cloves, mince them, and place them into a dark glass jar. Pour some olive oil over them—until the garlic is covered— shake, refrigerate for several days, strain the mixture and then use it. Keep it stored in a dark, cool place.

Garlic is available in tablet, capsule, fresh and liquid form. There is a form of aged garlic called kyolic garlic, which when fed does not have an odor to it. Garlic is good to use for dogs under stress or for those who live in a hot, humid climate where the chances of parasitic infestation are greater than in colder areas.

Supplements

Supplement:	**Digestive Enzymes.** Named after the food substances they digest, they end in *-ase*. Pancreatic enzymes are protease, amylase and lipase. Enzymes that digest sugar are called sucrase; those that digest phosphorus are phosphatase etc.
Purpose:	Found in all cells and fluids in the body, they are specialized protein substances that speed up and create chemical reactions. Killed at temperatures above 118–170 degrees fahrenheit, they are not available in commercial dog foods. They are necessary for all digestion to take place, particularly correct functioning of the stomach and the pancreas. Pepsin is the stomach's protein-splitting enzyme. Rennin, present only in puppies, causes milk to coagulate, changing the protein casein into a usable form in the body. Enzymes control, promote and guide all of life's vital processes including muscle movement, energy storage, breathing, digestion, reproduction, etc.

Degenerative disease, and cancer in particular, has been linked to enzyme deficiencies by researchers at the universities in London, Wales, Wisconsin, Loyola and Yale Medical School. *Cooked food is almost completely deficient in enzymes, which are destroyed during the processing.* The pancreas of rats increased in weight by 20–30 percent when fed cooked food. Cooked food makes the pancreas work harder. It passes through the digestive tract more slowly than raw food, tends to ferment and throws poisons back into the body, causing gas, heartburn, headaches, eye troubles and more serious illnesses. It begins to collect on the walls of the large intestine, which causes putrefaction and auto intoxication. Cooked foods rob the pancreas, stomach, salivary glands and intestines of enzymes. There seems to be a finite reservoir of enzymes in the body. If various organs and glands are continually robbed of their own enzymes, which must be utilized to digest food, the body eventually breaks down. Studies from the Center for the Advancement of Cancer Education have shown that pancreatic enzymes selectively destroy cancer cells. If the pancreas is provided with the correct enzymes by feeding the correct diet, those enzymes can protect the body against cancer.

A study done in Sweden clarifies the point about cooking food and digestion time. It showed that cooked, dry dog food took more than 15 hours to break down and clear the stomach and pass into the intestines. Semi-moist food took between 8 and 9 hours, and raw food was already passing into the intestines 20 minutes after ingestion, and cleared the stomach in $4^1/_2$ hours. This study shows that when the body is provided with the correct enzymes it can digest food in very little time. If the body's systems of enzymes are depleted, the stomach takes much longer to break down food. This study was done to see what time frame was required for it to be safe to anesthetize them for surgery after animals had eaten.

For dog feeders, this information is invaluable if you train, show or breed dogs. One third of the body's energy is required in the process of digestion. By supplementing with enzymes, the amount of time needed for digestion is reduced.

Raw foods contain enzymes and do not rob the enzyme-excreting organs of theirs in order to break down food reaching the stomach. Aging is directly related to enzyme depletion.

Protease, lipase, cellulase, and amylase are the enzymes that are necessary to break down protein, carbohydrates and fats for the body to digest them. Cellulase breaks down cellulose, the source of fiber in many dog foods. Pepsin and rennin are other enzymes found in the stomach. Rennin is present only in the stomachs of puppies. These enzymes break down protein from meat and milk sources into usable amino acid chains. Enzymes are catalysts, which means they cause an internal action without themselves being destroyed or changed in the process. Each enzyme acts on a specific food and one cannot be substituted for another. Enzyme deficiencies often mean the difference between health and sickness.

Credited with: Cancer prevention, weight gain, improved appetite, larger litters, increased milk production, lower puppy mortality, better recovery from surgery. Should be used when dogs experience stress, such as when they are boarded. Weight can be maintained in working, guard, sentry, hunting, breeding and showing animals by using digestive enzymes, as well as any time the dog is under extreme stress.

Experiments with enzymes are being conducted on autoimmune diseases, most notably the HIV virus and AIDS in humans, and these experiments will have some relevance to dog owners.

Digestibility: Enzymes can be sprinkled on food before eating, or put directly into the meal. Food must be consumed within $1/2$ hour after using enzymes; otherwise the enzymes will be deactivated by the stomach acid. If you travel with or show your dog it is wise to put enzymes on the food just before your dog eats, rather than packing up your food ahead of time with enzymes in it. Plant enzymes (protease, amylase, lipase etc.) break down food in the acidic environment of the stomach. Pancreatin—the pancreatic enzyme derived from an animal's pancreas—breaks down food in the alkaline environment of the small intestine. Other digestive enzymes are acidophilus (found in some yogurts, milk and kefir), bromelain (from pineapple), and papain (from papaya). Papaya and vitamin B_6 help some dogs overcome stool eating.

The action of bromelain and papain is different from other enzymes. They are best known as digestive aids that selectively digest tissue that is dead.

Especially useful in the recovery from injury or trauma, respiratory diseases, viral diseases, digestive disorders in general, certain cancers and degenerative diseases. Bromelain enzymes have been shown to reduce and eliminate swelling and inflammation in soft tissues and joints affected by diseases such as arthritis. Both bromelain and papain are helpful to get rid of scar tissue.

How much of the digestive enzymes should be used will depend on the life stage and the environment of your dog. Use kinesiology to test your dog (see Chapter 13). Young and old dogs, plus showing, working and breeding animals will need more than the household pet.

Deficiencies: Predisposition to bloat, cancer, underweight. Production of too much gas in the intestines, poor skin and coat, reproductive difficulties. Changes in vision, fatigue, depression, muscle pains, cramps in chest and back, change in the texture of the hair, brittle nails are all early cancer signs. Lysosomal storage diseases in dogs—abnormal facial characteristics—that have a genetic predisposition are caused by malfunctioning enzymes. Stool eating is a common sign of deficiency, as is scratching.

If, for example, a dog cannot break down fat in food, that dog would exhibit all the inherent signs of fat deficiency, including all the skin irritations.

Cravings: Raw foods, grazing on grasses and weeds.

Author's Note: If you added nothing else to the commercial dog food you feed except a balanced digestive enzyme product made **for dogs,** there would be an overall improvement in your dog's health. In the northern climates in winter this is important. There are no grasses or weeds for grazing. Without these natural enzymes, dogs may resort to stool eating, eating wood or even toys. Adding digestive enzymes to their food goes a long way to alleviating these problems.

Supplement: Hydrochloric Acid
Purpose: Found in the stomach, it is the first part of the digestive process. It improves the digestion and assimilation of all foods. Hydrochloric acid must be present

in the stomach in the right amount in order for food to be properly broken down before it enters the small intestine.

Credited with: Preventing diseases associated with poor assimilation of nutrients, especially calcium.

Digestibility: Tablets in the form of betaine hydrochloride are usually well tolerated. Check your dog frequently to see if this supplement is needed. Acid tablets are used for a short duration. Too many over a period of time can cause stomach and gastrointestinal tract ulcers, as well as mucousy stools.

Deficiencies: Pernicious anemia, system too alkaline, allergies of all kinds due to poor assimilation of food. Deficiencies of hydrochloric acid can be created by long-term stress. Gas, bloating, poor calcium and iron absorption, increase in intestinal bacteria, yeasts and parasites indicate a digestive system that is too alkaline. A dog that needs continuous worming needs to be tested for hydrochloric acid levels in the stomach.

Cravings: Apple cider vinegar, blackstrap molasses.

Supplement: **Lactobacillus Acidophilus,** the beneficial bacteria normally produced by the intestinal tract. Found in good quality yogurts, kefir and in tablet, capsule, powder and liquid form.

Purpose: Acidophilus is a natural bacterium that lives in the intestinal tract. It creates an environment that is undesirable for such things as fungi and microbes to grow in. It also contains a weak antibiotic substance called colicine. Acidophilus is killed when antibiotics are used, thus leaving an environment ideal for the growth of yeast and fungi. These grow and create diarrhea, flatulence and constipation. If the natural bacteria are not replenished, fungus can grow in the lungs, vagina, mouth and on the front and rear paws.

Credited with: Preventing bad breath caused by food putrefaction. Aids in digesting B-complex vitamins, some amino acids, fat and milk. Used to overcome yeast and fungus infections and to improve the functioning of the whole intestinal tract, including intestinal gas and inflammation of the digestive tract. Offers protection from contamination of food or water supplies when traveling to different areas (use with each meal). Rebuilds the "good" intestinal bacteria, which are killed when antibiotic drugs are used. Many years ago breeders successfully used acidophilus with their breeding animals during gestation and through lactation until puppies were weaned to prevent fading puppy syndrome, which has been associated with herpes infections.

Digestibility: Excellent—no known toxicity. In Europe, acidophilus and B vitamins are often prescribed along with antibiotics.

Cravings: Yogurt, soured milk products (kefir).

Supplement: **Brewers Yeast.** Commonly used in dog foods, it comes from the leftovers from the brewing industry. Some brewers yeast is grown on molasses.

Purpose: To provide extra B vitamins to the diet as well as protein, trace minerals and salts. One of the few sources of chromium and selenium.

Credited with: Repelling fleas. Contains low potencies of the B vitamins, which are credited with repelling insects. If the food being fed your dog is deficient in B vitamins (and most of them are—see section on B vitamins), then the addition of brewers yeast may not work as it will not be strong enough.

Digestibility: Generally well digested. If your dog is on antibiotics, which kill the good intestinal bacteria where yeast and fungi naturally grow, supplement with extra brewers yeast. Wait until you are through with medications. While brewers yeast used for any food purpose must have the live part of the yeast killed before being used, dogs can be allergic to yeast that comes from the brewing industry. Some yeasts are grown on molasses and are higher in B vitamins and show less allergy symptoms.

Deficiencies: Those common to the B vitamins. Infestations of fleas. May be found from feeding diets too high in grains, especially corn.

Cravings: Liver, eggs, green leafy vegetables and whole wheat bread.

Supplement: Kelp

Purpose: Provides iodine, needed for correct functioning of the thyroid gland, which in turn influences overall health, metabolism, skin and coat. Kelp contains some protein, and it is rich in iodine, calcium and potassium as well as some B vitamins.

One teaspoon of kelp contains the following:

$1/10$ grain organic iodine	$1/45$ grain organic iron
$3/5$ grain organic calcium	$1/1800$ grain organic copper
7 grains organic potassium	$1/6$ grain organic phosphorus
$1/2$ grain organic sulfur	$2^1/2$ grains organic sodium
$1/2$ grain organic magnesium	

According to researchers, kelp also contains vitamins A, E, B and D. It also contains something called mannitol, a gentle purgative and bile stimulant; small amounts of lecithin, a phosphorus compound thought to be of great importance in the knitting of broken bones, especially in the aged; and some carotin (precursor to vitamin A). (See *Folk Medicine* by D. C. Jarvis in the references.)

Kelp is used as an ingredient in many vitamin and mineral supplements and is credited with good pigmentation and healthy skin and coat as well as promoting proper thyroid function.

Supplement:	**Vitamin and Mineral Mixes**
Purpose:	To supplement diets that are deficient in vitamins and minerals.
Credited with:	All of those conditions common to vitamin and mineral deficiencies. A word of caution is necessary. Because of the needs of the dog at different life stages, a poor quality or unbalanced vitamin-mineral mix can create as many problems as it can cure. Overuse in puppies can create musculoskeletal dysfunction. While a good vitamin-mineral mix can do wonders for a dog suffering from deficiency diseases, use kinesiology (Chapter 13) to test to see if (a) your dog needs it, (b) if it is correct for your dog, (c) how much to give and (d) when to give it. Retest

frequently. The time of the year has a great influence on how much your dog will need. Our preference is to use one that is formulated from natural herbal ingredients, rather than one from a chemical base that may or may not be able to be broken down and assimilated by your pet. Nearly all dogs that we have tested using kinesiology and are fed commercial dog food have shown a need for extra supplementation. (See source list, Chapter 19, for recommendations.)

Supplement: **Coat additives**

Purpose: Since many of these products rely on vitamins A and E (fat soluble) as well as large doses of other vitamins, be very careful when you use them. *The body stores fat-soluble vitamins and it is easy to overdose on them.* Test, using kinesiology, to see if the product you have chosen is safe for your dog. Retest frequently to find the correct amount to use. A dog fed well with the correct food will not need these supplements.

Supplement: **Apple Cider Vinegar**

Purpose: "An apple a day keeps the doctor away" seems to have some veracity. Apples contain a large amount of potassium plus phosphorus, chlorine, sodium, magnesium, calcium, sulfur, iron, fluorine, silicon, and many trace minerals. In long-term studies done in Vermont on herds of cows, many benefits have been observed, e.g., lack of mastitis, itchy skin, influenza, respiratory diseases, easier freshening (whelping), lack of eclampsia and cramping after delivery of calves. Horses with ACV (apple cider vinegar) in their feed raced much better and never came down with distemper, even when exposed. ACV is credited with killing bacteria outright, and in fact was used in the late 1800's to prevent food poisoning. People carried flasks of ACV with them when they were invited to feasts. In those days the preserving of food was often done through salting or soaking in vinegar. People invited to eat away from their homes always put ACV into their drinking water to protect them against food poisoning. If you occasionally use raw fish in your dog's diet, use a little ACV. Fish even slightly "off" can create horrible gastric problems.

Credited with: Curing pyelitis, a condition caused by inflammation of the kidney. Chronic itching. According to Dr. Jarvis's book, itchy skin is a sign that the skin is too alkaline in nature. You can therefore soak your dog down with water and rub in ACV or make a wash and sponge it into the coat, allowing it to drip dry. It is amazing how quickly this stops itching. We have used it on beginning hot spots, which immediately dry up. If the skin is already broken, we dilute the ACV with water in a 1:1 ratio (think of Willard Water here), put it into a spray bottle and spray it onto the coat. This way, if you have a show dog, you do not need to shave the dog down. The hot spot dries up in 24 hours.

ACV is helpful to use internally when a dog's eyes run with clear watery discharge, or the nose runs, or when your dog is coughing a liquid kind of cough. Put a couple of tablespoonfuls in the food a day (for a dog 50 pounds or over), and you will immediately notice a difference. Use a couple of drops, diluted half and half with water, in your dog's ears at his weekly grooming session to avoid ear infections.

All of the above conditions relate to potassium deficiencies, so if your dog shows any of the following signs, such as lack of mental alertness, mental and muscle fatigue after exercise (agility participants and people who work their dogs take note), susceptibility to the cold, calluses on elbows and hock joints, constipation, itchy skin, cuts, bruises too easily, pimples on skin surface, twitching of the facial muscles, cramps in muscles, sore joints or the beginnings of arthritis, try some ACV in the dog's food and see the difference.

Try an ACV rinse in bathwater and let the dog drip dry. Fleas and ticks do not find an acidic-based skin desirable to live on, so it provides good protection against both of these parasites. Give an ACV dip when going into tick-infested country, and also before you show your dogs in the summer, where the stress of the shows seems to allow even the healthiest dog to pick up an occasional flea. ACV normalizes the pH of the skin and you get used to traveling with a dog that smells like a salad!

Supplement:	**Honey**
Purpose:	Contains iron, copper, manganese, silica, chlorine, calcium, potassium, sodium phosphorus, aluminum and magnesium. Can be used externally for treatment of skin disorders, especially effective with burns. Internally, for sinus problems, coughing, sore throats, digestive upsets, and most importantly, bringing a dog in shock around. Dark honey is more effective than light honey.
Credited with:	Honey has the ability to kill bacteria. You will notice that no matter how long you keep honey on the shelf, it doesn't change in consistency, and doesn't go bad. The Agriculture College in Colorado tried several experiments with honey in which a bacteriologist tried to grow certain diseases in honey. The honey killed all of the microorganisms. Typhoid, A and B typhosus, bowel bacteria, broncho-pneumonia bacteria, peritonitis, pleuritis and suppurative abscesses bacteria all died, as did dysentery-producing bacteria. These tests were duplicated in Canada and Washington, D.C., producing the same results.

Honey is a *must* in dog rearing. We keep some in the refrigerator at all times. If anything untoward happens with the dogs—a fight, for example—and one of the dogs goes into shock, we have honey in a hardened form that is easily administered to the dog in question. About a tablespoon brings around an 80-pound dog immediately and the color comes back into the dog's gums.

In breeding, we use it for females who slow down when whelping and the interval between puppies gets longer. It gives them a little pick-me-up and helps them go back into labor. It is wonderful for feeding orphaned pups. If dogs are sick for any length of time and have not eaten, a meal of honey and yogurt can do wonders to restore their appetites. It is especially important for those dogs that have weak digestive systems and are already being supplemented with enzymes. Honey contains the enzymes amylase and invertase, which aid digestion. Honey is not irritating to the lining of the digestive tract, it is easily and rapidly assimilated, it quickly furnishes the demand of energy, it helps recuperation from any stressful event—be it surgery or an athletic endeavor—it is handled well by the kidneys, it has a gentle laxative effect and it acts as a natural sedative to calm the body.

Every dog house should contain honey!

Supplement:	**Antioxidants. Vitamins A, C, D, E and Selenium**
Purpose:	Special nutrients that protect the body from invasion of pirate cells called free radicals. Free radicals are cells that act alone instead of in pairs as do normal cells in the body; they destabilize cells that keep the body in balance.

There are good free radicals and there are bad ones. The bad ones are responsible for the oxidization of body processes, something like the rusting of iron when exposed to air, or more commonly, turning ripe fruit brown. Acting like single bullets going toward a special target, when they get there, they generate more of themselves and create a chain reaction that disrupts many bodily functions. They compete in the body with *vitamin E and selenium (good free radicals)*, destroying them and many enzymes necessary for correct bodily function. Ethoxyquin used as a preservative in some dog foods is a bad antioxidant.

Credited with: Good free radicals act as vacuum cleaners in the body, mopping up the bad free radicals in a cell's interior. Clinical tests on animals show that by the use of antioxidants life spans can be increased dramatically. Activity levels increase as does the ability to reproduce longer, overall appearance of skin and coat and muscle tone, and the animals show higher energy levels.

Digestibility: Vitamins A and D are retained by the body and are oil soluble. They are found in most dog foods. Supplementing with these vitamins should be done carefully. Vitamin E, while being a fat soluble vitamin, is much less harmful in large doses, than A and D. Care should be taken in supplementing E in too high quantities if there is a history of heart disease. Selenium is also retained by the body, and should only be used in small amounts. Vitamin E, listed as dl-Alpha tocopherol, and Selenium, listed as sodium selenite on the dog food package, are used as natural preservatives and are both antioxidants. The addition of fresh liver to your dog food will provide Vitamins A and D in the correct, balanced quantities. Supplement with extra vitamin E and Selenium. Using enough Vitamin C in your dog's diet will not only safeguard health, it will make these antioxidants work better. Using the vitamin/mineral mix that we recommend, will provide all of the above vitamins and minerals.

Deficiencies: Cancer, weak hindquarters, muscular wasting, premature aging, respiratory diseases, autoimmune diseases, chronic fatigue, chronic ear conditions, gum disease, colitis, and some heart problems.

Cravings: Liver, milk, brewers yeast, fish, whole green leafy vegetables, yellow vegetables and organic wheat.

Author's Note: More research dollars are going into studies on antioxidants and free radicals than any other area of nutritional research. It is predicted that the 1990s will unravel the mysteries of these destructive cells. One area where you can make a difference is by keeping all cooking or vegetable oils refrigerated after opening. Nearly all oil, after being opened and exposed to light, becomes rancid—the breeding ground of free radicals. To keep your oil fresh after opening, put a few drops of vitamin E oil or a broken vitamin E capsule into the cooking oil and then refrigerate.

Summary

1. HUNDREDS OF SUPPLEMENTS ARE AVAILABLE TO THE DOG OWNER, AND UNLESS YOU HAVE A DEGREE IN NUTRITION OR CHEMISTRY, IT IS DIFFICULT TO KNOW WHAT IS CORRECT FOR YOUR DOG. A dog fed correctly will need minimal supplementation.

2. IF YOUR DOG IS A POOR EATER, OR GENERALLY UNTHRIFTY, USE KINESIOLOGY TO CHECK IF THE DOG'S STOMACH IS FUNCTIONING CORRECTLY. If you notice undigested food in your dog's stool, either the stomach or pancreas is not functioning well. Hydrochloric acid

tablets can put this in balance. Test frequently, and do not overuse this supplement. If it is not the stomach, test the pancreas. There are special pancreatic enzymes that can be added to your dog's diet to normalize this organ.

3. IF YOU HAVE A DOG THAT HAS BEEN SICK FOR A WHILE AND YOU ARE WORRIED ABOUT POOR EATING HABITS, CONSIDER OFFERING LIVER. Cook very lightly and save the water. Put into a blender and mix into a thin soup. You can use a turkey baster to suck up the liver mixture and gently and slowly squeeze it into the side of the dog's mouth. Be careful not to elevate your dog's head too high. When you need to get food into your dog this way, the animal's head should be almost parallel to the ground. If you bring the head up and force food down the dog's throat, you may activate the gag reflex and your dog may vomit. Liver has brought more dogs around after a bout of sickness than any other food.

4. ABOVE ALL, USE COMMON SENSE. Do not fall victim to the latest fads in dog foods or supplementation to your dog's food. If you find that you are putting in too many supplements just to keep your dog in good condition, or jumping around from one food to another, think about changing your dog's diet to one of higher quality or use the Natural Diet. Use kinesiology backed up by blood work to monitor your dog's health on a regular basis.

Chapter 8

Reading Labels and Making Choices

On the back of every dog food package is certain information that, if you understand it, can help you decide what food is correct for your dog.

It lists the *ingredients* by order of weight, with the heaviest items coming first. It contains the *guaranteed analysis* of the product in terms of crude protein, fat, fiber, moisture, ash and often calcium, phosphorus and magnesium ratios. It may also state that it is **nutritionally complete**, or provides *100% nutrition* for the dog. If it does the food has met the nutrient requirements of the Association of American Feed Control Officers (AAFCO), which guarantees some form of testing has been done on the product.

A company must also list its name and address and give a telephone number plus the date of manufacture; the weight of the food will be given, and usually the life stage for which the food is intended, for example, puppy, maintenance, adult, old age, or light ("lite") for less active dogs and so forth.

Ingredients—Dry Dog Food

"You get what you pay for" is not necessarily true for dog food. There is a surprisingly small difference between good and bad, and some bad are higher priced than good!

Ask yourself what your expectations are for your dog. There are more than 3,000 foods from which to choose. **Performance foods** provide your dog with a lot of energy to meet an active lifestyle. They contain animal protein sources as the first two ingredients, or list two sources of animal protein in the first three ingredients. Performance foods are intended primarily for working animals as well as dogs used for breeding. They have the highest amount of protein and fat but no soy.

The next category contains higher levels of protein from animal sources but usually uses an animal protein source first, and then two grain sources next. These are called **Super Premium I** foods, and are quite high in protein and fat. They provide more energy from the higher fat levels.

Super Premium II foods are similar in terms of protein content, but their fat levels are lower. Those listed do not contain soy.

Premium foods contain the higher levels of protein common to the Super Premium foods, but you need to check the sources of protein. They are midrange in fat levels—7–12 percent—and they may contain soy.

Foods listed as Regular, Econo, Low-Protein Fat or Lite and so on are so full of grains, they would only be useful if you wanted to make your dog into a semi-vegetarian or a couch potato. They are animal protein deficient. Reports from the industry state that some of these foods are so low in vital minerals that tails have fallen off dogs who have eaten them! They also produce large quantities of smelly stools.

Guaranteed Analysis

On the back of the package is a list of figures that give, in percentages, the levels of crude protein, fat, fiber, moisture, and in some instances the calcium and phosphorus levels. *Crude* means the sum total of these nutrients in all the ingredients. When you add these percentages, you may come up with a figure of only 35 to 55 percent, and this represents a rough guide to the nutrients and composition of the ingredients. What is left over is called *dry matter* and is composed of carbohydrates. Adding up those figures can be useful, since it will tell you how much of the food can be used by your dog. For example, the *"lite" foods*, containing large amounts of cereal grains and little fat, contain totals of dry matter much higher than the foods high in protein. These foods give your dog the feeling of being full, with a lot of bulk to digest, and provide a smaller amount of nutrients.

Digestibility

A simple test is to check the volume of what goes in and what comes out! If the volume of stool produced is greater than the volume of food eaten, the digestibility of the food is poor. A volume of stool equal to or slightly less than the quantity of food eaten means poor digestibility. A volume of around 25 percent of the food fed, with little odor, indicates good digestibility.

Quality

A dog food manufacturer buys ingredients from many sources. The quality of those ingredients reflects itself in the price. **Use a poor-quality food and you raise a poor-quality dog.** What we have learned from talking to the pet food industry is that there is no way under the Labeling Act for a company that is using top of the line, natural ingredients to differentiate itself from a company using cheap ingredients. Some companies buy their beef and chicken from federally inspected plants and have control over what is fed the source animal used in the food. This is rare in the industry. Others advertise that their grains come from sources free of chemical pesticides. We think that the consumer needs to have these facts clearly stated on the labels.

Testing

A label that says something to the effect that it is complete and balanced or 100% nutritionally complete reflects that the food meets the AAFCO guidelines. AAFCO does spot testing of products by taking them off the shelf and putting them through rigorous testing. To earn the stamp of approval the food must contain what the label states.

Evaluating a Food

To learn more about the food you use, telephone the company and talk to the nutritionist in charge. It has been our experience that they are very helpful. Ask what experiences they have had with dogs of your breed and if they know of any special needs that breed may have. Ask for their help in determining the kind of food best for your dog's lifestyle.

However, remember that the company is going to try and influence you to buy its brand. If the food contains a lot of preservatives, coloring agents, a preponderance of grains or such things as peanut hulls, eliminate that food from your list. None of those ingredients are good for your dog.

In evaluating the food best for your dog, remember that *crude protein* is the sum total of all the protein contained in the animal protein source, plus the protein found in grains. A high protein content is not necessarily a sign of quality. Check out the animal source proteins. The same goes for the fats. It is the sum total of the fat that is added, plus that found in the grains. *Crude* doesn't equal *available*. Our shoes are made from leather that is high in protein, but that doesn't make it available for our dogs, even when he chews up our favorite pair! *Fiber* means that part of the grain or plant that is not digestible. It is composed of cellulose, lignins, and gums. **Bio-availability, what our dogs can actually use and digest, comes from high-quality ingredients.**

Minimum Daily Requirement

Although there is no chart on the back of the package to indicate that the ingredients meet known minimums, AAFCO studies are in general based on those same National Research Council studies that have just been rejected in favor of the AAFCO guidelines. Confused? You should be!

The quantity of each nutrient in the food you have chosen is supposed to meet the levels required to sustain *minimum* life for a 24-hour period. This is what MDR means. As we have noted in the chapters on vitamins, minerals and amino acids, many levels for differing life stages have not been established by laboratory testing. So statements on the packages to the effect that the food is complete for all life stages or is complete and balanced are inherently untrue. What is true is that companies or individuals that have been in business for long periods of time have, by experience, developed foods that are adequate for the majority of dogs.

How Much to Feed

If you follow the feeding suggestions on the label of the food you have chosen you may notice that your dog is simply not eating the recommended amount. You think to yourself that the manufacturer is just telling you to feed that amount of food in order to sell more food. For a Newfoundland, the package may suggest 14 cups of food a day. We have never come across one that could eat that much, so what does that mean? *If the package says a 50-pound dog needs 4 cups of food, that amount is needed to get the minimum daily requirement of known nutrients.* The food meets those needs by providing those nutrients in the number of cups listed on the label. A dog eating substantially less than suggested is not receiving what is needed to maintain health. The dog will ultimately experience a deficiency disease, often expressing itself in skin, ear or eye conditions, as well as musculoskeletal disease.

Canned Food

Wet Weight versus Dry Weight

Canned foods measure their ingredients in wet weight, the actual amount of the raw ingredient as it goes in the can, versus a concentrated version with 90 percent of the moisture removed, as reflected in dry food. You cannot compare the 8 to 10 percent protein listed on the can to a dry food. A simple, approximate way to convert the protein level is to add 10 percent. If the can lists 10 percent protein, for example, 20 percent would compare to the dry form.

Canned food comes in many price ranges and in many qualities, from all beef to those that are primarily cereal based, and some cross-bred stew mixtures. For assurance that the food meets some guidelines or has been tested, look for the AAFCO statement on the can. Feeding canned food is much more expensive than feeding dry food. Canned food contains up to 78 percent moisture, so you are paying for only 22 percent actual dry ingredients.

Many people add canned food to their dry food to pep it up a bit, and dogs certainly seem to enjoy it. One large plus in favor of canned food is that by virtue of the processing it undergoes few companies feel the need to add preservatives. The heat and vacuum packing in the canning process makes it unnecessary. One drawback is that the integrity of the vitamins and minerals is in doubt because many are destroyed in the heating process.

Semi-Moist Food

Semi-moist food is "consumer friendly" and palatable to most dogs. It contains sweeteners or preservatives to give it a long shelf life and coloring agents to make it attractive. As the sole diet it may cause digestive upsets. Moisture content will range from 20 to 25 percent. Recently a very attractive semi-moist food in the shape of a sausage has appeared on the market. Made from natural ingredients and preserved with Vitamin E, the feeding suggestions are given by the inch. Fifty-pound dogs are said to need anywhere from $1^3/_4$ to 3 inches a day. It is a cute and attractive idea and the dogs love it. But if you look carefully, the *fourth ingredient is sugar*, listed as sucrose. Remember, that means by weight. Should we care?

Sugar stimulates the pancreas to produce insulin, which is needed to metabolize carbohydrates. The pancreas has to work overtime to produce additional insulin when simple carbohydrates (sugar) are ingested. The stress and the work overload to the pancreas sets the stage for pancreatic disease. Once this happens the body loses its ability to digest food properly. Poor digestion leads to dizziness, confusion, fatigue, headaches, restlessness, and a change in temperament. If at the same time the food has high levels of fat, your dog will feel tired, as the tissues of the body will not be receiving enough oxygen to function properly.

Salt can be used together with sugar or alone as a preservative and is found on the label as sodium chloride. Although some will always be present, check its position on the ingredient list. Excessive salt can cause fluid retention, heart disease and strokes. In high doses, salt disrupts mineral metabolism.

Frozen Food

The type freshest and closest to a natural food is frozen dog food. Not readily available, it has its drawbacks in distribution and storage. If it is available to you, and your dog enjoys it, it may be the best answer to the dog-feeding dilemma. Composed mostly of fresh, raw ingredients, its moisture content ranges from 40 to 70 percent.

If you do your own digestibility trial on fresh frozen foods, you will be amazed at how little stool is produced. As the dog is a partial carnivore, this should not be surprising. Frozen food provides food that the dog's system is geared toward digesting.

Recognizing Preservatives

It is hard to tell what is a preservative and what is not when you read the labels on dog food packages. Here are the most common preservatives used in dog food. There are five kinds:

1. **Antioxidants** such as BHA, BHT, ethoxyquin and propyl gallate, are used to preserve fats.
2. **Mold inhibitors** retard the growth of molds and yeasts such as potassium salts, sodium or calcium proprionate, sodium diacetate, sorbic acid, acetic acid or lactic acid.
3. **Sequestrants** prevent physical or chemical changes to the color, odor, flavor or appearance of the food. These are listed in the form of sodium, potassium or calcium salts or citric, tartaric, or pyrophosphoric acids.
4. **Humectants** are chemicals that prevent food from drying out or getting too moist. Calcium silicate is common as are propylene glycol (the same ingredient used in antifreeze), glycerine and sorbitol.
5. **Texturizers**, not preservatives as such, are used in meats to maintain their texture and color. The most common are sodium nitrite and sodium nitrate.

The **good preservatives** are vitamin C and vitamin E. Vitamin E is often listed as tocopherol. The **bad preservatives,** which cause side effects that accumulate over time, are ethoxyquin, propylene glycol, BHA, BHT, sodium nitrate/nitrite and many of the chemical salts.

Reading the Date Code

You can determine how fresh your dog food is by learning to read the bar or production code on the label. Often found on the top of the package, it will consist of a series of numbers and letters that indicate the date of manufacture, the factory where it was manufactured and the number of the batch. Each manufacturer has a different way of listing these, but what follows are the most commonly used codes.

International Date Code—160293, for example, means that this batch of food was made on February 16, 1993.

Month/Day/Year—021693 means that this batch was made on February 16, 1993.

Julian Calendar—10293 means the 102nd day of the year 1993. Sometimes the 9 of the year is left out and only 4 digits are used.

Best Before—3/15/94 means the food must be used before that date (March 15, 1994) because it was probably made one year prior to that date.

Lifestyle

In trying to choose just the right dog food, an important element is your own lifestyle. If you work all day and your dog is left alone for long periods of time, a high-performance food that provides loads of energy may be counterproductive. Left alone, the dog with nothing to do and lots of energy to spare finds ways of expending that energy without you. Your dog could become a chewer, digger, barker, or a combination of all of these. A food higher in cereal grains produces a calmer dog, one less likely to get into trouble. Many perfectly normal dogs are labeled hyperactive because they have nothing to do with their energy. If you are a committed exerciser and take your dogs for long walks daily, or work or train him, a high-performance food is for you.

If, like the majority of owners, your dog is a pleasant pet that keeps you company, and you do not have the time or interest to get involved in a great deal of exercise, then one of the super premium II foods may be the best choice.

Working Dogs

One third of your dog's energy goes into digesting food. When you are working a dog, it is helpful to understand how long food stays in the digestive tract so you can feed appropriately. The kind of food you feed determines this. For example, dry dog food stays in the stomach 15 to 16 hours before all of it is passed into the small intestine. Canned or semi-moist food stays in the stomach 8 to 9 hours. Raw foods stay in the stomach 4 to 5 hours; they break down the quickest and can be detected in the small intestine within 30 minutes.

Your Dog and Stress

Do remember that if your dog is exposed to stress, such as being put into a kennel, having surgery, going to dog shows, traveling, moving, accepting another pet or child into the household and so on, you need to increase the protein content to counteract that stress. Finding a line of foods that has differing protein levels is good, so the basic ingredients are the same but the protein contents are different. For example, if your dog is eating one kind of food that falls into the premium category, you could choose the performance food from that line during times of stress. It will contain the extra animal protein and fat your dog needs to counteract the stress. You could also add canned meat from that same company, instead of upgrading to the premium food. Adding the vitamin/mineral mix, vitamins B and C and a digestive enzyme, also helps your dog to adjust well to stressful situations.

Stress is also incurred when a dog is fed food that it cannot easily digest. Many German Shepherd Dogs and other European breeds cannot digest and utilize corn well, and they thrive on beef but not chicken. Feeding a chicken- and corn-based food to these dogs stresses their systems, which creates allergic reactions, an inability to gain weight, musculoskeletal problems, plus digestive system upsets.

The summary of this chapter will list several other guidelines for choosing the correct food for your dog. If you are feeding a commercial nonfrozen dog food, remember that it is a processed product, probably deficient in digestive enzymes and some vitamins and minerals. Most of the B vitamins, many of the minerals and all of the enzymes are killed by heat over 118 degrees.

Supplementation

Supplementation in the way of a good vitamin/mineral mix for adult, breeding and old dogs is crucial to good health. Young puppies will certainly need extra B-complex and C vitamins, or the Puppy Stress Formula as they progress through rapid growth, and to counteract the stress of the vaccines to which they are exposed at that age. (See the section on raising puppies in Chapter 14.) Adding fresh food in the form of raw meat, liver, fresh fruit and vegetables—in moderation—is always a good idea. Any additions should not total more than 10 percent of the complete diet.

Of the hundreds of dogs we have tested with kinesiology over the past 12 years, some common supplements were needed by all of them. These are vitamin B-complex, vitamin C (calcium ascorbate), a vitamin/mineral mix, plus some raw food in their daily meals. Others had greater needs such as amino acid complex tablets, digestive enzymes, vitamin E and selenium or fatty acids. Use kinesiology to test the correct supplementation for your dog.

Half and Half

Trying to mix a commercial balanced dog food with natural foods, half and half, is *not* a good idea. We tried this for six weeks, after which the dog's blood was drawn and tested. The results were not good. We found it to be extremely complicated, and the amount of supplements needed to balance out the whole diet was so complex and expensive it was not worthwhile. It could also prove to be dangerous in the long run. Many owners in the veterinary practice have tried this kind of feeding without success. Our advice is either to use the best commercial food for your dog with sensible supplementation or to follow the Natural Diet in the second part of this book.

Food and Behavior

There is a direct correlation between what your dog eats and how the dog behaves. If a dog is hyperactive or lethargic, chances are something in the food—or not in the food—is creating the behavior. Many behavioral disorders in children are traced to coloring agents and preservatives in food. In the last decade researchers have found a frighteningly similar pattern in dogs. Many of the most advertised and popular brands of food contain the highest number of food colorings and the greatest amount of preservatives. *Dog biscuits and treats can be the worst culprits.*

Behavior ranging from aggression to timidity, an inability to learn, being stubborn or hardheaded, obsessive-compulsive disorders, and uncontrolled barking, can be traced to improper feeding.

The charts below list some dry dog foods for comparative purposes. Due to the large number of foods available, many foods are not listed. We did not mention the regular, econo or "lite" foods as we feel they are dangerous to feed to dogs without proper supplementation. They lack animal protein, are generally too low in fat, extremely high in fiber, and many of them contain undesirable preservatives and food dyes. Part of these charts appeared in the popular magazine *Dog World* and the consumer magazine *Good Dog*. They are for your guidance only.

Product	Protein %	Fat %	Fiber %	Moisture Category
Performance: highest protein and fat; no soy				
Eukanuba Original	30	20	4	10
Pro Plan Performance[a]	30	20	3	12
Annamaet Ultra[a,b]	32	20	3	10
Eagle Power Pack	30	20	4.5	9
Super Premium I: high protein and fat; no soy				
ANF 30	30	18	3.5	10
Bil-Jac Select[b,c]	27	17	4	10
Dad's High Protein	30	15	4.5	12
Eukanuba Adult	25	16	5	10
Precise—Endurance[a,c]	28	18	3	10
Fromm Performance[a]	26	18	3.5	10
Pro Plan Turkey & Barley[a]	25.4	16.5	2	10.2
Nutro Max	26	16	4	10
Natural Life Condition[a,d]	28	18	3.5	10
Pet Guard-Lifespan[a,b,c]	26	15	4	12
Super Premium II: high protein, lower fat, no soy				
Annamaet Extra[a]	26	12	4	12
Precise Foundation Formula[a,c]	24	14	3	10
Nature's Recipe Maint.[a,d]	20	10	4.5	10
Nutro's Natural Choice[a,d]	21	12	5	10
Natural Life Lamaderm[a,d]	22	10	4	10
Premium: high protein, lower fat; may contain soy				
Alpo Protein Plus	28	11	4	12
Hill's Science Diet, Maint.	22	13	3	10
Kennel Ration Biscuit	24	7	3	10
Purina High Pro	27	10	4	12
Solid Gold Hund-N-Flocken[a,c,d]	22	8		

Code:
[a] Naturally preserved
[b] Animal protein first 2 ingredients
[c] Company controls source of ingredients
[d] No corn in ingredients

Where there is no code, or where the [b] appears without the [a] note, indicates a food that is p▸ with ethoxyquin, BHA, BHT or propylene glycol.

Following are the phone numbers of some of the companies that make naturally preserved foods.

Annamaet	(215) 453-0381	
Precise	(800) 446-7148	
Fromm	(800) 325-6331	
Nature's Recipe	(800) 843-4008	
Nutro	(800) 833-5330	
Natural Life	(800) 367-2391	
Pro Plan	(800) PRO PLAN	
Pet Guard	(800) 874-3221	This company also produces a
	(800) 331-7527	line of natural pet products.

There are two frozen foods that have control of their ingredients and that are preserved naturally. These are Bil Jac Frozen (800-321-1002) and Adaby (914-473-1900).

Summary

Choosing a dry food is an exercise in compromise. If you find the ingredients you want to feed in the correct ratio, the company has chosen to use BHA, BHT or ethoxyquin as a preservative. If you find a naturally preserved food, then the ingredients generally contain far too much cereal for the average dog. If you find a naturally preserved food with the correct ingredients, then often the distribution of that food is the problem. If everything else is correct, there is only one product put out by that company and so the various life stages have to be correctly supplemented—not an easy task for the average dog owner. The reader is left to make the compromise that he or she can accept.

1. IN CHOOSING THE CORRECT FOOD FOR YOUR DOG, LOOK FOR THE FOOD THAT WILL SUPPLY THE ENERGY NECESSARY FOR THAT DOG'S DAILY ACTIVITIES AND LIFE STAGE.
2. LOOK FOR A FOOD THAT HAS AT LEAST ONE IF NOT TWO ANIMAL PROTEIN SOURCES IN THE FIRST THREE INGREDIENTS. Remember that the sum total of the protein listed on the package is from both animal and cereal sources.
3. MAKE SURE THAT THE FOOD LABEL HAS THE AAFCO STATEMENT OF TESTING ON IT.
4. BUY YOUR FOOD FROM AN OUTLET THAT HAS A LARGE AND QUICK TURNOVER OF FOOD, ESPECIALLY IF IT IS PRESERVED NATURALLY.
5. IF THE BAG IN WHICH YOUR FOOD IS PACKAGED SHOWS GREASE ON THE OUTSIDE, DO NOT BUY IT.

6. WHEN YOU OPEN A BAG OF FOOD, IF YOU SEE MOLD, SMELL RANCID-ITY OR SEE THE INGREDIENTS BREAKING UP, RETURN IT AND GET ANOTHER BAG. *Do not feed food that is not fresh.*

7. ELIMINATE FROM YOUR LIST ANY FOOD THAT GIVES YOUR DOG EITHER LOOSE STOOLS OR A LARGE VOLUME OF STOOL WITH AN UNPLEAS-ANT ODOR.

8. SELECT A FOOD THAT GIVES YOUR DOG TWO OR THREE STOOLS A DAY THAT ARE SMALL AND WELL FORMED.

9. DO NOT "DOCTOR" UP A FOOD TO MAKE IT MORE PALATABLE. If your dog is refusing to eat, the food probably contains something that the dog is not able to digest or may be allergic to.

10. THE FOOD YOU CHOOSE SHOULD PROVIDE A HEALTHY, SHINY AND ODORLESS COAT.

11. ANY FOOD THAT CAUSES YOUR DOG TO LOSE WEIGHT SHOULD BE ELIMINATED FROM THE LIST.

12. AVOID FOODS THAT REQUIRE ENORMOUS AMOUNTS TO FEED. Look instead for a food that has more calories (energy) in a smaller amount of food. These are the foods higher in animal protein.

13. LOOK FOR A FOOD THAT USES CHELATED, OROTATE OR AMINO ACID–BASED MINERALS.

14. AVOID ANY FOOD THAT CONTAINS ETHOXYQUIN AS A PRESERVATIVE.

15. IF YOU ARE USING A CANNED FOOD, LOOK FOR AN ANIMAL PROTEIN SOURCE IN THE FIRST THREE INGREDIENTS.

16. CANNED FOODS SHOULD NOT CONTAIN MORE THAN 78 PERCENT MOISTURE.

17. CANNED FOODS SHOULD NOT CONTAIN PRESERVATIVES.

18. CANNED FOODS SHOULD CONTAIN THE AAFCO TESTING STATE-MENT ON THE LABEL.

19. AVOID SEMI-MOIST FOODS AS THE SOLE DIET FOR YOUR DOG. They contain the largest content of coloring agents and preservatives of all the foods.

—Chapter 9—

Allergies, Toxins and Vaccines

Just like people, dogs are subject to allergic reactions. The allergen can be natural or artificial, organic or inorganic. The effect can be immediate or delayed, dramatic or subtle. In most cases, there is something you can do about it.

Environmental

In *Pet Allergies: Remedies for an Epidemic*, Alfred Plechner, DVM, paints a dismal picture for the future of our pets: "Because many commercial foods are woefully deficient in key nutrients, the long term effect of feeding such foods makes the dog hypersensitive to its environment" (p. 6). Dr. Plechner notes "it's a dinosaur effect. Animals are being programmed for disaster, for extinction. Many of them are biochemical cripples with defective adrenal glands unable to manufacture adequate cortisol, a hormone vital for health and resistance to disease" (p. 7).

Allergies can be deficiency diseases that go unrecognized. We can often use the term *allergy* or *deficiency* interchangeably. A dog fed correctly should have a lifetime free of any allergies, especially allergies to parasites. Fleas and ticks are a good example; they rarely infest a really healthy animal. They are a sign that the dog's acid/alkaline balance is not correct and the dog's system is out of balance. Many skin allergies are deficiency diseases causing the surface of the skin to be too alkaline. Itchy skin can result only if the skin is too alkaline. (See Chapter 4.)

Many typical treatments for skin conditions contain sulfur. Sulfur is in meat and other animal proteins, and the amino acids that contain sulfur are often deficient in dogs who respond to sulfur drugs. These dogs often have a protein deficiency. Other allergies can be caused by the dog's environment and genetic predisposition.

Common allergens are the detergents and fabric softeners used to wash the dog's bedding. Softeners contain formaldehyde, which is associated with causing arthritis in people. Wormers can cause an adverse reaction in some dogs. Flea repellents of whatever kind, including medicated shampoos and dips, are all possible sources of allergic reactions.

What about all those lawn products our neighbors use? Within a few moments of a dog's walking on sprayed surfaces, these chemicals enter the dog's bloodstream through the footpads. A few minutes later the dog may show adverse reactions. Do you take your dog to the local park for a walk? Is that park sprayed for mosquitoes or the grass sprayed for weeds? Do you live in an area where the local county sprays your streets in the summer for mosquitoes? If you show your dog and the shows are held in parks, has your dog experienced a lack of appetite at the shows, developed hot spots or come home with fleas? All of these symptoms and many others may be the results of toxins in the environment.

Consider also *rawhide treats*, many of which contain *propylene glycol*, a preservative with a sweet flavor that is a component of antifreeze. Dogs get hooked on them, and we are then surprised when they lick up the antifreeze that drips out of our cars. Antifreeze is deadly to our pets. Today, dog treats come in new and exciting shapes like hooves and ears of pigs and horses. What makes them stand up to heat, light and contaminations from being chewed and left, without going moldy? Preservatives! How many different chemicals does *your* dog ingest?

Other allergens include dust, wool carpets and blankets, molds, cedar chips used in bedding, flowers, pollens, house and garden plants and weeds. Numerous bacteria that float around, especially on food that is left out, or rotten human food that is thrown to the dog, the water your dog drinks—all can contain contaminants. (See Chapter 8.)

If you have a kennel facility for your dog, what housing do you provide? Concrete, gravel, earth, grass? How do you clean your kennel? What sprays do you use on a regular basis for grooming, bathing? What kind of light do you use? (Yes, even light can be an allergen to some dogs.) Ordinary fluorescent lighting has been linked to depression, inability to breed and poor appetite in some dogs. (See Chapter 17.)

Pillows containing feathers, perfumes you wear, walking your dog where the leaves are on the ground and covered with mold, can all have an effect, as can pollens from trees, plants, flowers and bacteria that contaminate food or water.

Vegetables or fruits bought at the supermarket that have been exposed to frequent spraying during growth (grapes and apples go through 15 sprayings before they are picked and marketed), also can produce an allergic reaction. They need a thorough cleansing before you feed them to your dog. (See Chapter 19.)

Even the dog dishes you use can contain contaminants. Pottery is popular for gifts, and gaily colored dog dishes are frequently given as presents. These dishes can contain heavy metals in the bright paints that are used

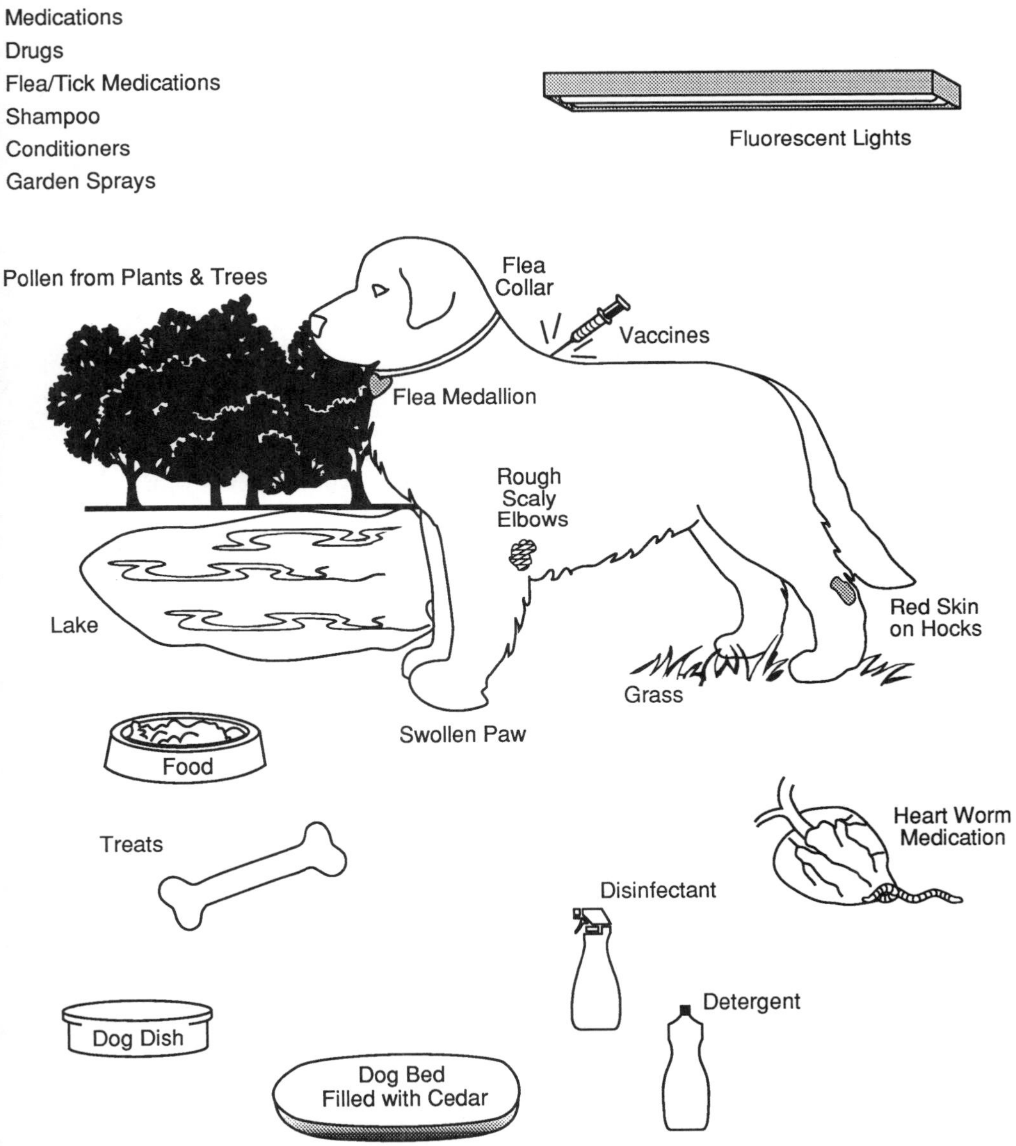

Medications
Drugs
Flea/Tick Medications
Shampoo
Conditioners
Garden Sprays

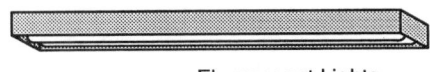

Fluorescent Lights

Pollen from Plants & Trees

Flea
Collar

Vaccines

Flea Medallion

Rough
Scaly
Elbows

Lake

Red Skin
on Hocks

Grass

Food

Swollen Paw

Treats

Heart Worm
Medication

Disinfectant

Dog Dish

Detergent

Dog Bed
Filled with Cedar

9–1: The Toxic Dog

to decorate them. If the pottery is not fired at a high enough temperature or for the right length of time, lead can leak out and mix with the food in the bowl, causing eventual lead poisoning. *Use stainless steel dishes to be safe.* Other sources of lead include batteries, linoleum, putty, tar paper, golf balls, fishing sinkers, drapery weights (puppies love these), shotgun pellets, and water from lead pipes in old houses or buildings and brass faucets found on sinks and tubs. Eating lead-based paints also creates toxic symptoms.

Lead poisoning is only now being recognized as more prevalent than was previously thought. It is difficult to diagnose. More commonly found in puppies, and for some reason more often between the months of June and October, according to a University of Pennsylvania study, it shows up as central nervous system depression, vomiting, abdominal pain, convulsions, muscular twitching, violent blinking of the eyelids, excesssive salivation, grinding of teeth and paralysis of the jaw.

Pressure-treated lumber contains arsenic, which can be deadly if your dog chews it.

Here is a list of common allergy or deficiency symptoms in dogs:

fatigue	rubbing face/head	slow learning
mood swings	headache	hyperactivity/lethargy
depression	aggression (common)	muscle aches/weakness
anxiety and fear	running away	stomach problems
vomiting	diarrhea	constipation
roached backs	dark circles under eyes	irritated, red eyes
discharges from eyes	dilated pupils	runny noses
sores in mouth	earaches	deafness
ear infections	coughs	change in bark
sore throat	itchy skin	hives
skin rashes	edema, joint swellings	infertility
false pregnancy	weight gain	no lactation
obesity	constant hunger	eating strange objects
swelling of paws	licking at feet	washing genital areas
swelling of testicles	ileitis	arthritis
sneezing	seizures	cancer
ulcerative colitis	bloating	kidney disease
improper growth	timid behavior	adrenal exhaustion
thyroid problems	liver disease	heart disease
		to name just a few!

A dog fed properly will be healthy and not react to the majority of the toxins in the environment. If your dog is experiencing any of the above symptoms, examine the dog's diet and all those chemicals you keep around the house.

Vaccines

Potential Problems

Vaccinations are also responsible for many allergic reactions we see in dogs. Because of the severity of some of these reactions, both short and long term, vaccines have become a hugely controversial subject. The veterinary community is becoming increasingly aware of the potential dangers of the combination vaccines and the routinely given annual vaccinations.

Our purpose here is not so much to question the underlying validity and benefits of vaccinations as to make the reader aware that the manner in which they are used may be detrimental to the dog's health—specifically, the kind of vaccine given, the practice of giving several vaccines at the same time, the timing of the inoculations and annual booster shots. Moreover, some breeds have extreme, sometimes fatal reactions to vaccines readily tolerated by other dogs.

Vaccines have the potential to cause allergic reactions in any dog. No two dogs are alike, and what may be tolerated by one may be extremely toxic to another. For some, getting yearly vaccines can produce a myriad of small reactions that build up and get worse each year they receive their vaccines. Giving several vaccines at once instead of spacing them out over a period of time can create reactions in many dogs. Symptoms will appear anywhere from 10 to 21 days after the vaccine has been given. These vary from lethargy, joint swelling, gastrointestinal upset, lameness, seizures, wasting, thyroid and adrenal gland diseases and general lack of vitality and energy.

Immunologists are finding a direct correlation between the increase in autoimmune and chronic disease states and the overuse of vaccines. Breeders have had entire litters wiped out after using Parvo vaccines. Some breeds, notably Rottweilers, who were subjected to weekly doses of Parvo vaccine in the late 1980s, were riddled with bone cancers and died around the age of 4 years. The Lyme disease vaccine is thought to have been responsible for the collapse of some dogs' immune systems, and a recent study at Cornell University suggests that treating the disease is less risky than getting the vaccine.

Some European veterinarians now believe that the benefit of many vaccines are outweighed by the risks and that the dog is better off either not being vaccinated or being vaccinated only for distemper and parvo. There is also a growing concern about the scheduling of shots. It is becoming recognized that bombarding a puppy with multiple vaccines several times during the course of a few months has an adverse effect on an immature immune system. For example, the young puppy bought at 7 weeks, having already received vaccines while with the breeder, goes to a new home and then visits a new veterinarian, who immediately vaccinates again.

The reason that puppies are vaccinated so heavily during the first few months of life is that the protection from disease they receive through their mother's milk wears off anytime from 6 weeks up to 20 weeks. They are then vulnerable to many diseases. Vaccinating puppies is supposed to protect them. The problem is that maternal antibodies interfere with the efficacy of the vaccines. Because there is no easy way to find out when these maternal antibodies stop working, multiple vaccines are given to puppies to protect them when maternal antibodies no longer provide the protection.

Jean Dodds, DVM, a noted veterinary immunologist, also challenges the number of vaccines used. She asks why a Toy Dog and a giant breed dog should get the same amount of a vaccine when the blood volume of each dog is so different? She also talks about the "shedding" of live virus vaccines. This means that if you have one dog in your household vaccinated with live vaccines, that dog sheds the virus through skin and feces for 10 to 21 days after receiving the shot. The other dogs in the household are exposed to this and pick up their own immunity from the vaccinated dog. If one of those other dogs has an autoimmune disease, exposure to the shedding can be extremely dangerous to that dog.

Dodds (1995, 26-31) asks, "Why are we causing disease by weakening the immune system with frequent use of combination vaccine products? After all vaccines are intended to protect against disease."

Modified Live versus Killed Vaccines

There are two types of vaccines used in veterinary medicine: (1) modified live (MLV) and (2) killed (inactivated). In MLV the viruses are altered to decrease their virulence or ability to produce disease yet retain their ability to stimulate the immune system. In order to produce enough antigen to cause immunity the MLV must replicate after your dog is vaccinated. Because the MLV do replicate, it is felt they produce a stronger and more durable immunity. Because a live virus is being used, there is a decrease in vaccine safety. MLV may cause immune suppression, be shed into the environment and return to a more active form and cause a "vaccine induced" disease. Immunologists agree that modified live vaccines are not always the best nor suitable for all animals.

Killed vaccines cannot replicate and they are not able to cause infectious disease in the vaccinated animal. As a result, they are much safer. It is now well recognized that a properly prepared killed vaccine is preferable to an MLV due to the increased safety for both the vaccinated animal and the environment.

There are some drawbacks to the killed vaccines. Although all licensed killed vaccines meet the current USDA efficacy and safety standards, they produce levels of protection that are lower and of shorter duration. They are more expensive because they contain adjuvants (a substance added to the vaccine to improve the response) and larger doses are needed to make them effective. Because of the use of the adjuvants, there is a greater chance of adverse reactions at the site of the injection (hard masses).

As the effectiveness of the killed vaccine continues to improve, the safety of killed versus MLV far overshadows its drawbacks. At this time the only vaccine that is not available in the killed form is distemper.

Tolerance

Vaccinating your dog has to be an individual decision on your part. Some people, prominent breeders among them, have experienced such dreadful side effects from vaccines that they are raising dogs without vaccines at all. Some have found that by not vaccinating, their puppies' mortality rate is lower than when they were vaccinating. They are, however, compensating by feeding their dogs naturally and boosting their dogs' immune systems with the appropriate homeopathic remedies. There are breeds of dogs that have a poor tolerance for vaccines—solid-colored dogs, those breeds with a lot of white coloration in the coat, giant breeds, Rottweilers and imported dogs.

What You Can Do

If you have a dog that has had a bad reaction to a vaccine, or you know for sure that you own one of the breeds that is susceptible to vaccinosis, get a veterinary certificate to this effect. In most cases this will be honored.

You don't have to give your dog any vaccinations except for rabies. There are drawbacks to this position. If you want to take your dog to an Obedience class, enter Matches or shows, go to seminars or take the Canine Good Citizen test, proof of vaccinations may be required. Leaving your dog in a kennel when you go on vacation or even having routine surgery done at your veterinarian may require having your dog vaccinated.

For the dog deficient in vitamin B it is possible that either a vaccine will not work properly, or if the dog is experiencing severe stress at the time the vaccine is given, side effects could develop. It is therefore advisable to give the dog some B complex several days before the vaccines and continue for the several weeks after the vaccine is administered. Remember that *vitamin B works better in conjunction with vitamin C*. Both of these are water-soluble vitamins and are flushed through the system in 4 to 8 hours. You can add a small amount of fresh raw beef or chicken liver, which contain vitamin B, to your dog's food during this time period. These supplements should be part of your daily routine with your dog if you are feeding commercial dog food.

You can also talk with your veterinarian and explain that you would like the vaccinations spaced out at least by 3 weeks, and where possible, for only single vaccines to be used. If your puppy or dog shows the slightest side effect from the vaccine anytime up to 10 to 21 days after the shots, bring this to the attention of your veterinarian. Do not get the vaccine until your dog's sensitivity has been checked out. Continuously using the same vaccine that has caused the symptoms can create enormous problems. This is particularly true in the case of the Parvo and Lyme disease vaccines. If your dog has experienced side effects, there are homeopathic remedies than can detoxify these side effects from some vaccines. (See Chapter 16.)

If your pet is not left in kennels on a regular basis or is around other dogs much, the use of the kennel cough vaccine is hardly necessary. Many veterinarians have come to the same conclusion about the corona vaccine. Sometimes the dog finds it easier to deal with the disease itself than the side effects from the vaccine. The continued use of leptospirosis and hepatitis vaccines is questionable. Both diseases are contracted from rat and deer urine, and unless you are in a rat-infested area or one that contains herds of deer, it is unlikely that your dog will come into contact with these diseases. If you do need to use them, do so at 9 and 15 weeks. Look at the suggested vaccination schedule below, which is provided by Jean Dodds, DVM.

Vaccination Schedule

6 weeks	DM	Distemper, Measles
7$\frac{1}{2}$ weeks	Parvo	killed
10$\frac{1}{2}$ weeks	Parvo	killed
12 weeks	DA$_2$P	Distemper, adenovirus, parainfluenza; kidneys are now mature enough to cope
14 weeks	DA$_2$P	
16 weeks	Parvo	killed
18 weeks	DA$_2$P	

cont'd

Vaccination Schedule

20 weeks	Parvo	killed
24 weeks	Rabies	killed
16 months	Booster DA$_2$P	you can do a titer test to see if the 16- and 17-month boosters are necessary.
17 months	Parvo	killed
18 months	Rabies	3 years—killed
All vaccines except distemper are killed.		

Code:
 D = distemper
 A$_2$ = adenovirus
 P = parainfluenza

Source: Jean Dodds, DVM. Genetic, Environmental and Nutritional Influences on Autoimmune Disease States. Holistic Study Group Seminar, June 3–4, 1994. VanderKamp Center. Cleveland, N.Y.

Care must be taken that when the DA$_2$P is given, the P is for parainfluenza and not Parvo. Leptosporosis should be given at 12 and 16 weeks, if you live in an area where this disease is endemic. Ask your veterinarian.

If you have a very healthy female who was up to date on vaccinations before she was bred, you may want to spread out the above schedule for the puppies over a longer period of time. Using kinesiology would help you to make the correct decisions. (See Chapter 13.)

In order to minimize the side effects of vaccines, homeopathic products can be used to build up the puppy prior to vaccinating and to detoxify any side effects after the shot. Supportasode should be used daily during the first months of the puppy's life all through the vaccination period, and Viratox for one week after each vaccine has been received. For more information, see Chapters 15 and 16.

Time to Vaccinate

The best time to vaccinate adult females is between seasons, when there are no hormonal changes going on in the body. Make sure you write down the day the bitch's season started, and count 12 weeks forward from that point. Blood work and hip X-rays, as well as any surgery, would be suggested during this time frame.

Annual Checkup

According to Robert Kirk, writing in *Kirk's Current Veterinary Therapy XI* -205, a textbook used in all veterinary schools, there is no immunologic reason that would necessitate annual revaccinations. He tells us that as a practice it lacks scientific validity or verification. Immunity to viruses persists for years or for the life of the dog, and revaccinating does not add to that immunity. Given the potential adverse side effects, it is best not to revaccinate. Presumably the practice developed as a means of bringing the dog owner into the veterinarian's office on an annual basis so the dog could get a checkup.

We strongly encourage an annual veterinary visit. If you choose not to vaccinate yearly, have your veterinarian check the titer or immune level of your dog with a blood test. If your dog shows immunity to distemper, parvo, kennel cough and so on, a vaccine isn't needed at that time. If the titer is low, the vaccine is needed.

When you take your puppy for the rabies vaccine, make sure that it is separated by at least a month from other vaccines. After the first shot, subsequent rabies vaccine lasts for 3 years. Numerous side effects from aggression to chronic long-term disease have arisen when dogs are exposed to yearly rabies vaccinations. Even though some states have legislated that puppies have to have a rabies vaccination at 3 to 4 months, try to wait until your puppy is 6 months old. A puppy's immune system is immature during the first months of life and cannot adequately deal with so many vaccines all at the same time.

When in doubt, talk to your veterinarian and find out his or her position on vaccines. Look for a veterinarian who is aware and up to date on current thinking and research being done on vaccines. Avoid the 5, 7 or 9 combination vaccines. When you get a vaccination for your dog, have your veterinarian write down on your dog's record the batch number of the individual vaccine so if there are problems with the vaccine, it can be traced back by lot to the manufacturer.

Heartworm

Capable of creating allergic reactions in some dogs, heartworm medication should only be used during those months when you have mosquitoes.

Heartworm medication comes in many forms. There are several drugs that can be used daily; others are used only once a month. Using kinesiology, check to see which drug is suitable for your dog. If your dog comes from a family of dogs that has an inherited autoimmune disease, thyroid or adrenal gland dysfunction, the once-a-month medication should not be given. The daily medication is safer for these dogs.

Summary

1. CHOOSE YOUR VETERINARIAN WITH CARE. ANY PRACTITIONER NOT AWARE OF THE CHOICES ALTERNATIVE TO TRADITIONAL TREATMENTS MAY NOT BE UP TO DATE.

2. WHEN RAISING A YOUNG PUPPY, MAKE SURE YOU HAVE TALKED TO THE BREEDER OF YOUR DOG AND FIND OUT WHAT HAS BEEN SUCCESS-FUL IN TERMS OF FOOD AND VACCINATION SCHEDULES.

3. USE STAINLESS STEEL DISHES IN FEEDING YOUR DOG.

4. WASH YOUR BLANKETS AND DOG BEDDING IN A DETERGENT OR SOAP PRODUCT USED FOR WASHING BABIES' DIAPERS IF YOUR DOG EXHIBITS SKIN SENSITIVITIES.

5. BE CAREFUL WHEN YOU USE SPRAYS ON YOUR GARDEN. Check to see if they could be dangerous to your dog.

6. IF YOU TAKE YOUR DOG SWIMMING, BATHE THE DOG AFTERWARD.

7. USE A MILD, HERBAL SHAMPOO FOR YOUR DOG. Fleas drown in soapy water.

8. WHEN YOU CLEAN YOUR HOUSE, KENNEL OR DOG AREAS, CHLORINE BLEACH AND WATER ARE BEST. SPRAY DOWN YOUR DOG AREAS WITH THIS MIXTURE (UP TO $1/4$ CUP PER GALLON) AND KEEP IT DISIN-FECTED. This is all that is necessary.

9. MANY DISINFECTANTS AND CLEANERS CAN BE TOXIC. Lysol is one of these.

10. USE AS FEW CHEMICALS IN THE FORM OF CLEANSERS OR FLEA SPRAYS, FLEA COLLARS, MEDALLIONS OR MEDICATIONS AS YOU CAN. If you are experiencing problems with parasites, internal or external, the problem is that your dog's immune system is weak. Start rebuilding the immune system by feeding your pet properly.

11. VISIT YOUR VETERINARIAN AT LEAST ONCE A YEAR. Learn to think preventatively and have your vet do a blood test (chemistry pro-file) to check to see if your dog is healthy.

12. WHEN YOU GIVE VACCINES: (a) Make sure that your dog needs them. (b) Make sure that the vaccines are spaced apart a mini-mum of 3 weeks. (c) If you know you are going on vacation with your dogs, or leaving them in a kennel, get your vaccinations at least 4 weeks prior to your trip. Putting a dog in a stressful situa-tion directly after receiving vaccinations needlessly stresses the immune system. Allow time to build immunity to the disease for which your dog was vaccinated (10–21 days) before inducing stress. (d) If your dog is not feeling up to par, or if you adopt a dog from an animal shelter, give the dog time to settle into a new

home before giving vaccinations. Check with the animal shelter to see if they vaccinated the dog before adoption. Feed the dog well, give a good vitamin/mineral supplement for a couple of weeks, put in a little raw food daily and when the dog is feeling and looking good, give those vaccinations that are necessary. (e) Check a dog's individual shot record before you rush off to get more vaccines. *MORE IS NOT BETTER!*

If your dog has experienced reactions to vaccinations, look in the chapter on homeopathy as to those remedies you can use through this time frame.

13. THINK NATURALLY! The fewer chemicals you use around or in your dog, the healthier the dog will be in the long run. *MORE IS NOT BETTER!*

14. REMEMBER THAT EVERY TIME YOU USE ANY FORM OF CHEMICAL, FROM FLEA SPRAYS AND SHAMPOOS TO CARPET CLEANERS IN YOUR HOUSE, FROM PREVENTATIVE MEDICATIONS SUCH AS HEARTWORM PILLS TO TOO MANY VACCINATIONS, YOU ARE CAUSING A BUILDUP OF TOXINS IN YOUR DOG'S BODY. Over time, the body cannot deal with them and starts to break down. In a study done at the Veterinary School at the University of Pennsylvania in the early 1980s, dogs were classified as geriatric at 5 years of age. Eighty percent of the dogs tested showed degeneration of the vital organs such as their liver and kidneys.

    Many breeds of dogs are only just full grown at that time (giant breeds in particular). Since many giant breeds have a life span of 7 to 8 years, they have an adult life of only 2 or 3 years. Accepting this is like expecting humans to die at 25 years of age.

15. IF YOU HAVE TO USE PARASITE CONTROL MEASURES ON YOUR DOG, USE NATURALLY BASED INGREDIENTS. There are many excellent products out that use substances that are not harmful to your pets. Write for a catalog to sources listed in the sources chapter.

Make a commitment to your dog. Educate yourself. There are high-quality foods out there, just as there are some superb veterinarians. Go out and have the courage to find them and learn to make intelligent decisions for yourself and your dog.

If for any reason your dog gets into something toxic, contact the **ANIMAL POISON CONTROL CENTER at (900) 680-0000. It costs $2.95 a minute and is available 24 hours.**

Chapter 10

The Digestive Tract

Digestion: What Is It All About?

For food to be properly digested, the digestive system must be healthy. When food reaches the stomach, it has to be broken down into something called chyme. Chyme is like a thick soup. Unless it has reached the proper consistency in the stomach, it cannot be passed down into the small intestine, where digestion and assimilation starts for the dog. Hydrochloric acid and pepsin must be present in the proper amounts for the chyme to reach the correct consistency. If for some reason such as sickness, incorrect food, use of drugs or lack of hydrochloric acid or pepsin the stomach does not function properly, the food will not be digested. Worse, it goes all the way to the large intestine or colon, where it sits and putrefies. It is easy to tell if this is happening to your dog. He will have a great deal of foul-smelling gas, burp frequently, pass large amounts of smelly stools, experience a lack of energy and his breath will smell.

Some studies show a link between improper digestion and cancer. The bacteria that are normally produced in the large intestine may multiply, causing putrefaction to take place, which in turn creates chemical reactions that provide an ideal environment for cancer.

How It Works

The **gastrointestinal system** is the body system responsible for taking nutrients in, breaking them down, absorbing them, eliminating the waste products and absorbing water. It is a system made up of many parts, each with its own specific job—all with the responsibility of getting nutrition to the rest of the body. Although digestion is a very complex process, a simplified tour down the GI tract will make it easier to understand how food is handled and why the type and quality of food is so very important.

The Oral Cavity

The mouth or oral cavity is one of the most specialized parts of a dog's body. Its purpose is to take in food and water, mechanically break it up and advance it to the esophagus.

The **lips** have few functions in the dog as they are relatively immobile. They form the buccal cavity, the area between the lips and teeth, which receives the saliva from two of the larger salivary glands.

The **teeth** of a carnivore are designed for tearing and cutting through tissue rather than chewing. Unlike humans and herbivores, the outer enamel layer of a dog's teeth is thin, probably because they eat nonabrasive foods and chew little. The adult dog has 42 permanent teeth and the puppy has only 28 deciduous or puppy teeth.

Table 1: Dental Table

Types of Teeth	No. in Puppy	No. in Adult	Eruption of Adult Teeth
Incisors	6	6	14–16 weeks
		12 Avg	
Canine	2	2	5$\frac{1}{2}$–6 months
Premolars	6	8	5–6 months
Molars	0	4 or 6	5$\frac{1}{2}$–6 months

Except for the lower first molar, the calcification of the permanent teeth does not begin until after birth. As a result, diseases and stress during the first 3 months of life can affect the tooth development, especially the enamel layer. This is often noted as discoloration (browning) of the enamel or irregularities and loss of enamel layers. Also make note of the root pattern of these teeth. A healthy, clean tooth has roots that are tightly seated in the bone of the jaw. Poor nutrition and/or poor care of a dog's teeth and gums causes tartar development or periodontal disease as well as bone resorption around the roots of the teeth, resulting in loosening and loss of teeth. This may explain incorrect or crooked bites.

The **hard palate** forms the front two thirds of the roof of the mouth. It separates the respiratory system's nasal tract from the digestive system's oral cavity. The abnormal development of the hard palate of the fetus results in a cleft palate, creating a communication between the oral and nasal cavities. Unless this defect can be corrected, the puppy cannot form an airtight oral cavity for sucking and will eventually starve or suffer aspiration pneumonia (sucking in milk to the lungs).

The **pharyngeal area** is the back third of the oral cavity. It is the crossroads of the nasal cavity, larynx (opening to the trachea), the back of the oral cavity and the esophagus. These pharyngeal muscles act as a sphincter that keeps the esophagus closed when nothing is being swallowed and

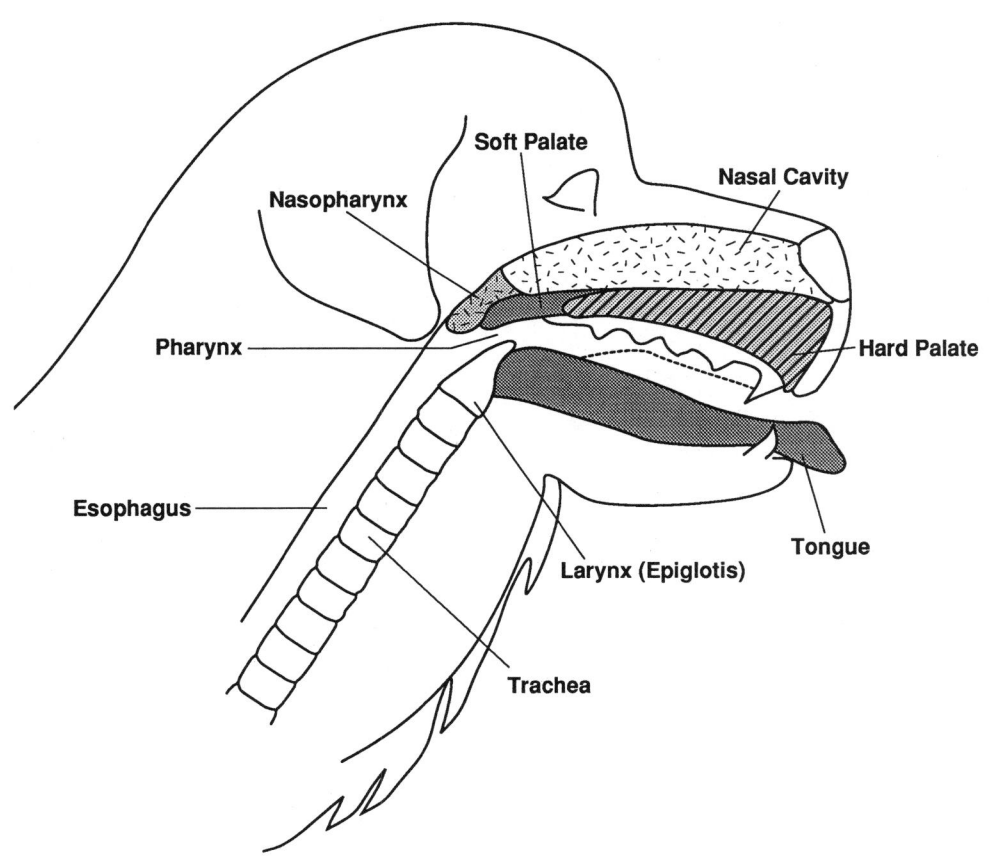

10–1: The Oral Cavity

protects against the backup of juices from the stomach. Paralysis and dysfunction of the pharyngeal area can result in an inability to swallow and food being pulled into or backed up into the trachea.

The **soft palate** forms the roof of the front of the pharynx and is the continuation of the hard palate, which separates the oral and nasal passages. The soft palate is pliable and forms a valve that when lowered closes the orapharynx, allowing air to enter, thus preventing food from entering the trachea. When raised, the soft palate closes the nasopharynx, allowing food to pass the tracheal entrance and enter the esophagus.

The **salivary glands** of the dog produce large amounts of saliva, which lubricates the food in the mouth. Unlike human saliva, which plays an important role in digestion, the saliva of a dog does not initiate digestion of food. Dog saliva does contain a number of bactericidal agents that help prevent oral infection. The continuous production of saliva helps prevent tooth decay by continuously "washing" the mouth and teeth. The major salivary glands that produce the majority of saliva are called the parotid, mandibular, sublinguals and zygomatic glands.

The **tongue** is a very muscular structure that lies on the floor of the oral cavity. It plays a vital role in lapping, sucking and in the process of swallowing. When food is brought into the mouth, it is pushed toward the pharynx by the tongue (see Fig. 10-1).

The first step in digestion is simple—the teeth grab and shear off the food. The salivary glands produce large volumes of saliva to lubricate the food. The tongue maneuvers the food and propels it toward the pharynx. The process of swallowing is initiated. The soft palate elevates to block off the nasopharynx. The larynx closes. Pharyngeal muscles contract to propel the food toward the esophageal opening. Esophageal sphincter muscles relax and allow the food to enter the esophagus, and the food is on its way. The next stop is the **stomach** via the esophageal thruway.

The Esophagus

The **esophagus** is the muscular tube that connects the pharynx to the stomach. It has a tough, slippery mucous membrane lining and a muscular wall that is capable of stretching two to three times its normal diameter. This ability to stretch is created by dogs' style of eating—swallowing large amounts of food at one time. There are four narrow areas to the esophagus that limit what can pass. After the food enters the esophagus, muscular contractions propel the food to the stomach. As the food approaches the stomach, the **esophageal sphincter** and the **cardiac region** of the stomach relax and allow the food to enter the stomach. Splash! The second stage of the food journey has been completed.

The Stomach

The stomach serves three important functions. First, it provides a rapidly adjustable reservoir for the intake of food. Second, it acts as a site for mixing stomach contents with stomach secretions (gastric juices). Third, it gradually passes the stomach contents into the small intestine for digestion and nutrient absorption.

The **fundus** is the first section of the stomach. It acts as a reservoir relaxing and expanding to accommodate the food taken in. The stomach secretes hydrochloric acid, electrolytes, pepsinogen, gastrin and mucous. (See Table 2.) As contractions begin (known as peristaltic waves), the food gets mixed with the gastric juices and the stomach wall contracts, physically breaking down the food, while the gastric secretions begin digestion of the food particles.

As they liquefy into gastric **chyme**, the stomach contractions move the food along into the **antrum** of the stomach. The antrum propels all sticky and solid materials back to the body of the stomach for further mixing, but it allows liquid material and fine food particles to pass on into the **pylorus**. The valvular action (sphincter activity) of the pylorus allows liquid and food particles less than 2 millimeters in diameter to pass on into the **duodenum**. Stage three of digestion is complete. The food has been physically broken down and is well on its way to being digested. Small intestine, here we come!

Table 2

Gastric Secretion	Function	Source
Hydrochloric Acid	Breaks down connective tissue to release nutrients, activates pepsin, kills ingested bacteria	Parietal cells of all parts of the stomach wall
Pepsinogen	Activated by acid pepsin, hydrolyzes protein	Fundus
Proteocytic enzymes	Protects stomach from self-digestion	All parts of stomach wall
Mucous	Lubricates food, protects stomach from damage by pepsin and gastric juice	All parts of stomach

The Small Intestine

The small intestine is the longest portion of the digestive system. It is approximately 5 times the length of the dog's body. It is divided into three sections: (1) the **duodenum,** (2) the **jejunum** and (3) the **ileum.** The primary function of the small intestine is the assimilation, digestion and absorption of nutrients. As food enters the duodenum it is mixed with secretions from the pancreas, liver and intestinal lining (mucosa). These secretions, containing enzymes, bile salts and colipase, break down the dietary nutrients into small molecules that can be absorbed by the cells lining the intestinal wall. (See Figure 2.) The small intestine contracts in segments, which mixes the food with the secretions and increases the amount of contact time with the absorbing microvilli cells. These contractions or peristaltic waves move the food and fluids along their trip through the long **jejunum** and short **ileum.** The digestion and absorption of carbohydrates, protein and fats continues to take place.

CARBOHYDRATES are readily digested and absorbed as single sugars of maltose, glucose, galactose and fructose. They are actively transported across the microvilli cell border.

PROTEIN is primarily digested in the duodenum and jejunum. It is digested and made into peptides, which are broken down into amino acids and then absorbed. This digestion is dependent on pancreatic enzymes and requires a pH of 7 for optimal activity.

FAT digestion and absorption is the most complex process of the three classes of nutrients. Approximately 95 percent of ingested fat is absorbed from the intestines. Fat digestion takes place entirely in the small intestine. The stomach's release of fats into the duodenum stimulates the pancreas to release lipase and the gallbladder to contract, which in turn releases bile into the duodenum. The intestinal movement mixes up and emulsifies the fat. Emulsified fat is then broken down by the lipase. This mixed-up (hydrolyzed) fat then combines with the bile salts so it can be absorbed across the cell membranes.

The fat-soluble vitamins A, D, E and K are incorporated into bile salt form and absorbed. The water-soluble vitamins C and B-complex—which includes biotin, choline, folic acid, inositol, nicotinic acid, thiamin and riboflavin—are also absorbed in the small intestine.

The small intestine is also capable of and responsible for the resorption of water, approximately 85 percent of the ingested fluids and gastrointestinal secretions. Half of the total amount is absorbed by the jejunum and the majority of the remainder by the ileum.

By the time food has passed through the small intestine and reached the ileo-cecal junction, most of the nutrients and fluid have been absorbed. The remaining food passes through and moves on to the colon. Stage four of the digestion is complete—on to the large intestine.

The Large Intestine

The large intestine consists of the **cecum, colon, rectum and anal canal**. The cecum in the dog is small and serves no known specific function. The colon is divided into the ascending, the transverse and descending colon. Its first major function is the absorption of water and electrolytes from the contents of the three parts of the colon. The second major function is the regulation of movement of the final food for maximum absorption. The colon stores fecal residue and is responsible for the final elimination of the solid wastes from the body. Stage five of the final step of digestion is complete. Food has moved from the mouth and has been digested and absorbed; water has been reabsorbed and undigested food has reached the final storage place in the colon awaiting one final step—oops! Time to go out. We will talk about the liver and pancreas when you come back.

The Pancreas

The **pancreas** is a V-shaped organ with both digestive enzyme (exocrin) and insulin (endocrine) functions. The left lobe of the pancreas lies near the stomach, and the right lobe lies next to the duodenum. The external or exocrine portion of the pancreas has two large ducts that collect the pancreatic juices from the glandular tissues and transport them to the beginning of the duodenum. The external portion of the pancreas produces three major pancreatic juice components: **digestive enzymes** or their precursors, **bicarbonate ions** and **colipase**. The digestive enzymes have the ability to **split starch (amylase), fats (lipase)** and **proteins (trypsin elastase), ribonuclease, dexoyribonuclease** and **collagenase**. These enzymes can potentially damage the pancreas and adjacent organs, so they are produced and stored in an inactive form. They are not activated until they enter the duodenum. The bicarbonate ions neutralize the stomach acids. This alkalizing of the intestinal contents allows pancreatic enzymes to function and promotes the digestion and absorption of triglycerides by fats.

The endocrine function of the *pancreas* is the *production of insulin*. Insulin is essential for the proper oxidization and utilization of blood sugar as it transports the glucose into the cells. Inadequate secretion of insulin results in diabetes mellitus.

This pancreatic reaction of secreting enzymes is not a constant process but rather the rapid response to the proper digestive stimulus. Upon the

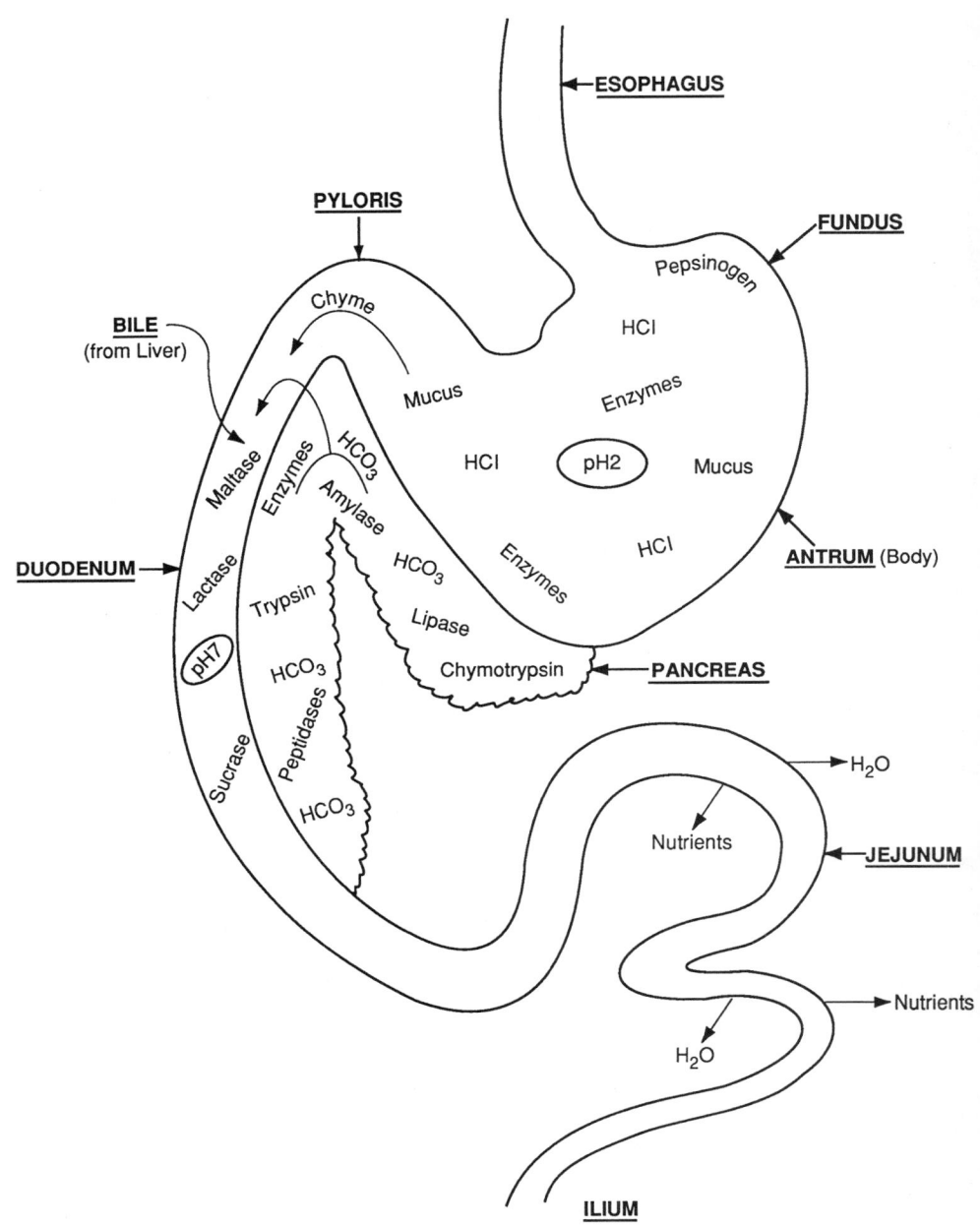

10–2: The Digestive Tract

release of the pancreatic juices into the duodenum, digestion goes into full gear. Obviously, without the pancreas the dog is in major trouble. *No pancreas means no digestion—no healthy puppy!*

Table 3: Digestive Enzymes

Class	Nutrient	Enzyme	Produces	Source
Carbohydrate	Starch	Amylase	Maltose	Pancreas, stomach
	Maltose	Maltase	Glucose	Intestines
	Lactose	Lactase	Glucose Galactase	Intestines
	Sucrose	Sucrase	Glucose Fructose	Intestines
Proteins	Proteins	Pepsin	Peptides	Stomach
		Trypsin	Peptides	Pancreas
		Chymotrypsin	Peptides	Pancreas
	Peptides	Peptidase	Amino acids	Pancreas Intestines
Fats	Triglycerides	Lipase	Monoglycerides Free fatty acids Glycerol	Pancreas
	Phospholipids	Phospholipase	Phosphoglyceride Free fatty acids	Pancreas
	Cholesterol	Cholesterol-lipase	Cholesterol Free fatty acids	Pancreas Pancreas

The Liver

The liver is the other primary organ associated with the assimilation process of the gastrointestinal tract. Most of the liver lies under and is protected by the dog's rib cage. It is next to the diaphragm and just ahead of the stomach. The main function of the liver is to synthesize many of the body proteins, especially albumin.

The liver controls carbohydrate storage, metabolizes many hormones and drugs and controls fat metabolism as well as the formation of bile salts and bile secretions. It detoxifies the blood returning to the heart from the intestinal tract. In the storage of carbohydrates, the liver forms and stores glycogen and converts it to glucose when the body needs energy. The production of glucose from non-carbohydrates also occurs in the liver.

Fat metabolism in the liver results in the formation of lipoproteins, enabling the body to transport the fats (lipids) to other body tissues to act as body fuel (fatty acids and triglycerides). The bile salts produced by the liver are stored in the gallbladder. Gallbladder contractions expel bile into the bile duct and out into the duodenum, where the bile salts are broken down to promote the digestion and absorption of fats in the small intestine.

The liver is also the "detox" house for the intestinal tract. All blood returning to the heart from the intestinal tract (about 30 percent of the total blood returning to the heart) passes through the liver. The primary toxins removed are ammonia and short chain fatty acids. If the portal blood bypasses the liver and contaminates the rest of the blood, this will interfere with brain function, often causing seizures and/or eventual death. The liver is an organ that plays many vital roles in both the use of nutrients and in their assimilation.

Summary

This is a somewhat simplified explanation of what happens in the dog's digestive tract. The complex interactions of the systems emphasize the importance of a healthy body. Without quality food the body cannot assimilate the nutrients it needs. Without proper nutrition the body systems cannot function optimally. When the body does not function at its optimum, nutrients are wasted. Simply stated, if there is one item that controls the quality of a dog's health more than any other, it is nutrition.

—Chapter 11—

Thyroid and Adrenal Gland Functions

The thyroid and adrenal gland are two of the most significant endocrine glands in the body. When functioning normally, they are major controllers of metabolism. When there are abnormalities, major metabolic problems occur.

The Thyroid Gland

An old medical saying states, "A few grams of thyroid medication makes the difference between an idiot and an Einstein." The thyroid gland is an endocrine gland with two lobes, one on either side of the trachea, just below the larynx. The thyroid hormone maintains optimal levels of metabolism of all cell functions. The thyroid gland, under the control of TSH (thyroid stimulating hormone), which is produced by the pituitary gland, produces all the T4 (thyroxine) in the body. T4 is converted to T3, which enters the cells and is used in cell metabolism. This conversion takes place primarily in the liver.

Although many thyroid function tests are available, we use the free T4 by dialysis test performed by Michigan State University. It is currently felt that this free T4 evaluation gives the most accurate evaluation of thyroid gland health. In cases where initial tests are inconclusive, a TSH response test is performed. This tests the ability of the thyroid gland to respond to stimulation.

Hypothyroidism

Thyroid dysfunction is the most commonly seen endocrine disorder in dogs. *Hypothyroidism* is a *deficiency* of the thyroid hormone. It is most frequently caused by destruction of the thyroid tissue or autoimmune thyroiditis. This autoimmune response has been linked to genetic predisposition, drug reactions, heavy metal toxicity, reaction to modified live vaccines and viral infections. Although hypothyroidism is seen in all breeds, there does appear to be a predisposition in certain breeds.

The clinical signs associated with hypothyroidism can involve many body systems. These signs usually become evident after age 4 in the majority of breeds and age 2 or 3 in giant breeds, although it is now found in increasing numbers in much younger dogs. Most dogs are hypothyroid for 6 months to 1 year before obvious clinical signs are recognized. See Table 1.

Table 1: Clinical Signs Associated with Hypothyroidism

Alterations in Metabolism	Skin
Lethargy	Dry, scaly skin
Mental dullness	Coarse, dull coat
Exercise intolerance	Hair loss both sides of body
Weight gain	"Rat Tail"
Cold intolerance	Soft, fuzzy, "puppy coat" in adult dog
	Hyperpigmentation (black skin on belly)
	Seborrhea, oily skin and coat
	Inflammation of the skin
	Pyoderma

Reproduction—Male	Reproduction—Female
Enlarged mammary glands	Infertility
Lack of libido	Prolonged estrus
Testicular atrophy	Failure to cycle
Decreased sperm production	Weak, silent cycles
Infertility	Long time between cycles
	Weak, dying, stillborn pups

Eyes	Heart
Corneal lipid deposits, ulceration	Bradycardia (slow heart)
Uveitis	Cardiac arrhythmias
Dry eye (keratitis)	Cardiomyopathy
Swelling of eyelids	

Gastrointestinal	Neuromuscular
Constipation	Weakness
Vomiting	Stiffness

Gastrointestinal (cont.)	Neuromuscular (cont.)
Diarrhea	Knuckling, dragging feet
Change in appetite	Droopy eyelids
	Muscle Wasting
	Megaesophaegus
	Laryngeal paralysis
	Facial paralysis
	Head tilt

Blood Disorders	Other Disorders
Bleeding, anemia	Separation anxiety
Bone marrow failure	Shying away from strangers
Low white blood cell count	Emotional instability
Low platelet count	Loss of taste sensation
	Loss of sense of smell

Treatment

Treatment of hypothyroidism is very successful and gratifying. Soloxine is used as a T4 replacement. Thyroid profiles should be done at 8- to 10-week intervals until free T4 levels are returned to mid- to high-normal levels. (We supplement all low-normal readings). Once these levels are reached and maintained, tests should be done every 6 months and the soloxine adjusted accordingly. All rechecking should be done 4 to 6 hours after the medication has been given.

In cases where liver disease or compromise occurs, conversion of T4 to T3 is often depressed or nonexistent. Soloxine supplementation can raise free T4 levels to normal or above normal but conversion cannot occur. When this situation arises, T3 supplementation (cytobin) is used. This determination can only be reached by your veterinarian after definitive testing.

Hyperthyroidism

*Hyper*thyroidism (excessive thyroid production) is unusual in the dog and is most often associated with thyroid tumors. A firm mass in the area of the thyroid glands on the neck should be checked. Thyroid tests will indicate very high T4 levels and normal to high T3 levels. Other clinical signs are an increase in thirst (polydipsia), excessive panting, preference for a cool location, restlessness and fatigue. Treatment consists of surgical removal of the tumor. T4 supplementation is needed if both lobes of the thyroid are removed. When the thyroid has been removed, there is a tendency for the body to store excess water, salt and protein, and the blood cholesterol levels rise.

Nutritional support is crucial in both cases. *The thyroid cannot function correctly without sufficient amino acids, minerals and vitamins in the diet.* The B vitamin riboflavin cannot convert to its active (coenzyme) form unless the thyroid is producing sufficient thyroxin. Massive doses of vitamin C—over 9 grams per day—can inhibit thyroid function.

About 50 breeds are currently affected by *hypo*thyroidism, and more are being discovered. Neutered dogs of either sex are frequently affected, regardless of age.

The Adrenal Glands

The adrenal glands are a pair of small endocrine glands located at the front end of each kidney. The hormones produced by these glands are steroids. Simply, the adrenal glands produce the sugar, salt and sex hormones. The removal of these adrenal steroids occurs primarily in the liver. The hormones produced by the adrenal glands are vital to the body. When oversecretion occurs (hyperadrenocorticism), an extremely debilitated state results. **Cushing's syndrome** is the result of excessive secretion of ACTH by the pituitary gland or tumors of the adrenal glands. The clinical signs, listed in Table 2, develop slowly and insidiously.

Clinical Signs Associated with Cushing's Syndrome

Increased thirst and urination (polydipsia, polyuria "Pd or Pu")
Increased appetite
Abdominal distention
Decreased exercise tolerance (muscle weakness)
Increased panting
Lethargy
Obesity
Symmetrical hair loss (alopecia)
Calcium deposits in the skin (may appear as small "whiteheads")
Dermatitis (skin infections)
Hyperpigmentation of the skin (black skin, often seen on the belly)
Dogs that appear to be heavy in the body but thin in the limbs
Swollen eyelids
Females with male characteristics ("doggy bitches")

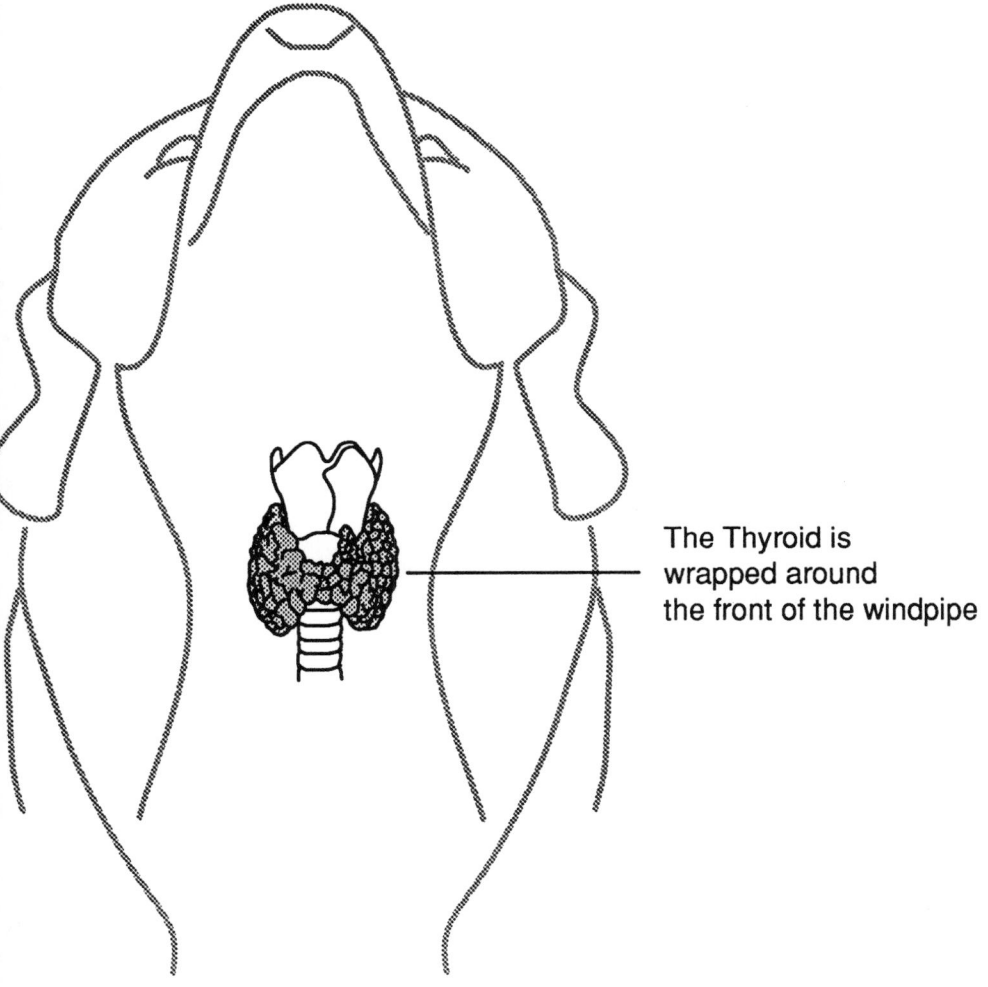

The Thyroid is
wrapped around
the front of the windpipe

11–1: The Thyroid Gland

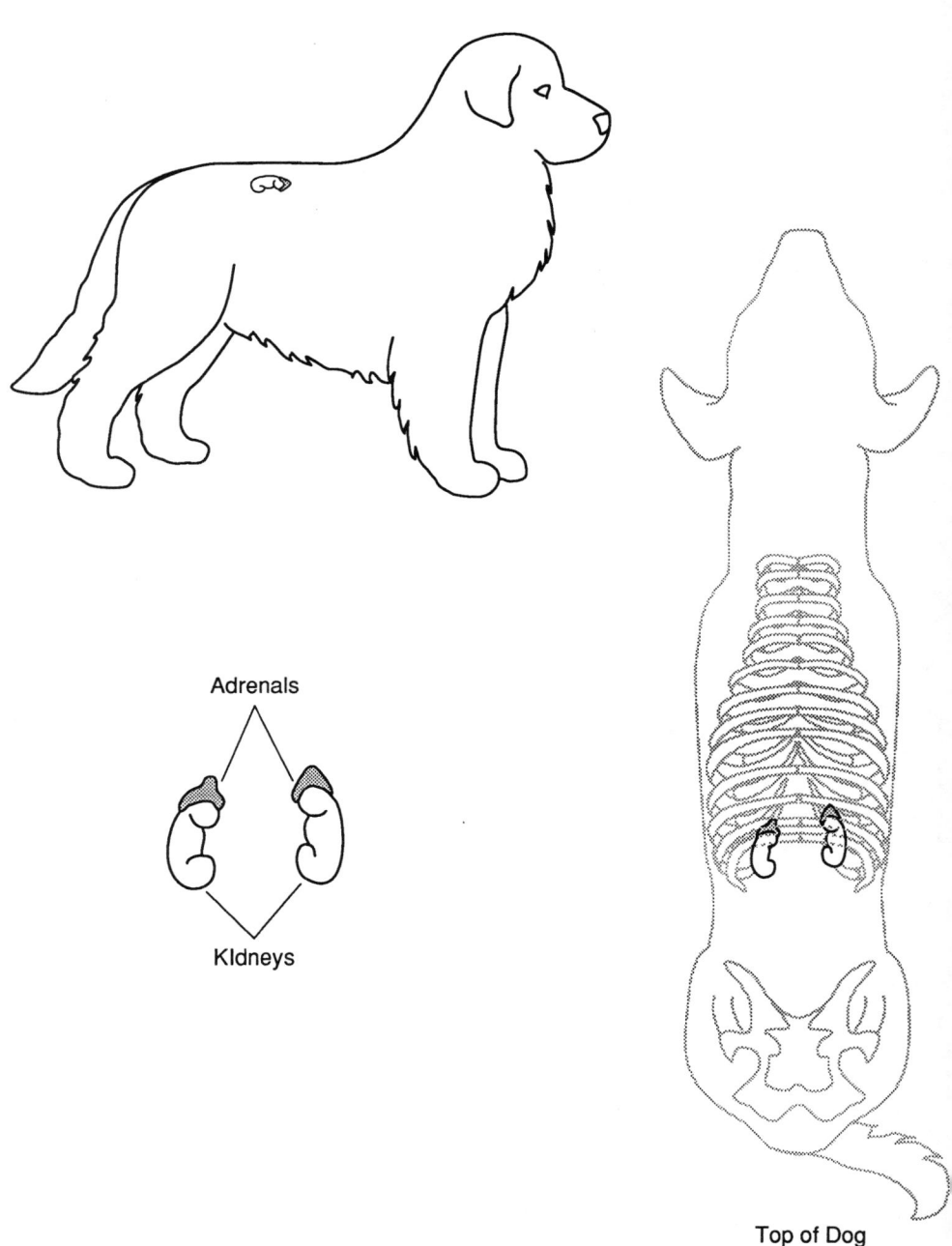

Adrenals

Kidneys

Top of Dog

11–2: The Kidneys and the Adrenals

Cushing's Syndrome

It is usually the increased thirst, urination and hair coat changes that indicate this disorder. Cushing's syndrome is diagnosed by a complete blood chemistry screen. The following findings are common to this disease:

CBC	increased neutrophils
	decreased lymphocytes
	decreased eosinophils
Glucose	increased
BUN	normal/decreased
SGPT	mild increase
ALK PHOS	increased
Cholesterol	increased
Sodium	mild increase
Potassium	mild decrease
Urinalysis	specific gravity decreased, often under 1.007
Cortisol	increased
ACTH Stimulation Test	Cortisol, increased
Dexamthasone Suppression Test	Cortisol, increased

Treatment of Cushing's syndrome (hyperadrenocorticism) depends on the cause of the disease. If adrenal tumors are confirmed, surgical excision followed by glucocorticoid supplementation is the treatment of choice. With pituitary-dependent hyperadrenocorticism, chemotherapy with O,P'-DDD is very effective. In all cases of treatment, continuous monitoring is important.

Addison's Disease

Addison's disease (hypoadrenocorticism) is usually the result of the atrophy of the adrenal glands caused by autoimmune disease. Unlike Cushing's syndrome, Addison's follows a waxing/waning course of illness. It is gradual and progressive, and often misdiagnosed as an allergy. It displays the following clinical signs:

depression
anorexia (no appetite)
diarrhea
vomiting
chronic ear infections
inability to cope with stress
loss of body hair
polyuria (with or without polydipsia)

weakness
shivering from cold
weight loss
abdominal pain
discoloration of skin on elbows, hocks, skin folds
slow heart rate

A clinical workup reveals:

CHEM PROFILE

CBC	increased eosinophils
Sodium	increased
Potassium	decreased
Cortisol	decreased
ACTH Response	decreased
BUN	cortisol increased

Treatment is based on replacement therapy of glucocorticoids (prednisone) and mineralocorticoids (DOCA).

The recognition and diagnosis of early changes is important. Observing your dog closely will allow you to pick up these early warning signs.

Nutritional supplementation is necessary for both Cushing's syndrome and Addison's disease. The adrenal glands will not function without adequate vitamin B complex, vitamin C, minerals and the amino acid tyrosine in the diet.

Chapter 12

Laboratory Tests—What Do They Tell?

Every dog needs a thorough yearly examination by a veterinarian. A good habit to form with your dog, this annual checkup will provide the following information. Your dog's temperature will also let your veterinarian know if your dog's health is within normal parameters.

Physical Examination

A complete and thorough physical exam will consist of evaluating the dog's general attitude and appearance. Eyes, nose, ears, mouth and skin will all be checked as will the musculoskeletal, respiratory, nervous, digestive, genitourinary and circulatory systems. During this physical examination, your veterinarian will probably be asking you for more details on your dog's history. Any abnormalities found during the examination will be explained to you.

Complete Blood Count

A CBC, or complete blood count, is a routine profile of tests used to describe the quantity and quality of the cells in the blood.

Serum Chemistry Profile

The Serum Chemistry Profile, sometimes called a *chem screen* or chem *scan*, is an extensive battery of tests that provide a broad database to evaluate your dog's general health. These tests confirm the results of the physical examination and provide early warnings of unsuspected problems. To ensure accuracy with these tests, the dog should be fasted for 12 hours prior to the blood being drawn.

Urinalysis

This test examines the urine of your dog, which not only reveals the health of the genitourinary system but also reflects a variety of disease processes that involve other organs in the body.

Fecal Analysis

The feces or stool of your dog can reveal not only the presence of parasites but also undigested food particles, which would indicate that your dog was not able to break down and digest food properly.

Blood Tests and Results

Once these yearly physical and blood chemistry exams are part of the routine health care you provide for your dog, they will give invaluable information for the future. They establish normal levels for *your* dog. If there is a deviation in those levels, your veterinarian will be alerted that trouble is brewing.

Every laboratory doing the blood work establishes its own level of what is normal. These values vary depending on the particular laboratory equipment being used. These norms are established by analyzing the blood of a certain number of dogs and then computing an average. If you are using the blood chemistry to work out a diagnosis, you need to stay with one laboratory for consistent results. Mailing blood chemistry from one side of the country to another is not helpful because the norms will be different. Always check how the norms are established for each laboratory and ask if the laboratory being used is for veterinary or human purposes. Human laboratories often perform tests that are less expensive than a veterinary laboratory, but they can be inaccurate because the instruments used are not calibrated for animal blood and may provide inaccurate results.

By working with your veterinarian on a yearly basis, you can determine what are normal results of blood chemistry tests on your dog. It may be that you have an individual or a breed that falls outside of the established norm.

You need to establish this prior to any health problems arising; otherwise the information may be incorrect and misleading. This is clearly evident in the taking of a temperature. Most dogs' normal temperature falls around 101.5 degrees fahrenheit. It is reasonable to assume that if your dog's temperature goes above 103 degrees you must get the dog to the veterinarian immediately. But if your dog's normal temperature was 102.5 degrees, a rise of one half a degree need not signify an emergency. Establish a norm while **your** dog is in a state of good health.

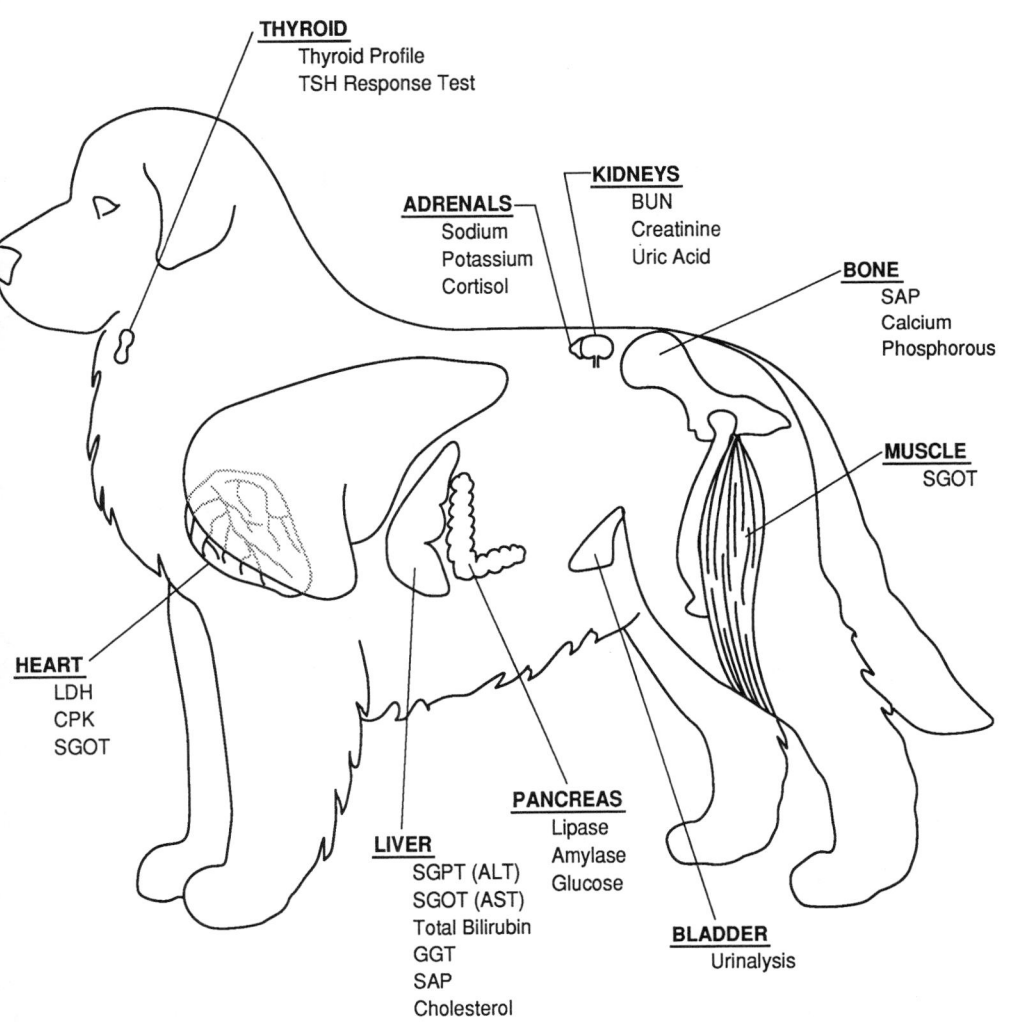

THYROID
Thyroid Profile
TSH Response Test

ADRENALS
Sodium
Potassium
Cortisol

KIDNEYS
BUN
Creatinine
Uric Acid

BONE
SAP
Calcium
Phosphorous

MUSCLE
SGOT

HEART
LDH
CPK
SGOT

PANCREAS
Lipase
Amylase
Glucose

LIVER
SGPT (ALT)
SGOT (AST)
Total Bilirubin
GGT
SAP
Cholesterol

BLADDER
Urinalysis

12–1: Chemistry Profile Dog

Normal CBC (Complete Blood Count) Values

RBC count × 10⁶/ul	5.57–7.98
Hematocrit (PCV count %)	36.8–54
Hemoglobin (Hb) g/dl	12–18
Reticulocyte count (%)	0–1.5
MCV (fl)	60–77
MCH (pg)	19.5–24.5
MCHC g/dl	32–36
Platelet count × 100000/ul	2–6
WBC count × 1000/ul	6.4–15.9
Neutrophils (seg) (%) × 1000/ul	(45–77) 3.0–11.4
Neutrophil bands (%) × 1000/ul	(0–3) 0–3
Lymphocytes (%) × 1000/UL	(12–30) 1.0–4.8
Eosinophil (%) × 1000/ul	(2–10) .1–.75
Monocytes (%) × 1000/ul	(3–10) .15–1.35
Basophils (%)	0.0–0.1

There may be a variation in the "norm" depending on the laboratory used.

Explanation of CBC Values

RBC—Red blood cell count. These cells transport oxygen and carbon dioxide between the lungs and body tissues. Red blood cells are produced in the bone marrow and are under the control of chemicals that are secreted by the kidneys.

HEMATOCRIT OR PCV—Pack cell volume is the most commonly used red cell number and is the percentage of blood composed of red blood cells.

Decreased levels of RBCs or PCVs is commonly termed anemia and has three basic causes: (1) Reduced bone marrow production, which can be from an iron deficiency, a vitamin B_{12} deficiency, or chronic kidney or liver disease. (2) Loss of blood from the body, such as from a hemorrhage or parasites. (3) Destruction within the body called hemolytic anemia (breaking down of red blood cells) or internal hemorrhage.

Increased levels of RBCs or PCVs are most often the result of dehydration. They can result from the bone marrow overproducing red blood cells, but this is rare.

HEMOGLOBIN (Hb)—Hemoglobin is the essential oxygen carrier of the blood. Found within the red blood cells, it is responsible for the red color of the blood. It is essentially equivalent to the hematocrit.

Decreased hemoglobin levels indicate the presence of hemorrhage and anemia.

Increased hemogloblin levels indicate a higher than normal concentration of red blood cells.

RETICULOCYTES—These are immature red blood cells that have been released from the bone marrow.

Decreased reticulocyte count—If associated with chronic anemia, it indicates a lowered red blood cell production by the bone marrow.

Increased reticulocyte count is associated with chronic hemorrhage or hemolytic anemia (destruction of RBC).

MCV, MCH, MCHC levels together are called Erythrocyte Indices. This count includes the total of the MCV (mean corpuscular volume), MCH (mean corpuscular hemogloblin) and MCHV (mean corpuscular hemoglobin concentration). They are calculated by using the RBC count, the PCV count, and the Hemoglobin concentration. These indices are used to classify the different kinds of anemia and their response to therapies.

PLATELET COUNT—Also called thrombocytes, platelets are derived from the bone marrow and play an important part in blood clotting.

Decrease in the number of platelets occurs in bone marrow depression, autoimmune hemolytic anemia, systemic lupus (a blood-clotting disorder), severe hemorrhage or intravascular coagulation (DIC).

Increase in the number of platelets occurs sometimes when there is a fracture or a blood vessel injury or if the bone marrow is overproducing (cancer).

WBC—The total number of white blood cells. WBCs are often called leukocytes. There are different kinds of white blood cells, and the figure shown on the chart is reached by combining the various kinds of white blood cells together. The different kinds of cells are called neutrophils, neutrophil bands, lymphocytes, eosinophils, monocytes and basophils.

Decreased levels of WBCs may indicate developmental or metabolic disorders, an overwhelming infection—especially viruses—or drug and chemical poisoning.

Increased WBC levels occur with infections, especially bacterial, as well as emotional upsets and blood disorders.

NEUTROPHILS—These are the white blood cells that function primarily in the face of inflammation. They act by consuming foreign material and destroying bacteria.

Decreased number of neutrophils would indicate viral infection, starvation, certain drug reactions or overwhelming bacterial infection.

Increased levels would indicate local bacterial infections and inflammation, stress, tissue destruction (such as abscesses or tumors) or the use of steroid drugs.

NEUTROPHIL BANDS—These are immature neutrophils that are released prematurely from the bone marrow when there is an immediate need for them, such as at the site of inflammation.

Increased number of bands together with mature neutrophils would indicate that the bone marrow has the infection or inflammation under control. If the band cells are greater than 10 percent of the mature neutrophils, and the total WBC is normal or low, this would show that the bone marrow is losing the battle.

LYMPHOCYTES—Their primary function is with the immune system. They recognize antigens (enzymes, toxins or foreign substances) and produce antibodies (protein substances), which fight the antigens.

Decreased numbers are seen during periods of stress or treatment with steroids or cancer chemotherapy drugs.

Increased numbers result from strong stimuli to the immune system, such as chronic inflammation, recovery from acute infections or underactive adrenal glands (Addison's disease).

EOSINOPHILS—They are the primary detoxifiers of histamine, a substance released by the body whenever tissue is damaged.

Decreased numbers occur with stress or the use of steroids and an overactive adrenal gland (Cushing's syndrome).

Increased numbers occur when the dog is showing an allergic reaction to something in the environment, when the dog has parasites in the system or when he has an underactive adrenal gland (Addison's disease).

MONOCYTES—These single cells are immature forms of the cells (macrophages) that "eat" foreign bodies and cellular debris.

Decreased numbers are not considered important.

Increased numbers occur with chronic fungus infections, dying tissue and chronic inflammatory and immune diseases, as well as a stress reaction from using steroid medications and Cushing's syndrome (overactive adrenals).

BASOPHILS—These cells contain both histamine and heparin, a blood-clotting *inhibitor*. These cells start the inflammatory response after the body is injured.

Decreased number of basophils can be an indicator of an underactive thyroid.

Increased number of these cells are associated with high fat levels in the blood, heartworm disease, Cushing's syndrome (overactive adrenal glands), thrombus formation (blood clot within the blood vessels) and ulcerative colitis.

The blood chemistry profile is a panel of tests that provide a broad database to evaluate your dog's general health. The panel results not only confirm abnormalities found on the physical examination, but also high-light unsuspected problems. The most accurate results are obtained if a 12-hour fast precedes the drawing of the blood sample.

What appears on the following chart is what you normally receive from the laboratory. Some laboratories include other chemistries on their list. Numerous other tests, some of which are shown at the end of the chart, can be requested if you are looking for a specific disease.

Calcium	9.0–11.5
Phosphorus	2.7–5.7
Sodium	139–153
Potassium	3.7–5.2
Chloride	103–121
Cholesterol	137–275
Triglycerides	20–80
LDH	20–250
SGPT (ALT)	10–75
SGOT (AST)	25–105
Bilirubin, total	0.0–0.6
Gamma glutamyltranspeptidase (GGT)	0–10
Alkaline phosphatase (SAP)	20–200
Total protein	4.9– 9.6
Globulin, total	2.2–3.9
Albumin	2.1–4.0
A/G ratio	0.50–1.68
BUN	5–24
Creatinine, serum	0.5–2.0
BUN/Creatinine ratio	individual
Uric acid	0.0–1.0
Glucose, serum	50–120
Amylase, serum	400–2000

Sometimes listed:
  CPK
  lipase
  magnesium

CALCIUM—Blood calcium levels are influenced by diet, hormone levels and blood protein levels. Calcium readings represent a balance between bone formation and bone reabsorption and are regulated by the hormone parathormone.

Decreased levels indicate acute damage to the pancreas or an under-active parathyroid gland. The parathyroid is a small endocrine gland attached to the thyroid. It secretes the hormone *parathormone* to regulate the calcium/phosphorus metabolism in the body.

Increased levels may indicate the presence of certain cancers, an overactive thyroid gland, too much protein in the blood or too much Vitamin D in the system.

PHOSPHORUS—Blood phosphorus levels are affected by diet, parathormone levels and kidney function.

Decreased levels show an overactive parathyroid gland and malignancies that cause the appearance of an overactive parathyroid gland, malnutrition, and malabsorption.

Increased levels develop with an underactive parathyroid gland and kidney failure.

SODIUM—Found in both bone and the body fluids outside of individual cells, the concentration of sodium is controlled by a naturally occurring steroid produced by the adrenal glands. This steroid (aldosterone) promotes excretion of sodium by the kidneys.

Decreased levels can be caused by lack of sodium in the food, diarrhea, vomiting, kidney disease and diabetes mellitus as well as an underactive adrenal gland (hypoadrenocorticism).

Increased levels are rare but can occur with salt poisoning and dehydration.

POTASSIUM—Found in fluid inside cells, it is excreted by the kidneys, influenced by the adrenal gland steroid aldosterone.

Decreased levels of potassium are the result of prolonged vomiting or diarrhea, an overactive adrenal gland (hyperadrenocorticism) and an increased alkaline pH level in the blood.

Increased levels can be caused by kidney disease, urethra blockage, dehydration and underactive adrenal glands. If pH levels get too high (acidosis) the death of large amounts of tissue will result and cardiac arrest *may* result.

CHLORIDE—These levels are measured to ascertain the acid-base balance of the body as well as the water balance.

Decreased levels of chloride often result from vomiting with a loss of gastric juices and hypoadrenocorticism.

Increased levels result from dehydration or the body being too acid (acidosis).

CHOLESTEROL—Produced by the liver, it is excreted in the bile. *Blood cholesterol levels tend to be inversely related to thyroid function.*

Decreased levels are found in an overactive thyroid gland.

Increased levels can occur when there is obstruction in the bile duct, kidney disease, dietary intake, diabetes mellitus, an overactive adrenal gland and an underactive thyroid gland.

TRIGLYCERIDES—This measurement shows the levels of fat in the blood. High levels will be found in the blood 4 to 6 hours after eating regardless of diet. Twelve-hour fasting is needed to produce accurate test results.

Decreased levels appear not to be a problem.

Increased levels may indicate diabetes mellitus, starvation, underactive thyroid and acute (sudden onset) of pancreatitis.

Liver

SGPT (ALT)—Alanine aminotransferase is an enzyme present in large quantities in liver cells. This enzyme is very specific for liver disease and increases of three times or more indicates cell damage in the liver. Increases do not necessarily correlate, however, with the *seriousness* of the disease.

Decreased levels are usually not significant.

Increased levels may indicate circulatory problems in the liver, trauma to the liver, active liver disease, degeneration of the liver (cirrhosis), obstruction to the bile duct, death of liver tissue, liver cancer and acute pancreatitis.

ALKALINE PHOSPHATASE—SAP is an enzyme found in high concentration in the liver and bone. Levels will be higher in young growing dogs. SAP of bone origin is normally elevated in puppies of less than 8 months of age. In adult dogs a steady increase in the levels may indicate cancer.

Increased levels indicate obstruction or congestive liver disease, overactive adrenal glands and drug treatments including steroids, anticonvulsants and barbiturates.

SGOT (AST)—This is an enzyme present in high concentration in liver, heart and skeletal muscle. It is not as specific to liver injury as in an increase of ALT.

Decreased levels are considered insignificant.

Increased levels are seen in liver damage, heart problems (myocardial infarction), inflammation of skeletal muscle, tissue damage and rupture of red blood cells. More tests should be considered when diagnosing liver disease.

BILIRUBIN—This is the orange or yellow bile pigment that comes from the breakdown of hemoglobin from old or damaged red blood cells. It is chemically changed in the liver, secreted into the bile and delivered to the small intestine. As it passes through, it is converted into a waste product excreted mostly through the feces and is responsible for their brown color.

Increase in "direct bilirubin" indicates bile duct obstruction or liver disease.

Increase in "total bilirubin" indicates disease in the liver, bile duct obstruction or destruction of red blood cells.

GAMMA-GLUTAMYLTRANSPĒPTIDASE—GGT is a protein enzyme produced by the liver and circulated in the blood. The body's resistance to disease is related to the concentration of these proteins in the blood.

Increased levels may indicate *pancreatitis*, blockage of bile excretion.

TOTAL PROTEIN—This measurement shows levels of a combination of various proteins produced by the liver and lymphoid organs.

Decreased levels occur with kidney disease, liver disease, starvation and malabsorption syndromes.

Increased levels occur with severe dehydration, cancer of the lymph nodes (lymphosarcoma) and bone marrow tumors (myeloma).

GLOBULINS—They come in three types. Alpha globulins transport fats, beta globulins transport iron and gamma globulins function as antibodies. Globulins total on the chem scan measures *a combination* of all three globulins.

Decreased levels indicate deficiencies in the immune system.

Increased levels can be due to infections involving the whole body (systemic), cancer of the lymph nodes, bone cancer, parasites in the system and liver disease.

ALBUMIN—This blood protein, which transports fatty acids, affects the pressure of the fluid in the cells (osmotic pressure).

Decreased levels indicate low production of blood protein associated with chronic liver or pancreatic disease, malabsorption, hemorrhage, burns and kidney disease.

Increased levels are the result of dehydration.

Kidney

BUN (Blood, Urea, Nitrogen)—Urea is an end product of protein breakdown. Proteins contain large amounts of nitrogen that are found mostly in the urine as well as in the blood and lymph glands. Urea is formed in the liver from ammonia derived from amino acid breakdown. The amount of urea excreted through urine is less when your dog is on a low-protein diet. Expect low readings from dogs being fed special diets or dogs that are being fed the "lite" foods.

Decreased levels are seen with low protein diets, liver insufficiency and the use of anabolic steroid drugs.

Increased levels (azotemia) occur from any condition that reduces the kidneys' ability to filter body fluids in the body or interferes with protein breakdown. Before kidney problems arise diseases such as renal azotemia can be seen. Heart disease, low adrenal gland function and shock can create azotemia. If more than 75 percent of the kidney tissues become nonfunctional through aging or kidney disease, the

BUN will increase. As the urea nitrogen cannot be eliminated, it builds up in the body. This extremely dangerous condition can kill the animal if not taken care of *immediately.*

CREATININE—This is a nonprotein nitrogen waste product of muscle metabolism.

Decreased levels are not significant and rarely seen.

Increased levels would indicate poor kidney filtration. This poor filtration results from the same pre-renal and post-renal causes that produce an increased BUN. An increased BUN and normal creatinine would suggest an early or mild problem. An increased creatinine and increased BUN with elevated phosphorus would indicate a long standing, severe kidney disease (kidney failure).

URIC ACID—This is the end product of purines, which are another end product of proteins. Purines mainly come from the nuclei of cells.

Increased levels show marked cellular destruction in such diseases as leukemia, pneumonia and toxic states often associated with pregnancy. Elevated levels may point to severe kidney disease and would elevate the levels of uric acid, but should not be taken alone as an indicator.

GLUCOSE—The metabolism and concentration of blood glucose is affected by many disease states. It is greatly influenced by diet, the ability of the liver to handle the diet and the rate at which it is excreted.

Decreased levels can result from an overdose of insulin or the presence of tumors or abnormal growths on the pancreas. Low levels may also come from a malfunctioning liver, underactive adrenal glands, excessive exercise or long-term starvation.

Increased levels can be caused by diabetes mellitus, recent feeding, an excess of the hormone progesterone, an overactive adrenal gland or stress.

AMYLASE—This pancreatic enzyme is released into the small intestine and allows starch to convert to sugar.

Increased levels show up in certain types of pancreatic disease or duct obstruction. Sometimes stomach problems, obstruction in the intestines or diseases of the salivary glands can create elevated levels.

Other routine tests that are sometimes shown on laboratory reports

LIPASE—This is a pancreatic enzyme that chemically changes fatty-acids in the body. It is used most often to confirm acute pancreatic disease.

Increased levels indicate acute pancreatitis, kidney disease (decreased excretions) and upper intestinal inflammation.

CPK—Creatine phosphokinase is an enzyme that is found both in heart and skeletal muscle.

Increased levels are caused by heart muscle damage (myocardial infarction) or death of skeletal muscle tissue.

CARBON DIOXIDE is used to measure blood levels of bicarbonate, which plays a major role in maintaining the body's acid-alkaline balance and changes in cases of respiratory insufficiency.

Decreased levels occur when the body pH is low (metabolic acidosis) and in kidney failure. This is often the result of shock, severe diabetes, diarrhea and underactive adrenal glands.

Increased levels are most often seen when there have been severe bouts of vomiting. The rise in body pH often results in low potassium and low chloride levels.

Urinalysis

The examination of the urine is an absolute necessity in the evaluation of your dog's health. Not just a measure of kidney and lower urinary tract problems, it also reflects a variety of disease processes that involve other organs. A urinalysis consists of the physical characteristics of the urine as well as the chemical and sediment present.

Physical Characteristics

Color:	Normal urine is yellow to amber
	Abnormal color can be caused by:
	• blood = red
	• bilirubin = dark yellow to brown with yellow foam
	• hemoglobin/myoglobin = reddish brown
Transparency:	Normal urine is clear
	Abnormal urine is cloudy, which can be caused by
	• crystals, cells, blood, mucous, bacteria or cast.
Volume:	Normal output is 12 to 20 ml of urine per pound of body weight in 24 hours

Increased levels (polyuria) come from an increase in water intake and may indicate sudden kidney disease, long-term kidney disease, diabetes mellitus, liver failure, overactive adrenal glands, too much calcium in the body, diabetes associated with kidney dysfunction, diabetes associated with pituitary gland dysfunction, excesssive thirst or uterine infections (pyometra).

Decreased levels of urine output indicate dehydration, which in turn may point to the sudden onset of kidney disease, shock, end stage of kidney disease and urinary tract obstruction.

SPECIFIC GRAVITY—This measure is an indication of how well the kidneys are able to concentrate or dilute urine. Normal levels should be greater than 1.030.

Decreased levels—1.007 to 1.029—occur with diabetes mellitus, insipidus, overactive adrenals, excessive thirst (polydipsia) and pyometra.

Increased levels—greater than 1.040—are associated with high fever, dehydration, diabetes mellitus, vomiting, diarrhea and severe hemorrhage.

PH LEVELS (hydrogen-ion concentration)—A dog's diet should be on the acidic side, making the pH of the urine 6.2 to 6.5. If the diet is too alkaline, the urine pH may be greater than 7.0. A fresh urine sample is needed to obtain an accurate pH, as urine becomes more alkaline the longer it stands. Urine pH should not be used alone to determine the acid-alkaline status of the body.

Chemical Characteristics of Urine

PROTEIN—The level of protein is tested by using a test strip with a scale of 0 to 4+. Normal urine = 0–1+ protein level.

Increased levels of protein are 2 to 4+. A temporary increase (false positive) may result from very alkaline pH urine, muscular exertion, being in season or excessive protein intake.

Decreased levels of protein are associated with dilute urine (low specific gravity, –1.020), chronic kidney disease, infection, inflammation or tumors in the lower urinary tract. Pre-renal disease will show a high protein level with normal to high specific gravity.

GLUCOSE—This sugar is not normally found in the urine.

Increased levels may be temporarily seen when the dog is stressed or on cortisone therapy as well as in cases of hyperglycemia caused by diabetes mellitus, overactive adrenal glands and acute inflammation of the kidneys.

KETONES—These acids represent the end product of fat metabolism and have a scale of 0 to 3+. Normal is 0.

Increased levels indicate excessive fat in the body and occur when fat provides the bulk of energy in the diet. It is highly suggestive of diabetic problems. Starvation diets will also increase urine ketones, especially in young, immature dogs.

BILIRUBIN—Reagent strips are used to detect direct bilirubin. Range falls between 0 and 3+. Trace quantities (0–1+) are considered **normal.**

Increased levels or high-normal levels (2+–3+) would indicate the obstruction of bile flow and the reflux of direct bilirubin. *Severe liver disease is often present before elevated bilirubin is detected in urine.*

OCCULT BLOOD—Red blood cells apparent in the urine give it a red, cloudy appearance. In the absence of anemia or muscle disease, it is evidence of urinary tract disease. A urine color of reddish brown with no red blood cells present indicates loss of hemoglobin from red blood cells. Brownish urine with an absence of red blood cells in the sediment indicates muscle damage.

SEDIMENT—The evaluation of the sediment in the urine must be interpreted considering the specific gravity and how the sample is collected. Samples collected by the owner may yield cells and bacteria from the dog's urethra and genital tracts as well as the bladder, ureter or kidneys.

RBCs—Presence of red blood cells results from inflammation or trauma to the urogenital tract (kidneys, ureter, bladder, urethra).

WBCs—White blood cells are few in number in normal urine. Large numbers in collected samples indicate inflammation of the urinary or urogenital tract and possible kidney infections.

EPITHELIAL CELLS—Originating in the ureters, bladder wall and urethra, they are increased in numbers with inflammation and tumors.

CRYSTALS—These are formed by precipitation of minerals present in the urine. The pH of the urine will determine the kind of crystals formed. Crystals may indicate the presence of stones (calculae) in the bladder.

Fecal Analysis

To check for intestinal **parasites,** a fecal analysis should be run at least twice a year. Internal parasite eggs that can be detected under a microscope are *roundworms* (ascarids), *hookworms* and *whipworms. Tapeworms* are noted on the surface of the stool or around the anus as small flat ¹/₄-inch white segments that may stretch to a full inch in length. These segments are filled with eggs. *Coccidia* and *giardia* are simple, single-celled parasites (protozoa) that can also be detected in the stool.

Undigested food material, muscle, fat and starch granules may indicate that the food is passing through the digestive tract too quickly, or that there is a pancreatic enzyme deficiency, which results in malabsorption syndrome.

Occult blood, detectable only under a microscope, indicates hemorrhage into the gastrointestinal tract. *Gross blood,* which can be seen by the naked eye, presents a dark, tarry stool when it comes from bleeding in the upper gastrointestinal tract (mouth to upper part of the small intestine). Bleeding in the colon and rectum produces bright red blood in the stool.

Heartworm Testing

Heartworm is a disease on the move. With our mobile society, we have spread the disease by transporting infected dogs to areas where heartworm has not been known. Mosquitoes transfer the infection through their bite. Heartworm is an insidious disease that shows no clinical signs until the adult worms have been present in the dog's heart for 3 to 4 years. By the time clinical signs are seen it is often too late to treat the disease. Yearly testing can detect heartworm disease early.

Two basic diagnostic tests procedures are used. The *Knotts test* detects young heartworms (microfilaria) that are circulating in the blood. This test will give false negatives if the dog has been receiving heartworm medication. It may also give false negatives at certain times of the day. Microfilaria seem to be more active in the blood at peak mosquito activity hours. The *occult test* has become much more accurate and reliable than the filter test. If you are in an area where heartworm is common or if you have been using a heartworm preventative, this test is a must for you.

Summary

1. YOUR VETERINARIAN IS ONE OF THE MOST IMPORTANT PEOPLE IN YOUR DOG'S LIFE. You should choose your veterinarian just as you select your own doctor, by reputation and quality of service. You and your dog should feel at ease with this professional. You need to feel that you can trust your veterinarian, especially in an emergency situation.

2. BE SURE THAT YOU HAVE STATED YOUR OWN GOALS AND YOUR INTENTIONS WITH YOUR DOG SO THAT YOUR VETERINARIAN CAN KNOW WHAT YOU ARE EXPECTING. *Your dog's health depends on your being able to work together with your vet.*

3. WHEN YOU HAVE A PUPPY, YOU WILL BE VISITING YOUR VET MANY TIMES THE FIRST YEAR. After that, establish a routine by visiting every six months for fecal and physical examinations and once a year for a complete work up, including blood tests. Use this as a

preventative measure. Dogs cannot tell you where it hurts or if they are not feeling very well. Preventative medicine can put years on your dog's life.

4. WHEN HAVING BLOOD WORK DONE, MAKE SURE YOUR DOG HAS FASTED AT LEAST 12 HOURS BEFORE THE TEST.

5. BLOOD WORK AND URINALYSIS NEED TO BE HANDLED VERY CAREFULLY. IN SOME OF THE TESTS, THERE IS A TIME FACTOR INVOLVED.

6. SOME DIFFERENCES IN CLINICAL CHEMISTRIES EXIST BETWEEN THE BREEDS. German Shepherd Dogs, for example, tend to be lower than other breeds in glucose, LDH, alkaline phosphatase, BUN and uric acid. Their amylase and transaminase may be higher. Phosphorus and SGPT were found to be higher in Beagles and Labrador Retrievers.

7. YOUR BEST GUIDE IS THE COMPARISON OF YOUR OWN DOG'S TEST RESULTS. Establish what is normal and be sure that the tests are run always using the same laboratory.

8. IF YOU HAVE MADE THE DECISION TO CHANGE YOUR DOG'S DIET FROM COMMERCIAL DOG FOOD TO A NATURAL DIET, HAVE BLOOD DRAWN BEFORE YOU CHANGE. You should have a CBC, a chemistry screen or profile and also a fecal analysis done. One month after putting your dog on the new diet, have the same tests run. This will give you a basis for comparison. Changing to the natural diet often puts a dog who had health problems back into balance.

Glossary of Terms for Lab Profile

Following is a glossary of terms that are helpful for you to know. These are terms you will see and hear frequently. Knowing them will help you to understand and better communicate with your veterinarian.

Acidosis:	A physiological state in which the body's pH becomes too low (acid range).
Alkalosis:	A physiological state in which the body's pH bcomes too high (alkaline range).
Cardiac:	Refers to the heart.
Hepatic:	Refers to the liver.
Hyperadrenocorticism:	The state of an overactive adrenal gland (Cushing's syndrome).

Hypoadrenocorticism:	The state of an underactive adrenal gland (Addison's disease).
Hypoglycemia:	Low blood sugar levels.
Hyperthyroid:	An overactive thyroid gland.
Hypothyroid:	An underactive thyroid gland.
Necrosis/Necrotic:	Dying or dead tissue.
Polyuria:	Increased urination.
Polydipsia:	Increased thirst.
Pyometra:	An infection of the uterus.
Renal:	Refers to the kidneys.

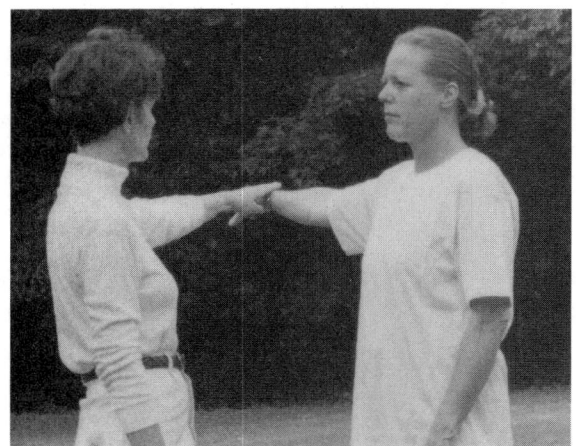

13-1: How to stand to test the strength of the deltoid muscle. (See page 147.)

13-2: Testing weak.

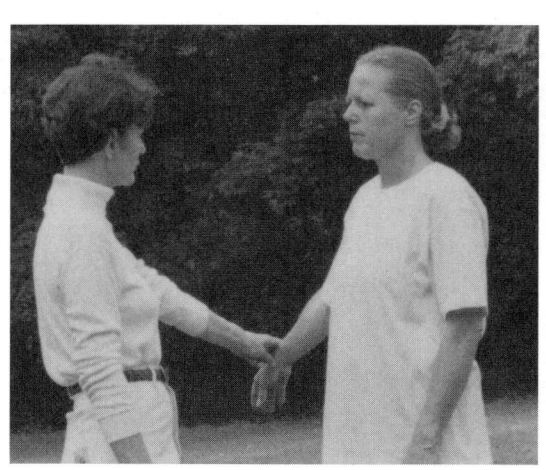

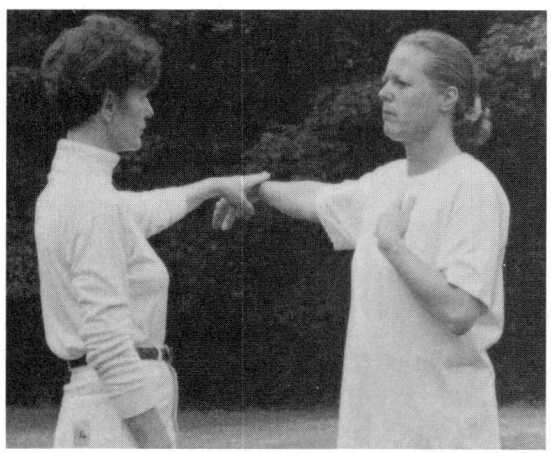

13-3: Holding Finger over the Thymus gland.

—Chapter 13—

What Is Kinesiology?

"It's quackery, Wendy, please don't teach it!" This is what my staff told me in the early 1980s, when I tried to introduce kinesiology into the nutrition and health curriculum at our training camps. But because I had had so much success in using it, I felt driven to continue.

Case History

Bobby was a 6-month-old German Shepherd puppy that came to Training Camp with his owner, Jean. In some sense they didn't know why they had come. As Jean explained it to me, she had attended obedience classes in her area, but Bobby was not able to learn the lessons because he was so hyperactive. Jean gave her dog huge amounts of exercise, visited a veterinarian, who prescribed various medications, all to no avail. Bobby couldn't settle down at home and at night needed to go out several times. They were both exhausted. With pupils dilated and not wanting to be touched, Bobby appeared to be in a state of perpetual anxiety.

Before I worked with Bobby, I asked Jean to sit down and as carefully as she could, write out the medical history of this puppy. What she recorded was shocking but typical. The medical record revealed that Bobby had been subjected to combination vaccinations every two weeks since he was 7 weeks old, resulting in violent attacks of diarrhea and skin problems, which were taken care of by antibiotics, steroids and stool hardeners. His ears had been taped and glued inside in order to develop erect ears. Because Jean had obtained Bobby at the age of 7 weeks, there had been no time when the dog was not on medication of one type or another. Thinking that the vomiting and diarrhea were diet related, Jean tried Bobby on various foods. Everything shot right through him. Only the use of stool hardeners worked. Jean was desperate and willing to try anything.

Using kinesiology, it was determined that Bobby's system was toxic. He was allergic to the food, antibiotics, steroids and especially the stool hardeners. The glue in his ears had made red, irritated patches where the hair had fallen out. The puppy was allergic to that, too. What a sad little guy!

After testing that it was safe to withdraw Bobby from all of the medications, it was suggested to Jean that she fast Bobby for a day, giving nothing but distilled water and honey. She agreed. By the end of that first fast day, we all noticed that Bobby was calmer and slept the whole night through for the first time that Jean could remember. Bobby was tested the following day to see what he could eat. A diet of fresh home-cooked foods, including a vitamin-mineral supplement, was formulated. Digestive enzymes and acidophilus were added to restore the good bacteria in his digestive system, which had been wiped out with the overuse of antibiotics. That next day Bobby was allowed about half the amount of food he would normally eat, and the third day, he was allowed his full quota. Bobby was perfectly calm, did his obedience lessons, played, had fun, slept and became "normal"—so normal, in fact, that Jean thought he might be sick! She had never seen her dog the way he should have been. They had a lovely week and returned home happy.

Jean, full of excitement from what she had learned, went back to her veterinarian, who made it very clear that if Jean did not follow his program, he would not want her as a client. For a while, Jean stood her ground, but then she left Bobby in a kennel while she and the family went on a week's vacation. On her return, Bobby had mange. Her veterinarian told her to dip the dog and put him back on dog food. Jean was reminded that Bobby's vaccinations were overdue. The call for help came very soon afterward. Bobby had had a relapse.

The testing and the fasting had to be done all over again. This time it took much longer for Bobby to bounce back.

This dog will always have to be on a special diet to maintain his health. Bobby stresses badly when left alone, refuses to eat and returns to hyperactivity if left for any length of time. Like many German Shepherd Dogs, and other dogs that have autoimmune problems, Bobby cannot tolerate the monthly heartworm medication. Jean has decided not to vaccinate Bobby again, knowing that she may lose him the next time. She does give the 3-year rabies vaccine. If she has to leave home, she places Bobby with a friend and he lives in the house. Although this is not ideal, Bobby is much less stressed upon Jean's return.

Was Bobby genetically predisposed to ill health, or were his problems a result of bombarding an immature immune system with too many vaccines? What effect did all the drugs have on his young growing body? We believe that knowledge of kinesiology put Bobby on the right track.

History of Kinesiology

In human medicine the concept of biofeedback, that is, controlling the body through the mind by the use of a special machine, is old. This is a mechanical kind of kinesiology. The newest energy concepts are being explored by research companies in this country, Austria, Russia and Japan. Successful experiments have been conducted where electrodes are attached to the head to access the energy of the brain and thought processes, which is then used to drive machinery. This concept has already been used experimentally by people in wheelchairs, who have no use of their bodies. (*ABC News*, October 25, 1993.) In Russia, a plane has been piloted by using the energy from the pilot's brain waves.

Kinesiology is an early form of biofeedback without the machine, whereby the body's energies can be tested through the muscle system. It was first developed by Wilhelm Reich, a psychoanalyst and disciple of Freud, who introduced the idea that the body was influenced by the flow of what he called bio-energy.

Chiropractic practitioners have developed a special technique of muscle testing known as applied kinesiology. This combines both Indian and Chinese medical concepts of energy to look at the body as an integrated system of muscles and nerves. Kinesiology uses the muscle system as a source of information about the state of balance of the organism. The founder and researcher of this technique was Dr. George Goodheart, whose student Dr. John Diamond, an Australian psychiatrist, wrote the book *Your Body Doesn't Lie* (originally titled *Behavioral Kinesiology*) in 1978. That book is the basis for much of the following research and use of the technique.

In simple terms, the knowledge of kinesiology gives us a way to communicate with the body—be it our own *or* our dogs'. It has opened the doors for asking questions pertaining to health and nutrition. It is in these fields that we have worked and have had the greatest success. Our introduction to the subject first came with a visit to Deva Khalsa, DVM, a holistic veterinarian, and secondly through the late Richard Kearns, DVM, also a holistic veterinarian with whom we studied.

Einstein's theory of mass is energy ($E = mc^2$) goes a long way to explaining the concept of energy fields present in all matter. Our bodies, our dogs' bodies, the food we eat, the medicine we take, the environment in which we live all have energy fields. Energy fields are measured by frequencies using an oscilloscope or wavelengths using a frequency meter. The secret to good health with harmony and balance in our lives is in the synchronicity of all of these energy fields. Dis-harmony and dis-ease, as the energy medicine texts put it, are caused by an imbalance in one or more of these energy fields. For example, we all experience a lack of energy when we don't feel well, but when we feel good, we feel full of energy.

Dr. Diamond said that the food we eat, what we drink, the clothes we wear, the music we listen to, the pictures or photographs we look at, the people with whom we associate, where we live, where we work—*all* these have a direct effect on our energy fields and therefore our health. Our total environment affects how we look at life. Here, we will describe only how kinesiology can be used to work with our dogs' diets and health, although it has much broader application as well.

Food Energy

Eating correctly energizes us and eating incorrectly can decrease our energy. This decrease in energy can manifest itself in many ways, such as feeling tired, a skin outbreak, digestive or respiratory upset or an allergy. When we experience decreased energy, we often crave certain foods knowing that they give a pick-me-up. How many of us eat candy bars mid-afternoon to get over the slump in energy that often occurs? This can be explained by using the energy concept. That candy bar is full of sugar, and after eating it, we experience a short burst of energy. Unfortunately, after the burst of energy has gone, we are left feeling less energetic than before. Other cravings, such as a need for a cucumber salad, for example, would tell us that our body needs the energy from the cucumber to put itself in balance. It also means that we are low in vitamin A and in order to function correctly we need to increase our intake of vitamin A. The body is seeking to be in balance.

The opposite is true too. If we know we don't like something—for example, mushrooms—what the body is saying is that if it eats mushrooms, that energy will be bad and it will suffer the consequences by experiencing nausea, vomiting, skin problems, an allergic reaction or digestive upset.

How to Use Kinesiology

Dr. Diamond's concept is that when the body is stressed with the wrong form of energy from something in the environment or the food or drink we ingest, the thymus gland producing the T-cells in charge of our immune systems shrinks. When the thymus shrinks our immune system is impaired, our resistance to disease is compromised and we are out of balance. *To be in balance, the thymus gland needs to be working correctly.* The same is true for the dog.

Are You in Balance?

To test to see if we are in balance, Dr. Diamond found that by using the deltoid muscle of the body as an indicator muscle, he could test the balance of energy in any subject. Any muscle or set of muscles could be used, but the deltoid muscle is easy to test since it locks into the shoulder joint. A machine called a kinesiometer showed that the average healthy muscle can withstand around 40 pounds of pressure, and a weak muscle can withstand only 15 pounds of pressure. The deltoid muscle shows the strength and weakness of muscles well, and it is obvious to the tester and subject when that muscle is strong or weak.

The first step in using kinesiology is to make sure that both the people doing the testing are in balance. The energy field around a well person is usually 6 to 8 inches. Stand in an area with 16 inches of clear space around you (this is the combined measurement of both of your energy fields). Stand away from the walls and furniture. The subject has her left hand at her side and right hand out and parallel to the ground. The tester faces the subject and places two fingers of the left hand on the subject's right wrist. The subject is told to "brace" and the tester presses firmly down **without jerking.** The deltoid muscle will lock and it will be impossible for the tester to make the arm go down. Do not use so much force that it hurts!

Rebalancing

A person who is not feeling well has a much smaller energy field around his or her body. In this case, the arm would go down easily when pressed, indicating that the person is out of balance. Before testing can be done, that person needs to be brought back into balance. Have the testee place two fingers of the left hand over the thymus gland which is found just below the "v" in the breastbone (see illustration). Push down on the testee's right wrist, and it will go down. Have the subject thump this thymus point three times and then have him or her place the tongue behind the front upper teeth and keep it there. Test again, and the testee will have a strong right arm. The thymus gland has been temporarily stimulated and the testee is back in balance.

Once both the tester and subject are in balance, kinesiology can begin.

How to Test Food

Prepare the items to be tested. Place a small amount of the product, approximately 1 tablespoon, into a plastic bag. Securely knot the bag. A small glass container, without the lid, can also be used. You can test vitamins or minerals with the capsule or tablet held in the left hand. If in powder form, place a small amount into a plastic bag and prepare as above. If liquid is being tested, put a small amount into a glass or plastic bottle, without the lid. In the case of vegetables or fruit or any food, you can take the whole item in your hand.

Line up the products. In order to "feel" the difference between those food items that test strong and those that test weak, include some refined white flour or white sugar (which test weak for almost everyone) into your test items. You can also check a food that you know you don't like. Check these first and then test a small amount of honey in a container, and see how strong it feels in comparison. Also test a piece of natural whole wheat bread and then a piece of white bread.

1. Have the subject stand in the middle of the room with at least 16 inches of space all around.
2. With the left hand at rest, have the subject put out the right arm parallel to the ground. The product to be tested goes into the left hand and placed into the solar plexus area (see illustration). This area is a powerful center of the body's energy.
3. The tester stands directly in front of the subject and places two fingers of the left hand on the testee's wrist.
4. Subject is told to brace against tester, who presses down on the wrist.
5. The arm should not move very much.

Everyone has different strengths in the deltoid muscle, so some people may experience a little "give" in the muscle. This would be the norm for that person.

The foods that test strong will be showing the same energy frequencies as your body, meaning that they are in harmony with you. Foods that are not on the same wavelength will cause weakness in the deltoid muscle and the arm will go down, thus decreasing energy. This gives us a tool with which to test the food we eat to see if it agrees with us and if it will give us energy. Conversely, foods that are eaten that create weakness may cause allergies.

Balancing

In order for kinesiology to work, the person doing the testing and the subject have to be in balance. Things that cause imbalance are necklaces, earrings, watch bands or anything else that is metal and circles the body or a part of it. All of these should be removed before testing. If the body is out of balance a false reading can result. Another disruption to testing is if the person being tested has scars in the area where the product is being tested. Scars disrupt energy. In that case, another energy center can be

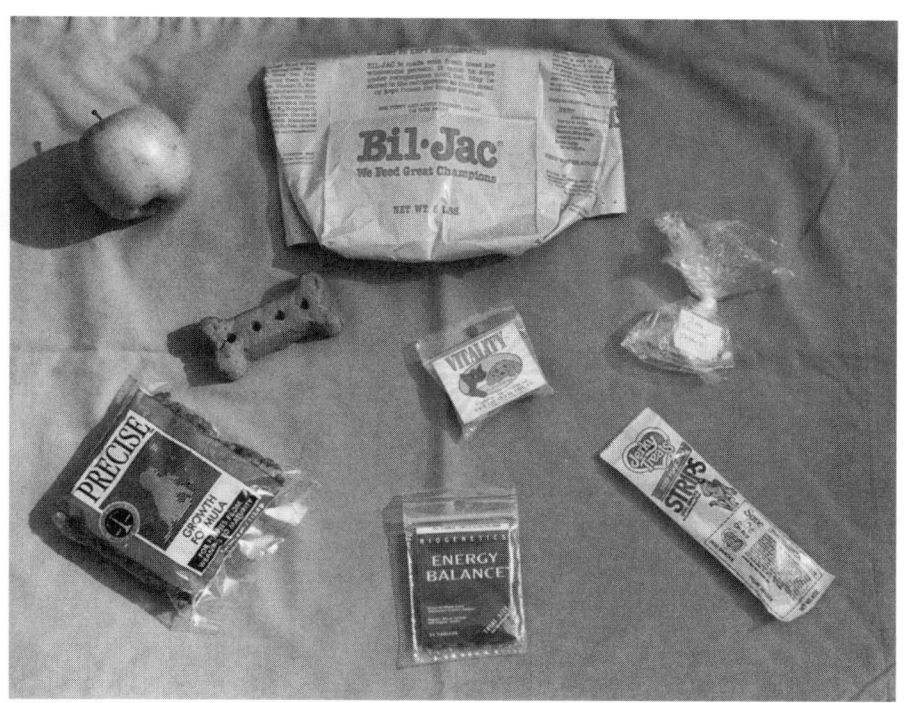

13-4: Items to be tested.

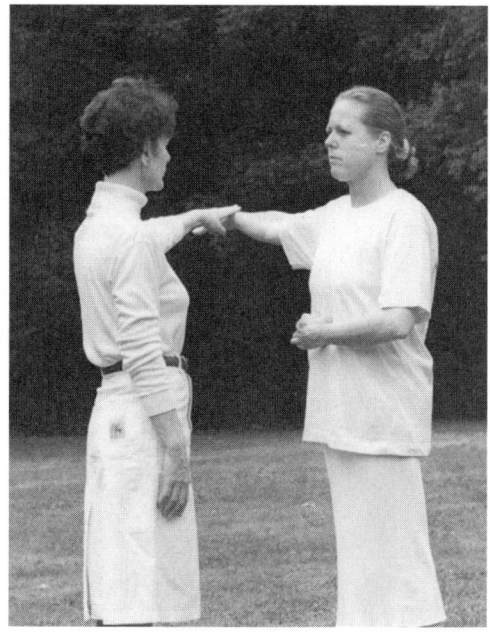

13-5: Testing an apple.

149

used (see illustration "Seven Major Chakras or Energy Fields"). While Diamond put food into the subject's mouth, we have found that it is equally effective—and less messy—to put the food in the hand and hold it in the solar plexus area. Since Diamond's book was written, Dr. Kearns found that the results were most effective and accurate if the food was put into the left hand and the right deltoid was tested. Kearns maintained that energy came into the body through the left side and went out through the right side, and subsequent testing seem to bear this out.

All the foods we eat can be tested for compatibility, as well as vitamin and mineral supplements. In fact the exact doses of supplements our bodies need can be worked out. For example, have the subject hold a 1-gram tablet of vitamin C in the left hand on the solar plexus and have the tester test the deltoid muscle of the right arm. If it tests strong, add another vitamin C tablet and test again. Keep adding vitamin C until the muscle tests weak, then take back one tablet and test again. This will tell you exactly how much vitamin C the subject's body needs. Do this with all vitamin and mineral supplements.

Kinesiology is somewhat like a blood test. It tells you the condition of the body at the time the test is done. In order to work out correctly the doses of daily supplements, it is best to check several times during the day until a supplement program has been worked out. The same goes for those foods that are found to be incompatible with the body's energies. Check several times during the day and over several days to see if a particular food shows a strong or weak response. For example, if you test weak for oranges right after drinking a glass of orange juice, what in fact your body is saying is that it doesn't need oranges *right now*. That does not mean to say that four hours from now a glass of orange juice or an orange won't be good for you. In order to get true results, test over several days and different times of the day.

When working with someone who is not feeling well, testing should be done on a weekly basis. What the body needs at the point of weakness will be different from what it will need as it rebalances. Keep testing until the same results come up several weeks in a row.

We suggest that you get used to working with someone and feel comfortable with kinesiology before you go to the next step, which is called Surrogate Testing and where the energy concept can be used to work with our dogs.

Testing Our Dogs

Dr. Goodheart's experiments showed that energy can be transferred from one person *through* another. If he had a patient who was unconscious, Goodheart found that the spouse, close friend or relative of that person could transfer energy. It also worked with someone who was not associated

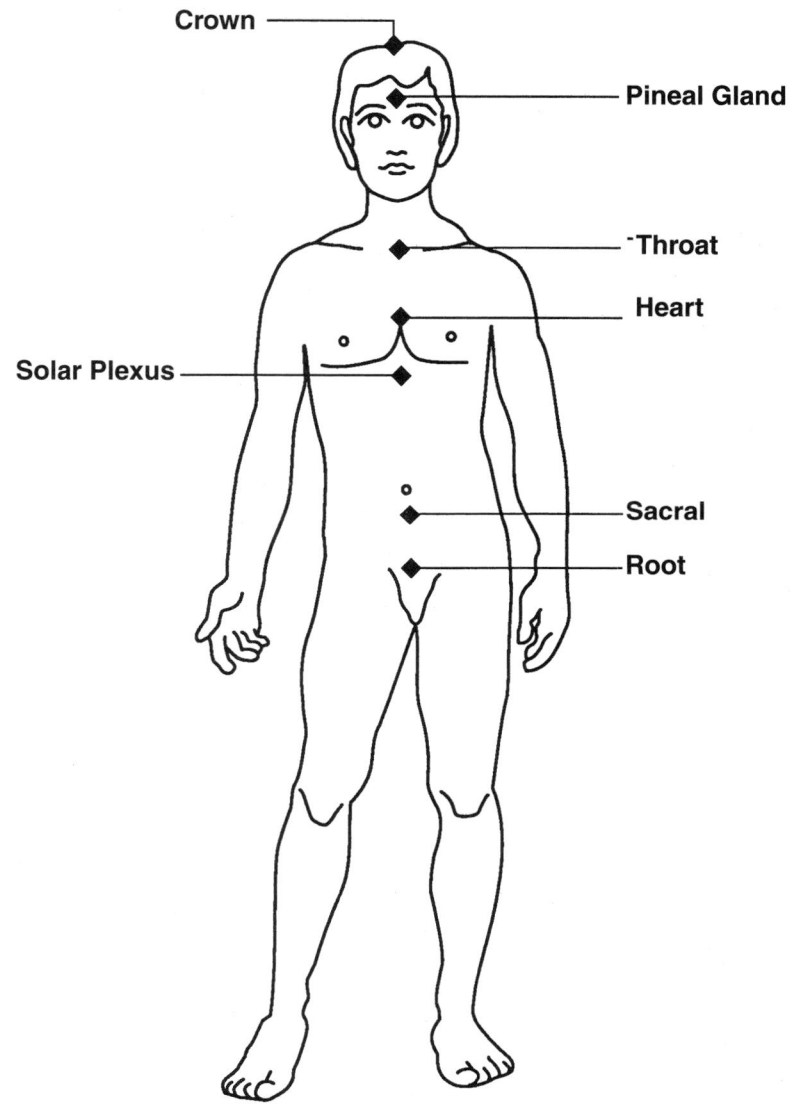

Crown

Pineal Gland

Throat

Heart

Solar Plexus

Sacral

Root

Energy centers are associated with either an endocrine gland or major nerve plexus.

13-6: Seven Major Chakras or Energy Fields

with the patient, like the office nurse. The surrogate would put her hand on the body of the unconscious person, and the tester could test the unconscious person's energy level through the surrogate.

In that sense, our dogs are like the "unconscious" person. The dog is lying by the owner's left side, with the handler on the floor next to the dog. A small portion of the dog's food should be placed either in a plastic bag or glass jar and held on the dog's body—anywhere except the head area. The owner's right arm is extended parallel to the ground. The tester pushes down on the wrist of the surrogate to see if the deltoid muscle tests strong. If it is weak, it means that the dog food is not "in tune" with the dog. In other words, the food is not compatible with the dog. Test several dog foods until you find one that tests strong.

There are more than 3,000 brands of dog food available in this country. Dogs all have their own individual body chemistry. It is not possible to have one food that tests strong for all of them.

Geographic Origins and Breed Heritage—Does It Matter?

Our testing clearly shows that food is ethnic. Many dogs that have been imported from Europe show allergies to corn. Corn, until recently, has not been used in European dog food and is not indigenous to the heritage of the dog. Test a food that is oatmeal based on an import Border Collie and it will test strong. The same applies to the Rottweilers and German Shepherd Dogs imported from Germany. Our Newfoundlands and German Shepherd Dogs have been imported from Germany, and both breeds experienced digestive and skin problems using the dog food in this country. Corn was the ingredient that created the most problems. *Rice-based foods created as many digestive difficulties for our dogs as the corn-based products. On a diet of oats and wheat they thrived.* We have worked with Labrador and Golden Retrievers, Boxers, Rottweilers and numerous other breeds who test the same.

Some dogs find beef, chicken or lamb incompatible with their bodies, and many dogs tested weak to the preservatives used. See the next section on how to test the ingredients in your dog food.

Using kinesiology allows us to find a food suitable for each of our dogs. We don't have to become Ph.Ds in nutrition to figure out what is best for our pets. It doesn't matter which food ingredient our dogs cannot tolerate, what is important is to *find a food with which the energies of our pets are in tune.*

How to Test Your Dog

The most accurate results are obtained when you work with a hungry dog. Prepare plastic bags each containing a small amount of different kinds of food—for example, a beef base, chicken base, lamb base, a mixture of beef and chicken base, and fish meal–based food. All the supplements used for the dog should be put into separate bags as well. Also include any kind of medications, for example, heartworm tablets.

Sit the owner and the dog on the floor with the dog lying on the left side of the owner. There should be a clear space around the handler and dog of about 16 inches, **and the food to be tested should be several feet away.** Have the owner hold a bag containing the dog food on the dog's body and test the owner's deltoid muscle. If the owner's arm registers a strong response by staying parallel to the ground, then that food would be compatible with the dog. Put those foods to one side and out of the 16-inch energy circle. Test all the foods and separate them out into groups of strong and weak. Results will be more accurate if the owner doesn't know which foods are being tested. Sometimes all of the foods show a weak response and the owner's arm will go down. Some foods test more weakly than others. This will be felt by the testee as the arm not going completely down, but not totally strong. This is when we know that the dog can tolerate the food, but will need supplementation.

When testing different products, make sure that the energy field around the dog and handler are clear. For example, many people put the items to be tested on a chair or on the floor in front of them. They are in effect in the same energy field as the dog and handler. They must be kept out of it and should be at least 16 inches away to get a clear reading. Make sure other animals or people are out of the 16-inch radius too. It is a strange phenomenon that when you start to test, other animals in the household will be extremely attracted to the energy field and want to get inside it. If you are testing one dog, another dog or cat in the household will come running and want to be in the same place! Remove the other animals to another room when you are testing.

Nearly all dogs test strong for one or more of the following supplements: vitamin C, vitamin B complex, vitamin E, selenium, a multi-vitamin-mineral supplement, an amino acid complex tablet or digestive enzymes. Put these supplements into separate plastic bags. Put the plastic bag containing the vitamin C, 1 gram (1,000 mg) at a time, or 500 mg for small dogs, in your hand on the dog's body and have the tester press down on your arm. If it is strong, add another tablet and check again. Continue adding more tablets until the arm goes weak. Take out the last tablet and check again. Let's say you are working with a large dog, and you have reached 4 grams of vitamin C and he tests strong, but then, when you put in another tablet and test again, the arm goes weak. This is a clear indication that 5 grams is too much, and that 4 grams is what the dog needs.

Progress through all the supplements until you get the correct dosage for that dog. Then take the food that tested the strongest, add the

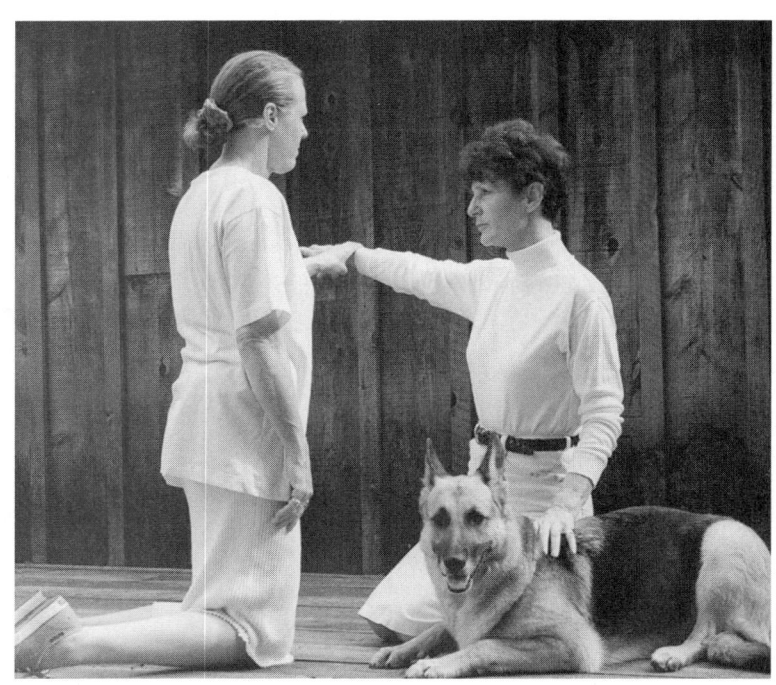

13-7: Testing our dog.

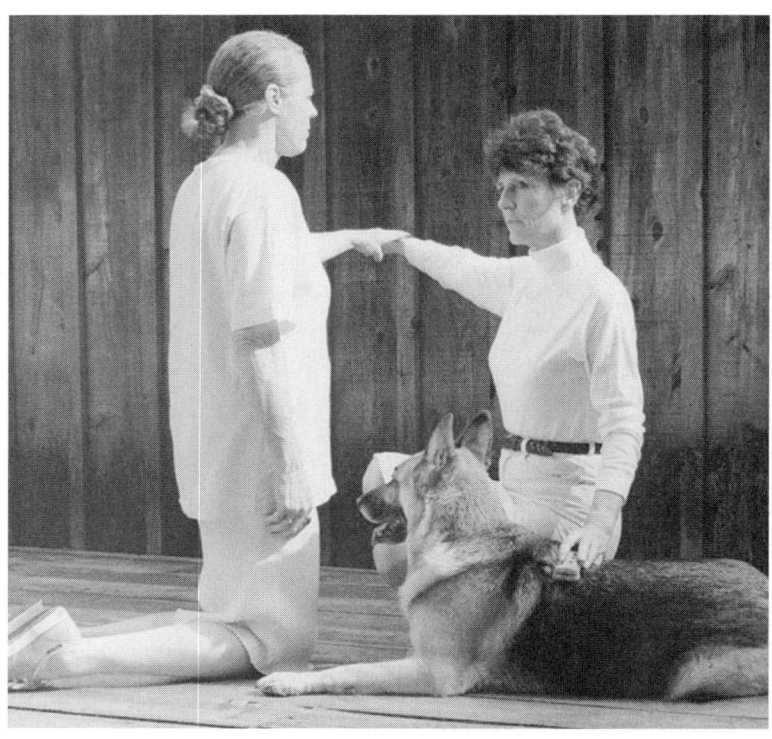

13-8: Holding food on the dog and testing.

vitamin-mineral supplements, combine them and put the whole lot on the dog and check again. The arm of the testee should be strong as a rock. Remember what we said in the beginning: kinesiology is like a blood test. It is checking the body's needs at that moment in time. Those results will be different before and after meals.

Since most of the vitamins used for our dogs are water soluble, which are washed through the body in a matter of a few hours, dosages need to be repeated in order to keep the levels constant in the body. This will be true of vitamins C and B as well as of enzymes used to break down the food into a more digestible form.

Most dogs test for needing vitamins C, B complex, the vitamin-mineral mix and enzymes in their food twice a day and vitamin E, selenium, and the amino acid complex once a day. Dogs are all individuals, and their dietary needs are affected by their environment. Long-haired dogs will have different needs from short-haired dogs, and the dog that lives in a hot climate will test differently than a dog of the same breed and age in a very cold climate.

When you are working out your program it is best to test your dogs two different times in a day. Test again in a week.

Working With the Out-of-Balance Dog

If your dog has been on a food and supplement program that now tests poorly, the dog has then been out of balance for some time. He needs to be rebalanced, and this is not accomplished over night. The foods and supplements that now test strong to create balance for that dog may change once the dog actually is in balance. It appears that in the process of rebalancing, the quantities of vitamins and minerals are greater than those for a maintenance diet. Frequently the amounts of vitamin C and B decrease as well as the need for the other supplements as the dog is brought into balance. If you are working with a very sick dog, you may have to test every week for several weeks until you find the maintenance diet for that dog.

Environmental Factors

Other things to test that can affect your dogs' health are the detergent you use to wash your dog's bedding and the fabric softener you use in the dryer. Test the cleansers used in your house, on the floors, in the bathroom, and on the carpet too. Check garden sprays, weed killers you use on your lawn (and those your neighbor uses), the food dish (stainless steel is best) and your water supply. Wal-Mart carries a small test kit that allows you to test the chemicals in your water supply.

Check the heartworm medication you use. There are many different brands on the market and you will find one that tests strong for your dog. The same goes for all medications. If your dog has a problem that requires antibiotics, see which brand tests the strongest for your dog. Veterinarians will have two or three medications that could be used for any given condition and it is through experience that their choice is made. To take the guesswork out of this decision process, check with your dog to see which medication would be most effective. Put each of the products you want to test either in a small plastic bag or a clean glass container. If something tests weak, do not use it.

For more toxic substances that may cause allergic reactions in your dog, check the list contained in the Allergies, Toxins and Vaccines chapter.

Stress

The irony of knowing how to do kinesiology is that when you need it the most—when your dog is sick, or when there has been an accident—the stress levels we experience may then affect the outcome of the testing. If you are under stress for whatever reason and you feel agitated, have a friend hold the food or medication on the dog instead. Our own energies can affect the results, if we are out of balance. When experiencing extreme stress, thump your thymus a few times and put your tongue on the roof of your mouth behind your front teeth to put yourself back in balance. Dr. Diamond explains that this centers and balances the body temporarily.

When you get comfortable with testing and have done it frequently, you will notice that the dog's body you are testing moves in such a way that tells you what is on his wavelength and what is not. When you get close to your dog's body with a compatible product, the dog will be quiet or curious to smell whatever it is that you are testing. When you enter the energy field with something not on the dog's wavelength, the dog may try to struggle away from you or actively get up and try to run away. You can also see from the dog's expression whether or not what you are testing is correct. Dogs that are stressed by the product being tested can show the following facial expressions—mouths pulled back, ears and whiskers pulled back and wrinkles on their forehead. When the product *is* on their wavelength, they often turn over onto their backs and stretch out, wagging their tails! They make it so easy for us.

Working Dogs—How Nutrition Affects Them

After teaching kinesiology for the last 12 years we have found it to be a simple and effective diagnostic tool in the field of nutrition. Many of the dogs that we see in a year—and we see hundreds—are not as energetic as they could be. They have dull eyes, poor coats and dry skin. Working and training dogs when they are not feeling up to par can be a frustrating experience. Many behavior problems, in particular aggression and the opposite, timidity, can be solved by feeding the correct food. We always follow up our kinesiology testing with diagnostic blood work.

Poor nutrition will affect the ability to learn and to retain what is taught, resulting in a dog that cannot recall an exercise at the appropriate time. We see this often at dog shows, when the owner has no idea that the dog food does not supply enough nutrients to help the dog overcome the stress of the show.

Nothing gives us more pleasure than putting the team of owner and dog in balance by teaching them kinesiology.

Choosing the Person to Work With You

Healthy skepticism when learning anything new is natural. Most people don't believe kinesiology can work until we show them that it does work. They are quite astonished. These people are skeptics *with open minds*. Do not try to work with someone who ridicules you and tells you that it cannot possibly work. Nothing that you do can convince them. Find someone who thinks it's fun to learn new things. Children are terrific learners and usually very good at kinesiology. You will give them a tool that will last them a lifetime.

Indicator Points

In the chapters describing protein, vitamins and minerals, there are illustrations of the indicator points for those nutrients. To test your dog for these nutrients, place one finger of your left hand on the proper point on your dog and have someone press down on your right arm. If the arm is weak it could mean that your dog is deficient in that nutrient, or conversely, that there is too much of that nutrient in your dog's diet. It could also indicate that your dog is not assimilating that nutrient properly, and it would need to be fed in a different form. Or it could show that your dog has a genetic predisposition not to assimilate that nutrient correctly.

When a weakness is detected, we suggest following up with blood work.

Often there are physical signs on the indicator points. It could be a patch of hair missing, a pimple or lump, discoloration of the skin, a disturbance in pigmentation or crooked whiskers or nails.

The Written Word

A more advanced way of doing kinesiology is by writing down the name of the food or supplement on a plain piece of paper and holding it on the dog's body. Incredibly, it works the same way as the product itself. While there is much speculation on how or why this works, it is another of those mysteries that science as yet cannot explain. The fact is that it does work, and our philosophy has always been to use things that work, even if we don't understand them. I confess that I don't know how the engine in my car works, nor do I understand the inner workings of the computer that I use on a daily basis, but that does not prevent me from using them. We would advise trying this technique after you are used to and feel comfortable with the first method of testing.

Do a test for yourself. Take some dry dog food kernels, put them in a plastic bag and place them on your dog. Have someone press down on your wrist and note the result. Then write down on a plain piece of paper the exact name of the food—for example, Brown's Mini-Chunks for Puppies—and hold that piece of paper on the dog and check it out. It will test the same. This is an easy method of testing many foods and supplements without actually having them on hand.

When using the written word for testing, it is important to be specific. It is not enough to write down the name of a line of products—for example, Purina Dog Food or Science Diet—it must be exact: Science Diet Adult Maintenance or Purina Puppy Chow, for example. When choosing supplements for your dog, the exact name and form of the supplement needs to be used. For example, vitamin C comes in many forms, so you would write down 1 gram of vitamin C in the form of ascorbic acid, or 1 gram of vitamin C in the form of sodium ascorbate and so on.

When you have formulated the correct ingredients for your dog, including supplements, then take all of the separate pieces of paper and hold them together on the dog and test for the results. Your arm should be strong.

We have developed a card file for the different ingredients in dog food. The cards are separated into food groups—protein, fat, carbohydrates, vitamins, minerals and so forth. I can use these cards over and over again when working with large numbers of dogs. It saves the time of writing down all the different ingredients.

Using the written word in a sense is a good way to see if your kinesiology testing is working well. If you experience differing results from the product to the written word, it would suggest that you are out of balance. In the beginning, more accurate results can be obtained if the surrogate

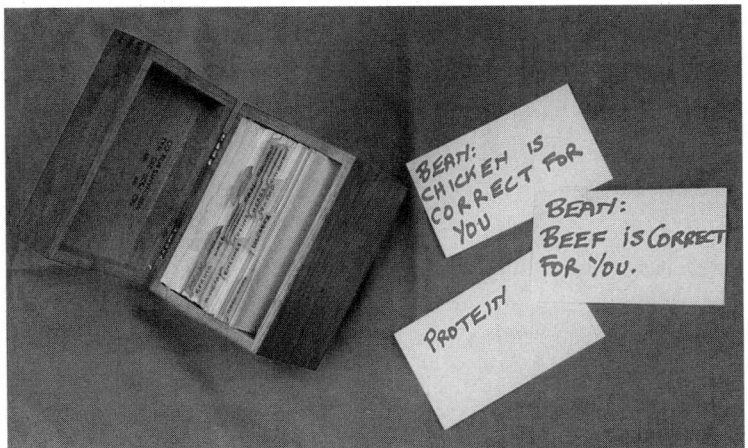

13-9: When using the written word, it is important to be specific.

13-10: Using a card on Bean—weak response.

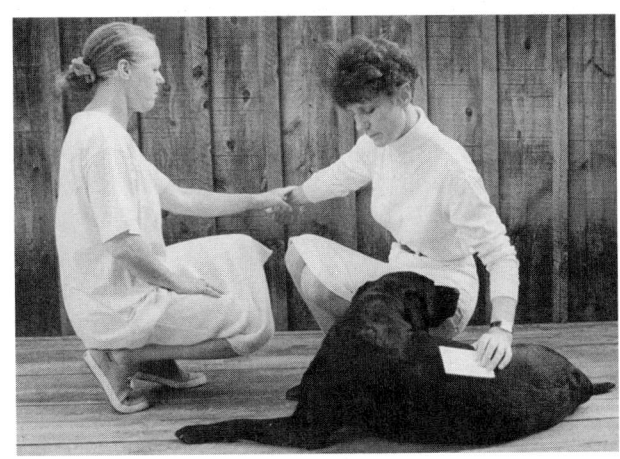

13-11: Using a card on Bean—strong response. (Photos by Brigitte Volhard)

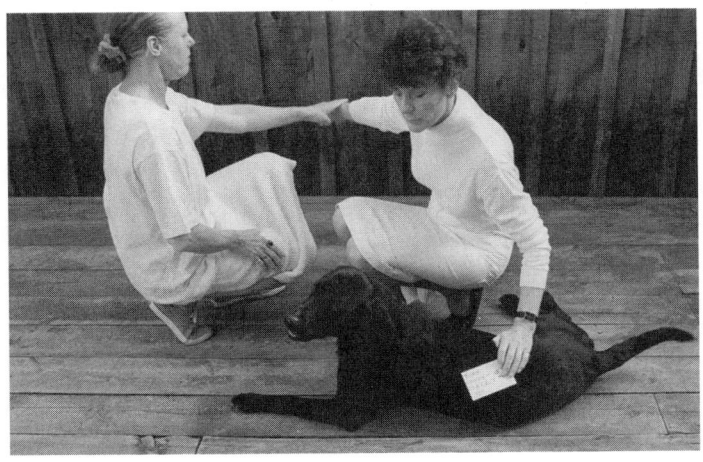

does not look at the name of the food in the plastic bag or written on the card.

Accepting the Answers

One word of warning for all testing: If you start to test with preconceived ideas of what the answer should be, kinesiology will not work for you. You have to be able to accept whatever answer you get. This is sometimes harder than it sounds. If you have been using a certain kind of food or medication for your dog and you are convinced it is correct, you will want the answer to be yes. If it is no, you won't believe it. It is these times when it is better to have someone else test the product. Or, if you are the kind of person who can close your eyes, take a deep breath, relax for a moment and clear your mind of prejudicial thoughts, test again and see which answer you get.

Time

There is a time of the day when you feel more energetic than other times. Everyone experiences what we have learned to call biological down times. (See Circadian Rhythms in Chapter 17.) Find the time of the day when you feel most energetic and do the testing then. For example, I am a morning person and I find that my testing is most accurate before one P.M. After that, I experience my biological "down time," and testing in the afternoon is not as accurate. I try to do all my testing in the morning.

Testing is tiring. It uses a lot of your energy. Do not try to do too much at one time. Testing more than two dogs in a row or more than one hour at a time without taking a break is not a good idea and can produce inaccuracies.

Kinesiology as a Diagnostic Tool

Perhaps the most important use of kinesiology is the use of the technique as a diagnostic tool. It allows us to ask questions of our dogs. Recently four of my nine dogs were not feeling well. They were picking at their food, and a couple of them were not eating at all. One had red spots on her skin, another was not moving well, another was overexcited and another was having difficulty breathing. Using kinesiology, I finally worked out that the problem was with the raw meat that I was using for their dinner meal. (I feed a natural, home-made, balanced diet to my own dogs—see Chapter 14.) Apparently, the batch of meat was contaminated and contained a high bacterial count. Each dog tested for a bacterial infection, and that bacterial infection manifested itself differently with each dog.

160

Those dogs needed a specific antibiotic, and after a short course they all got well. The other dogs were not affected.

How to Ask Questions

In order to diagnose any situation correctly, the questions asked must be specific. Use the dog's name and ask a question that has a definite yes or no answer or phrase your question as a positive statement. In the above example with the contaminated meat, I had to ask several questions to get to the right answer. For example, in the case of the dog that was experiencing bright red spots on her skin I asked, "Katharina, is there something in your food that is causing red spots on your skin?" When the answer was yes, it was merely a process of elimination to find the offending ingredient. It was the meat. When I asked the other dogs that were unwell the same questions, the answer was also the meat.

Another way to get an answer is to make a positive statement, for example, "Fido, you are limping on your right front leg." If the answer is yes, then you state, "Fido, you are limping on your right front leg because you fell when running after your ball this morning."

Once you have diagnosed the problem, questions can be directed toward the most effective treatment. For example, "Fido, the best way to treat the limp on your right front leg is to rest for 4 days" or "Fido, the best way to treat the limp on your right front leg is to take you for an acupuncture treatment" or "Fido, the best way to treat the limp on your right front leg is to get medication from the veterinarian," and so forth. Make sure that the questions are specific. It is not good enough to say to your dog, "Do you need supplements in your dog food?" You would more correctly state, "You need 50 milligrams of vitamin B complex twice a day."

When testing for the correct medication for your dog, you can either hold the medication on your dog to see if the dog reacts positively or write the name of the medication on a piece of blank paper and hold it on your dog. If the medication tests strong, then you would write a question that, for example, might say, "Bean, you need 50 milligrams of this medication twice a day for two weeks," or "Bean, the bacterial infection you have will be cured by using 50 milligrams XYZ antibiotic for two weeks," and so on.

Another use of kinesiology is when you take your dog for an annual physical exam, when vaccinations are normally given. You can ask your dog whether he needs the vaccination or if it is safe to have it at that time. This is very important with puppies, who are in the vulnerable state of growth and teething. It seems that there are veterinarians who give many vaccinations all at the same time, including rabies, and send their patients home with heartworm pills before 6 months of age. The assault to the immune system is something from which many young dogs never recover. (See the section on vaccinations, Chapter 9.)

Common Problems in Testing

If you are running into problems when you test and you feel you are not getting accurate readings, consider the following:

1. Are you on medication of any kind? If you are, when do you take it? Kinesiology should be done when that medication peaks in your system. If you take medication every 12 hours, test after it is in your body for 6 hours. Testing just before you need medication may give you inaccurate readings. Try testing at different times of the day to find the correct time for you.

2. Do you have scars on your body that cross the solar plexus, where you are holding the ingredients? Scars disturb the energy flow. Look at the different energy centers on the map on page 151 and put the item to be tested on a different energy field. I once tested a woman in an audience who had scars literally all over her body from a car accident, and the only unscarred energy center was on the top of her head. It provided great amusement to the rest of the audience when each item was placed on that location. It didn't matter—it worked for her.

There are a few people who simply cannot make kinesiology work for them. These are people whose minds are so active they simply cannot calm themselves long enough to do testing. Learning relaxation techniques helps these individuals.

Like anything else, learning to do kinesiology is a skill. The more you practice, the better you get. It can be enormous fun, and even if it only works part of the time for you and your dog, you are that much better off than if you didn't use it at all. As you will see in the second part of the book, it is used extensively for diagnostic and treatment purposes.

Sample Questions

Take a moment, sit down with some 3-by-5–inch index cards and write out the questions you need to ask your dog. You will need to have a protein, carbohydrate, fat, vitamin, mineral and water section. So you may have five cards with different proteins with the following question or statements:

"Bear, is beef the correct protein for you?"

"Bear, lamb is the correct protein for you."

"Bear, chicken is the correct protein for you."

"Bear, fish is the correct protein for you."

"Bear, a combination of beef and turkey is the correct protein for
   you."

If you get a positive and strong response to one or more of the proteins, put those on one side of the table. Put the cards that test weak on the other side of the table.

Do the same for your carbohydrates and other food groups. At the end you will have cards that may say beef, wheat, safflower oil, a particular brand of vitamin-mineral mix, vitamin C and digestive enzymes.

You can double check this test by actually putting those items in small amounts in containers on your dog's body and testing them. Then take all of the cards containing the positive responses and hold them all on the dog at once. This will ensure that there is no antagonistic response among the ingredients. Once you know the items for which your dog tests strongly, you will have to ascertain how much to use. The statements would then be:

"Bear, your diet needs to contain 25 percent protein."

"Bear, 10 percent fat in your diet is correct for you."

Look at the dog food packages to find a brand that comes the closest to the needs of your dog.

Remember that kinesiology can be used to test any form of medication, including wormers you use. In ascertaining the health of your dog, phrase your questions or statements exactly the same way. If, for example, you suspect your dog is harboring some sort of bacterial infection, your written question should be:

"King, do you have a bacterial infection?" If yes, then write down:

"King, do you need an antibiotic?" If yes, then you could visit your veterinarian, and you could test the antibiotics to find out which one would be suitable for King. You could also ask how long King needs to take the medication:

"King, do you need to take ampicillin for 2 weeks?" If no:

"King, do you need to take ampicillin for 3 weeks?" and so on.

If you suspect that your dog may be suffering from a thyroid disorder, you would write your questions the same way:

"Josie, do you have a malfunctioning thyroid gland?" If yes, then write the question:

"Josie, do you need to have a thyroid medication?" If yes, then you would go to your veterinarian and request that he run a thyroid test on your dog.

There are many veterinarians who are using kinesiology routinely in their practices. The address for the American Holistic Veterinary Association, which lists by state veterinarians who have been holistically trained, is in the sources chapter.

Summary

1. USE EITHER THE PRODUCT OR THE WRITTEN WORD TO TEST YOUR DOG.
2. BE VERY SPECIFIC IN YOUR QUESTIONS.
3. MAKE SURE YOUR QUESTIONS OR STATEMENTS ARE PHRASED IN SUCH A WAY TO ELICIT A YES OR NO ANSWER.
4. MAKE SURE THAT THERE ARE AT LEAST 16 INCHES OF "CLEAR" SPACE AROUND YOU AND THE DOG WHEN TESTING.
5. REMOVE ALL METAL ARTICLES SUCH AS JEWELRY FROM YOURSELF AND A CHAIN COLLAR FROM YOUR DOG WHEN TESTING.
6. IF THE ANSWERS ARE OBVIOUSLY NOT CORRECT, CHECK YOUR OWN BALANCE AND THAT OF THE PERSON WITH WHOM YOU ARE WORKING. Also recheck at another time during the day.
7. FIND THE TIME OF DAY THAT WORKS BEST FOR YOU AND YOUR TESTING. If you are emotionally upset, have someone else do the testing for you. Your emotions can affect the outcome of the testing.
8. AVOID PUTTING TEST PRODUCTS ON THE AREAS OF THE BODY WHERE THERE ARE SCARS.
9. ALL OF YOUR TESTING SHOULD BE CONFIRMED BY WORKING WITH YOUR VETERINARIAN AND TAKING BLOOD TESTS. This is exactly how we confirmed that kinesiology did in fact work. We diagnosed first by kinesiology, then took blood from the dog to double-check our diagnosis. We did kinesiology again, then formulated a diet with supplements, which the dog was fed for a month. We then did more blood work. We did this for many dogs at different life stages and for different illnesses. We have had enormous success.

    Kinesiology can't cure the dog that is dying. What it can do is improve the quality of life at the end, so whatever food or medications that dog is taking are correct *at that time* and are not causing more harm to that dog.
10. NO DIAGNOSTIC TOOL IS FOOLPROOF. Always confirm your testing with follow up blood work or appropriate veterinary testing.

Dogs have life spans that are all too short. What kinesiology has done for our dogs is to provide them with quality of life right up to the end. Our dogs no longer go through long, miserable times at the end of their lives. If this were the only thing that we have been able to gain from the use of kinesiology, it all would have been worth it.

CHART FOR 5LB DOG

A.M. INGREDIENTS

DAY	1	2	3	4	5	6	7
Grain Mix (dry/oz)	.75	.75	.75	.75	.75	.75	.4
Molasses (t)	1/4	1/4	1/4	1/4	1/4	1/4	-
Safflower Oil (t)	1/4	1/4	1/4	1/4	1/4	1/4	-
Vitamin E (IU)	20	20	20	20	20	20	-
Vitamin C (mg)	20	20	20	20	20	20	20
Vit B Complex (mg)							
Vit/Min Mix (t)	1/16	1/16	1/16	1/16	1/16	1/16	1/16
5-min egg with shell (small)	1/4	-	1/4	-	1/4	1/4	-
Yogurt/Kefir (t)	1	1	1	1	1	1	1
Honey (t)							1/2

P.M. INGREDIENTS

DAY	1	2	3	4	5	6	7
Vitamin C (mg)	20	20	20	20	20	20	-
Cod Liver Oil (t)	1/8	1/8	1/8	1/8	1/8	1/8	-
Apple Cider Vinegar (t)	1/2	1/2	1/2	1/2	1/2	1/2	-
Kelp (t)	1/16	1/16	1/16	1/16	1/16	1/16	-
Brewers Yeast (t)	1/8	1/8	1/8	1/8	1/8	1/8	-
Garlic Capsule (325 mg)	1/2	1/2	1/2	1/2	1/2	1/2	-
Bone Meal (t)	2/3	2/3	2/3	2/3	2/3	2/3	-
Wheat Germ (t)	1/4	1/4	1/4	1/4	1/4	1/4	-
Wheat Bran (t)	1	1	1	1	1	1	-
Dry Herbs/Greens (t) **or**	1/4	1/4	1/4	1/4	1/4	1/4	-
Fresh Herbs/Greens (T)	1	1	1	1	1	1	-
Fruit (t)	-	2/3	-	2/3	-	2/3	-
Beef Muscle Meat (oz)	2	2	2	2	2	-	-
Beef Liver (oz)	.45	.45	.45	.45	.45	-	-
Cottage Cheese (oz)	-	-	-	-	-	2.5	-

Code: T = tablespoon; t - teaspoon; IU = International Units

—Chapter 14—

The Natural Diet

Homemade dog food is becoming a popular option, although hardly a new one, for many dog owners. Every dog alive today can be traced back to dogs who were raised on homemade natural diets. The dog food industry, in comparison to dogs themselves, is young—maybe 50 to 60 years—although canned meat was sold as dog food at the turn of the twentieth century. Originally, the commercial foods were meant to supplement homemade food.

With few exceptions, commercially made dry food is primarily cereal based with the major portion of the protein coming from grains and a dash of animal protein in the ingredients. An amazing number of dogs have been able to exist and adapt to these diets, which have made the dog into a partial herbivore instead of a carnivore. Canned diets, which usually contain more animal protein with a dash of cereal, are also popular, especially among toy breeds. Some people successfully combine these two.

Why Feed Naturally?

Many dogs cannot thrive on commercially prepared rations. They exhibit disease states, often mistaken for allergies, which are deficiency diseases caused by cereal-based foods. Dogs in a natural state would eat meat. Their teeth are formed to tear flesh from the bone, and they would share a carcass with a pack of other dogs.

The carcass would be that of a grass-eating animal—an herbivore. Along with the internal organs dogs would eat the predigested grasses and plants of the carcass. Those grasses and plants would consist of no more than 20 to 25 percent of the dogs' total diet. They would raid nests from ground-breeding birds and eat the eggs, and they would catch the occasional insect. These dogs might forage on certain weeds and grasses.

In formulating the Natural Diet we have stayed within these boundaries—with the exception of the insects! The Natural Diet follows as closely as possible what the dog would eat if still in the wild state. It takes into account the limitations of the dog's short digestive tract, strong stomach acid and the enzymes the canine system produces to break down food. It consists of two meals: One is a cereal meal plus supplements, which makes up 25 percent of the total diet, and the other is a raw meat meal plus supplements, which is 75 percent of the total diet.

Benefits of the Natural Diet

The advantages of a natural diet are many. Health and longevity are increased, there is resistance to disease and the diet can be tailored to individual needs. This is crucial for some breeds of dogs, especially imported dogs or relatives of imported dogs, who have difficulty in digesting corn, which is in the majority of prepared commercial diets. The diet allows individual ingredients to be substituted.

Dogs are able to digest and utilize the Natural Diet well, and the stool volume is less than 25 percent. The diet contains a lot of moisture in the natural ingredients and therefore the dog drinks little, if any, water, which makes it easier to travel. Young dogs raised naturally grow more slowly than dogs raised on commercial food and therefore fewer musculoskeletal problems are observed. Fleas, ticks and worms are almost unheard of on the Natural Diet. Skin, ear and eye problems are rare, as is bloat. Teeth rarely, if ever, have to be cleaned. Overall vitality and energy are unequaled and dogs love to eat it.

Drawbacks

The disadvantages of making a homemade diet cannot be minimized. It takes a commitment on part of the owner to the dog. It means stocking up on ingredients, buying in bulk and finding storage space. An investment in a freezer is a must if there are more than two or three dogs being fed. While no actual cooking is involved, the diet requires boiling a pot of water, which some people find too much. It also means sticking to the diet without alterations, the stumbling block for many people who try the diet.

The Natural Diet makes no attempt to appeal to the owner of the dog. It looks and smells like raw meat. It doesn't contain coloring agents or other visual enhancers. The most popular comment from owners who didn't like the smell of the meat, the cod liver oil, or handling the liver, is "Oh, I left that out!" The diet was thus depleted of proper nutrients.

Many people find it impossible to fast their dogs when starting the diet. Some find fasting the half day a week that is necessary for adult dogs too upsetting, and they don't do it. If these owners understood the digestive system of the dog, they would not experience these qualms. The diet is formulated to provide the dog his weekly calories in six and a half days. *The commitment to this diet requires that all the ingredients are used*, or if substitutes are made to meet individual requirements, that they equal the nutritional content of ingredients they replace. Our advice to prospective dog food makers is, if you find you can't follow the philosophy or you don't like handling the ingredients, this diet is not for you. It is safer for your pet to be on a commercial food with supplements. Each and every ingredient used is in the diet for a purpose. Leaving one of the ingredients out unbalances the diet and will be dangerous for your dog in the long run. Even worse is using part of the diet and part commercial food. We tested this concept and the blood work showed that dogs fed this way were nutritionally unbalanced.

Origins and Testing

The Natural Diet is based on Juliette de Bairacli Levy's book, *The Complete Herbal Book for the Dog and Cat* plus updated information from many sources. It was tested on all life stages of dogs over a 12-year period before it was first published in 1979.

The testing consisted of complete blood work using serum chemistry profiles as well as feces and urine analysis. We personally are now on the fifth generation of dogs raised this way and some breeders are on their seventh generation of Natural Diet dogs. From time to time we have tried other natural diets or combinations of commercial foods and natural feeding, plus one experiment where all the dogs were put on commercial food. Nothing comes close to producing the health, vitality and longevity of the Natural Diet.

Through the veterinary practice, as well as seminars and camps where we teach a nutrition and health course together with behavior and training, we have seen hundreds of owners, breeders and exhibitors who have used this diet successfully. People who work their dogs and exhibit them have had great success, and they enjoy the extra stamina and endurance their dogs exhibit when being fed the Natural Diet.

Guaranteed Analysis
Percentage by Dry Weight Basis

Protein	34.7%
Fat	17.2%
Carbohydrate (including fiber)	33.7%

Ash (mineral content)	8.6%
Linoleic acid	2.7%
Calcium	1.8%
Phosphorus	1.3%
Calories per pound	2,172

Ingredients

In descending order by wet weight:

Beef muscle meat, water, cereal grain, milk (kefir, yogurt), cottage cheese, beef liver, egg, bone meal, apple cider vinegar, greens and herbs, molasses, wheat bran, safflower oil, fruit, honey, cod liver oil, wheat germ, kelp, eggshell, brewers yeast, vitamin-mineral mix, garlic, vitamin B complex, vitamin C and vitamin E.

The Natural Diet meets and exceeds the Minimum Daily Requirement of all known nutrients. What follows are diet sheets, by weight, for **normal, healthy, active** pets at differing stages of life. Special needs of older dogs or sick dogs are addressed later on in the chapter.

Transfer Diet

Changing a dog's diet from one food to another has to be done slowly. The intestinal bacteria that govern absorption need time to make the adjustment to the new food. Normally this process takes 11 days, but by fasting the dog, the process can be reduced to 4 days. If this timetable is not followed, the dog may experience an upset stomach or diarrhea. Fasting with water and honey flushes the digestive system and prepares it to accept the new food.

Fasting is more difficult for you than it is for your dog. When you are fasting your dog, at the normal feeding time, take him for a walk, play ball, or go for a drive in the car. The anxiety over food will last around 15 minutes.

FRESH WATER MUST ALWAYS BE AVAILABLE TO YOUR DOG.

The following is based on the needs of a 25-pound dog .

Day 1		No food, fresh water available.
Day 2	**a.m.**	No food, fresh water available
	p.m.	$^1/_2$ cup of raw milk, yogurt or kefir, 1 teaspoon honey.
Day 3	**a.m.**	$^1/_2$ cup raw milk, yogurt or kefir, 1 teaspoon honey.
	p.m.	$^1/_2$ cup raw milk, yogurt or kefir, 1 teaspoon honey, $^1/_2$ teaspoon dry herbs or 2 tablespoons fresh herbs.

Day 4	a.m.	1 cup raw milk, yogurt or kefir, 1 teaspoon honey, $1/2$ teaspoon dry or 2 tablespoon fresh herbs, $1/2$ ounce (cooked weight) oatmeal.
	p.m.	same as above, but use 1 ounce of cooked oatmeal, 1 garlic capsule.
Day 5	a.m.	$1/2$ normal ration for cereal and supplements as listed on the adult dog charts.
	p.m.	$1/2$ normal ration of meat meal and supplements as listed on the adult dog charts.
Day 6	a.m.	normal amount of food as listed on the Day 1 of the adult dog charts.
	p.m.	same as above.

How to Prepare the Diet

CEREALS: Seventy-five percent of the cereal can be made up from flaked oats. Twenty-five percent can be made from other grains. Barley grits, buckwheat, cracked wheat, brown rice and millet are good choices. To find out what mixture of grains is correct for your dog, use kinesiology. You will not only need to know the correct combination of grains, but also how much of each to feed. We have found 75 percent flaked oats and 25 percent buckwheat to be a good combination for most dogs. The acid grains are oats and wheat, and the alkaline grains are millet and buckwheat. Corn, depending on the part used, and brown rice fall somewhere in the middle. We suggest you use organically grown grains free of fertilizers, insecticides and pesticides.

The weights in the charts are dry weights. Weigh the grain on a scale, then put it into a cup measure to establish a measurement for convenient use. Use 3 times the amount of water to 1 part grain. Put in a selection of raw vegetables and bring the water to a boil. Add the grain, mix well, bring back to a boil and turn off the heat. Leave for at least 2 hours or overnight before using. This produces a finished product that is runny rather than sticky, which makes it easier to handle. See chart below for vegetables that are used at differing times of the year. Place the cereal into the food bowl and add the appropriate supplements. Mix well, add yogurt, kefir or raw milk and feed at room temperature.

Grains that are not well digested will be observed in your dog's stool. The cereal meal produces a stool that is less formed than that of the meat meal and is relatively pale in color. This is normal.

MEAT MEAL: Meat is fed raw, together with liver, five times a week. Put all the supplements into the dog bowl, add a little hot water and make into a sticky paste. Add the meat and liver, mix well and serve. On the sixth day the cottage cheese is substituted for the meat and on the seventh

CHART FOR 10LB DOG

A.M. INGREDIENTS

DAY	1	2	3	4	5	6	7
Grain Mix (dry/oz)	1.3	1.3	1.3	1.3	1.3	1.3	.7
Molasses (t)	1/2	1/2	1/2	1/2	1/2	1/2	-
Safflower Oil (t)	1/2	1/2	1/2	1/2	1/2	1/2	-
Vitamin E (IU)	40	40	40	40	40	40	-
Vitamin C (mg)	40	40	40	40	40	40	40
Vit B Complex (mg)	12.5	12.5	12.5	12.5	12.5	12.5	12.5
Vit/Min Mix (t)	1/16	1/16	1/16	1/16	1/16	1/16	1/16
5-min egg with shell (small)	1/2	-	1/2	-	1/2	1/2	-
Yogurt/Kefir (cup)	1/8	1/8	1/8	1/8	1/8	1/8	1/4
Honey (t)	-	-	-	-	-	-	1

P.M. INGREDIENTS

DAY	1	2	3	4	5	6	7
Vitamin C (mg)	40	40	40	40	40	40	-
Cod Liver Oil (t)	1/4	1/4	1/4	1/4	1/4	1/4	-
Apple Cider Vinegar (t)	1	1	1	1	1	1	-
Kelp (t)	1/8	1/8	1/8	1/8	1/8	1/8	-
Brewers Yeast (t)	1/4	1/4	1/4	1/4	1/4	1/4	-
Garlic Capsule (325 mg)	1/2	1/2	1/2	1/2	1/2	1/2	-
Bone Meal (t)	1.33	1.33	1.33	1.33	1.33	1.33	-
Wheat Germ (t)	1/2	1/2	1/2	1/2	1/2	1/2	-
Wheat Bran (t)	2	2	2	2	2	2	-
Dry Herbs/Greens (t) **or**	1/2	1/2	1/2	1/2	1/2	1/2	-
Fresh Herbs/Greens (T)	1.5	1.5	1.5	1.5	1.5	1.5	-
Fruit (t)	-	1.25	-	1.25	-	1.25	-
Beef Muscle Meat (oz)	3.7	3.7	3.7	3.7	3.7	-	-
Beef Liver (oz)	.8	.8	.8	.8	.8	-	-
Cottage Cheese (oz)	-	-	-	-	-	3.10	-

Code: T = tablespoon; t - teaspoon; IU = International Units

CHART FOR 25LB DOG

A.M. INGREDIENTS

DAY	1	2	3	4	5	6	7
Grain Mix (dry/oz)	2.5	2.5	2.5	2.5	2.5	2.5	1.4
Molasses (t)	1	1	1	1	1	1	-
Safflower Oil (t)	1	1	1	1	1	1	-
Vitamin E (IU)	100	100	100	100	100	100	-
Vitamin C (mg)	100	100	100	100	100	100	100
Vit B Complex (mg)	25	25	25	25	25	25	25
Vit/Min Mix (t)	1/8	1/8	1/8	1/8	1/8	1/8	1/8
5-min egg with shell (small)	1	-	1	-	1	1	-
Yogurt/Kefir (cup)	1/4	1/4	1/4	1/4	1/4	1/4	1/2
Honey (t)	-	-	-	-	-	-	2

P.M. INGREDIENTS

DAY	1	2	3	4	5	6	7
Vitamin C (mg)	100	100	100	100	100	100	-
Cod Liver Oil (t)	1/2	1/2	1/2	1/2	1/2	1/2	-
Apple Cider Vinegar (t)	1.5	1.5	1.5	1.5	1.5	1.5	-
Kelp (t)	1/4	1/4	1/4	1/4	1/4	1/4	-
Brewers Yeast (t)	1/2	1/2	1/2	1/2	1/2	1/2	-
Garlic Capsule (325 mg)	1	1	1	1	1	1	-
Bone Meal (t)	3.5	3.5	3.5	3.5	3.5	3.5	-
Wheat Germ (t)	1	1	1	1	1	1	-
Wheat Bran (T)	1.5	1.5	1.5	1.5	1.5	1.5	-
Dry Herbs/Greens (t) **or**	1	1	1	1	1	1	-
Fresh Herbs/Greens (T)	2	2	2	2	2	2	-
Fruit (T)	-	1	-	1	-	1	-
Beef Muscle Meat (oz)	7	7	7	7	7	-	-
Beef Liver (oz)	1.5	1.5	1.5	1.5	1.5	-	-
Cottage Cheese (oz)	-	-	-	-	-	8	-

Code: T = tablespoon; t - teaspoon; IU = International Units

CHART FOR 50LB DOG

A.M. INGREDIENTS

DAY	1	2	3	4	5	6	7
Grain Mix (dry/oz)	4	4	4	4	4	4	2.3
Molasses (t)	2	2	2	2	2	2	-
Safflower Oil (t)	2	2	2	2	2	2	-
Vitamin E (IU)	200	200	200	200	200	200	-
Vitamin C (mg)	200	200	200	200	200	200	200
Vit B Complex (mg)	50	50	50	50	50	50	50
Vit/Min Mix (t)	1/4	1/4	1/4	1/4	1/4	1/4	1/4
5-min egg with shell (small)	1.25	-	1.25	-	1.25	1.25	-
Yogurt/Kefir (cup)	1/2	1/2	1/2	1/2	1/2	1/2	1
Honey (t)	-	-	-	-	-	-	4

P.M. INGREDIENTS

DAY	1	2	3	4	5	6	7
Vitamin C (mg)	200	200	200	200	200	200	-
Cod Liver Oil (t)	1	1	1	1	1	1	-
Apple Cider Vinegar (T)	1	1	1	1	1	1	-
Kelp (t)	1/2	1/2	1/2	1/2	1/2	1/2	-
Brewers Yeast (t)	1	1	1	1	1	1	-
Garlic Capsule (325 mg)	1.5	1.5	1.5	1.5	1.5	1.5	-
Bone Meal (T)	2.5	2.5	2.5	2.5	2.5	2.5	-
Wheat Germ (t)	2	2	2	2	2	2	-
Wheat Bran (T)	3	3	3	3	3	3	-
Dry Herbs/Greens (t) **or**	2	2	2	2	2	2	-
Fresh Herbs/Greens (T)	4	4	4	4	4	4	-
Fruit (T)	-	2	-	2	-	2	-
Beef Muscle Meat (oz)	12	12	12	12	12	-	-
Beef Liver (oz)	2.5	2.5	2.5	2.5	2.5	-	-
Cottage Cheese (oz)	-	-	-	-	-	14	-

Code: T = tablespoon; t - teaspoon; IU = International Units

CHART FOR 75LB DOG

A.M. INGREDIENTS

DAY	1	2	3	4	5	6	7
Grain Mix (dry/oz)	6	6	6	6	6	6	3
Molasses (T)	1	1	1	1	1	1	-
Safflower Oil (T)	1	1	1	1	1	1	-
Vitamin E (IU)	300	300	300	300	300	300	-
Vitamin C (mg)	300	300	300	300	300	300	300
Vit B Complex (mg)	50	50	50	50	50	50	50
Vit/Min Mix (t)	1/2	1/2	1/2	1/2	1/2	1/2	1/2
5-min egg with shell (small)	1.5	-	1.5	-	1.5	1.5	-
Yogurt/Kefir (cup)	1/2	1/2	1/2	1/2	1/2	1/2	1
Honey (T)	-	-	-	-	-	-	2

P.M. INGREDIENTS

DAY	1	2	3	4	5	6	7
Vitamin C (mg)	300	300	300	300	300	300	-
Cod Liver Oil (t)	1.5	1.5	1.5	1.5	1.5	1.5	-
Apple Cider Vinegar (T)	1.5	1.5	1.5	1.5	1.5	1.5	-
Kelp (t)	3/4	3/4	3/4	3/4	3/4	3/4	-
Brewers Yeast (t)	1.5	1.5	1.5	1.5	1.5	1.5	-
Garlic Capsule (325 mg)	2	2	2	2	2	2	-
Bone Meal (T)	3.5	3.5	3.5	3.5	3.5	3.5	-
Wheat Germ (T)	1.5	1.5	1.5	1.5	1.5	1.5	-
Wheat Bran (T)	4.5	4.5	4.5	4.5	4.5	4.5	-
Dry Herbs/Greens (T) **or**	1	1	1	1	1	1	-
Fresh Herbs/Greens (T)	6	6	6	6	6	6	-
Fruit (t)	-	3	-	3	-	3	-
Beef Muscle Meat (oz)	15	15	15	15	15	-	-
Beef Liver (oz)	3.4	3.4	3.4	3.4	3.4	-	-
Cottage Cheese (oz)	-	-	-	-	-	18	-

Code: T = tablespoon; t - teaspoon; IU = International Units

CHART FOR 100LB DOG

A.M. INGREDIENTS

DAY	1	2	3	4	5	6	7
Grain Mix (dry/oz)	7.5	7.5	7.5	7.5	7.5	7.5	3.8
Molasses (t)	4	4	4	4	4	4	-
Safflower Oil (t)	4	4	4	4	4	4	-
Vitamin E (IU)	400	400	400	400	400	400	-
Vitamin C (mg)	400	400	400	400	400	400	400
Vit B Complex (mg)	75	75	75	75	75	75	75
Vit/Min Mix (t)	1/2	1/2	1/2	1/2	1/2	1/2	1/2
5-min egg with shell (small)	2	-	2	-	2	2	-
Yogurt/Kefir (cup)	3/4	3/4	3/4	3/4	3/4	3/4	1.5
Honey (T)	-	-	-	-	-	-	2.66

P.M. INGREDIENTS

DAY	1	2	3	4	5	6	7
Vitamin C (mg)	400	400	400	400	400	400	-
Cod Liver Oil (t)	2	2	2	2	2	2	-
Apple Cider Vinegar (T)	2	2	2	2	2	2	-
Kelp (t)	1	1	1	1	1	1	-
Brewers Yeast (t)	2	2	2	2	2	2	-
Garlic Capsule (325 mg)	2	2	2	2	2	2	-
Bone Meal (T)	4.6	4.6	4.6	4.6	4.6	4.6	
Wheat Germ (T)	2	2	2	2	2	2	-
Wheat Bran (T)	6	6	6	6	6	6	-
Dry Herbs/Greens (t) **or**	4	4	4	4	4	4	-
Fresh Herbs/Greens (T)	8	8	8	8	8	8	-
Fruit (T)	-	4	-	4	-	4	-
Beef Muscle Meat (oz)	20	20	20	20	20	-	-
Beef Liver (oz)	4.4	4.4	4.4	4.4	4.4	-	-
Cottage Cheese (oz)	-	-	-	-	-	24	-

Code: T = tablespoon; t - teaspoon; IU = International Units

CHART FOR 125LB DOG

A.M. INGREDIENTS

DAY	1	2	3	4	5	6	7
Grain Mix (dry/oz)	9.3	9.3	9.3	9.3	9.3	9.3	4.7
Molasses (t)	5	5	5	5	5	5	-
Safflower Oil (t)	4.5	4.5	4.5	4.5	4.5	4.5	-
Vitamin E (IU)	500	500	500	500	500	500	-
Vitamin C (mg)	500	500	500	500	500	500	500
Vit B Complex (mg)	75	75	75	75	75	75	75
Vit/Min Mix (t)	3/4	3/4	3/4	3/4	3/4	3/4	3/4
5-min egg with shell (small)	2	-	2	-	2	2	-
Yogurt/Kefir (cup)	1	1	1	1	1	1	1.5
Honey (T)	-	-	-	-	-	-	3

P.M. INGREDIENTS

DAY	1	2	3	4	5	6	7
Vitamin C (mg)	500	500	500	500	500	500	-
Cod Liver Oil (t)	2.5	2.5	2.5	2.5	2.5	2.5	-
Apple Cider Vinegar (T)	2.5	2.5	2.5	2.5	2.5	2.5	-
Kelp (t)	1.25	1.25	1.25	1.25	1.25	1.25	-
Brewers Yeast (t)	2.5	2.5	2.5	2.5	2.5	2.5	-
Garlic Capsule (325 mg)	2.5	2.5	2.5	2.5	2.5	2.5	-
Bone Meal (T)	6	6	6	6	6	6	-
Wheat Germ (T)	2.5	2.5	2.5	2.5	2.5	2.5	-
Wheat Bran (T)	8	8	8	8	8	8	-
Dry Herbs/Greens (t) **or**	5	5	5	5	5	5	-
Fresh Herbs/Greens (T)	10	10	10	10	10	10	-
Fruit (T)	-	5	-	5	-	5	-
Beef Muscle Meat (oz)	25	25	25	25	25	-	-
Beef Liver (oz)	5	5	5	5	5	-	-
Cottage Cheese (oz)	-	-	-	-	-	30	-

Code: T = tablespoon; t - teaspoon; IU = International Units

CHART FOR 150LB DOG

A.M. INGREDIENTS

DAY	1	2	3	4	5	6	7
Grain Mix (dry/oz)	11	11	11	11	11	11	5.5
Molasses (T)	2	2	2	2	2	2	-
Safflower Oil (T)	2	2	2	2	2	2	-
Vitamin E (IU)	600	600	600	600	600	600	-
Vitamin C (gram)	1	1	1	1	1	1	1
Vit B Complex (mg)	100	100	100	100	100	100	100
Vit/Min Mix (t)	1	1	1	1	1	1	1
5-min egg with shell (small)	3	-	3	-	3	3	-
Yogurt/Kefir (cup)	1.25	1.25	1.25	1.25	1.25	1.25	2
Honey (T)	-	-	-	-	-	-	4

P.M. INGREDIENTS

DAY	1	2	3	4	5	6	7
Vitamin C (gram)	1	1	1	1	1	1	-
Cod Liver Oil (T)	1	1	1	1	1	1	-
Apple Cider Vinegar (T)	3	3	3	3	3	3	-
Kelp (t)	1.5	1.5	1.5	1.5	1.5	1.5	-
Brewers Yeast (T)	1	1	1	1	1	1	-
Garlic Capsule (325 mg)	3	3	3	3	3	3	-
Bone Meal (T)	6	6	6	6	6	6	-
Wheat Germ (T)	3	3	3	3	3	3	-
Wheat Bran (T)	8	8	8	8	8	8	-
Dry Herbs/Greens (T) **or**	2	2	2	2	2	2	-
Fresh Herbs/Greens (T)	12	12	12	12	12	12	-
Fruit (T)	-	6	-	6	-	6	-
Beef Muscle Meat (oz)	28.8	28.8	28.8	28.8	28.8	-	-
Beef Liver (oz)	5.7	5.7	5.7	5.7	5.7	-	-
Cottage Cheese (oz)	-	-	-	-	-	32	-

Code: T = tablespoon; t - teaspoon; IU = International Units

day the dog is fasted in the afternoon. It may be more convenient to make these supplements weekly and keep them refrigerated.

It is possible to substitute half the amount of dicalcium phosphate for bone meal. Use kinesiology to test your dog. Since DCP is deficient in magnesium in comparison to bone meal, you need to add either apples or apricots, which are high in magnesium content, to rebalance the diet.

The stool produced from the meat meal is very small, dark and well formed.

VEGETABLES FOR CEREAL MEAL: Use root vegetables such as carrots, parsnips and beets as well as broccoli, Brussels sprouts, cauliflower, garlic and any variety of squash from late fall to early spring. In the late spring, summer and early fall use green leafy vegetables such as collard greens, kale, mustard greens and any variety of green or yellow beans as well as asparagus garlic and radishes. Lettuces, radishes and garlic can be used year round. Cabbage, turnips and peas should be avoided for dogs who have diagnosed thyroid problems.

Herbs and Greens for Meat Meal

Fall and Winter: We mix a selection of herbs that dogs need in winter. If you wish to make your own the following herbs are recommended: mullein leaves, angelica root, marshmallow root, parsley, nettles, comfrey root or leaf, corn silk, burdock root, ginger root, golden rod, raspberry leaves, watercress, rosemary, sage, cayenne pepper, dandelion root and alfalfa. These can be used on a rotational basis. Mix three or four together and use them for one week at a time. Cayenne, which together with ginger root stimulates the circulation and digestive tract, are used in moderation. Add a pinch to each herbal mix. Do not isolate herbs and use them by themselves unless you are using them medicinally.

Spring and Summer: We mix herbs for this season. If you want to make your own mix use the following herbs: dandelion leaves and flowers, borage, peppermint leaves, sorrel, goldenrod leaves, golden seal, licorice root, rosemary, watercress, comfrey leaves, alfalfa and milk thistle. Use on a rotational basis.

In the winter it is almost impossible to obtain fresh herbs so we usually use dried herbs. In the summer we use our own herbal mix but make use of what we can obtain fresh at the market. We add a small amount to each meal. Many herbs such as alfalfa, garlic, comfrey, watercress, dandelion, licorice and rosemary can be used for all seasons.

CAUTION: Comfrey contains ingredients that interfere with the kidneys when they are not functioning correctly and should not be used when kidney disease has been diagnosed.

FRUITS: Apples, apricots, bananas, dried unsulfured raisins, prunes and dates are some of the fruits that can be used. Use fresh fruits that are in season. In general, dogs do not like citrus fruits, but if they have a craving for oranges or lemons, let them have a small amount.

BONES: Every two to three weeks your dog can have a bone. *The kind of bone is important.* The large femurs or leg bones from a cow are safe, as well as large knuckle bones. These do not splinter. *Rib bones should not be used.* Neck bones from chickens can be used occasionally in the food, as these do not splinter. Never feed bones to your dog without supervision. Dogs love bones and they keep them happy for hours at a time. They are invaluable in raising puppies. If puppies have bones to gnaw on, especially during the teething process, they will be less likely to chew furniture or clothing. Bones satisfy the craving to chew, especially strong in young puppies. Giving your dog bones to chew on has the added advantage of keeping his teeth spotlessly clean. Cabbage stumps and carrots provide an alternative to fresh bones.

Fasting

The concept of fasting to cleanse the body is older than Hippocrates, who employed nutrition and fasting in his medical practice. Animals in the wild regularly fast because their food supply is not reliable. If lucky, wild dogs eat three times a week. They will gorge on as much food as they can eat, and then sleep that off for the next three days. Animals who are sick will fast in order to divert the energies needed for digesting food into the healing process.

Fasting with the Natural Diet consists of a half-day fast every week, and one full-day fast once a month for the healthy, adult dog. Young puppies and old dogs are not fasted. On the fast day they are given two cereal meals instead. Anytime a dog shows digestive upsets, from vomiting to diarrhea, they are fasted for 24 hours. This allows the system to calm down from whatever caused the problem. *If clinical signs continue, seek veterinary help immediately.* Water must always be available to the dog.

The Older Dog

Older dogs have different needs from those of a younger dog. After reaching the age of 8 years, most dogs need to adjust diets to aging and less efficient digestive systems. Cut back the amount of food. Most older dogs are less active and will need fewer calories. The *ratio* of 25 percent grain to 75 percent meat does not change.

Older dogs need vitamin and minerals in quantities similar to that of the growing puppy as the aging body does not break down and utilize the vitamins and minerals as well as a younger body. Increase the vitamin-mineral mix by one third in the breakfast meal.

Old dogs being transferred to the Natural Diet may object to the texture of the diet. They have been used to eating dry, crunchy food and acceptance of the diet can be difficult for some. Inevitably, they will like the meat meal and will refuse the cereal meal. In this case, mix the two meals together and divide them in half, feeding half in the morning and half at night. Later on, once the dog is used to the texture, you can experiment separating the two meals.

The Sick Dog

The sick dog needs to be changed slowly over to the Natural Diet. *Before you start the diet, have your veterinarian do a complete examination including blood work.* This is an invaluable tool with which to work, if the diet needs to be tailored to your dog.

Following the transfer diet. After your dog has been on the adult diet for a month, do the blood work again. If any adjustments need to be made, you will have guidelines to follow from the chem scans. Use kinesiology to test each ingredient that you change and be sure to test the total diet so that it is complete for your pet.

Raw meat can contain a high amount of bacteria, which under normal circumstances presents no problem to a healthy dog. When starting a sick dog on the Natural Diet, cook the meat to kill any bacteria. Bring a small amount of water to a boil in a saucepan and put in the meat and liver. Return the water to a boil and turn off the heat. The water in which the meat and liver has been cooked can be used for gravy to mix the supplements. As the dog gets used to the new diet, mix some raw meat with the cooked, gradually changing the proportions until the raw meat is accepted.

Exercise

The Natural Diet presupposes a degree of exercise daily for dogs. Aim for 2 hours of exercise a day. No diet, however superior, will provide the kind of health needed for your dog to live a long life without adequate daily exercise.

Recipes

Homemade Dog Biscuits

8 cups whole wheat flour
2 tablespoons molasses (optional)

2 tablespoons honey
2¹/₂ cups (approximately) warm water
2 tablespoons safflower oil
1 cup raisins or other dried fruit

Warm the flour in the oven for a few minutes. Make a well in the center of the flour. Pour in the molasses, honey and water and mix to a fairly sticky dough. Cover and leave for 15 minutes. Make a well in the center of the dough and add the oil and raisins. Mix the dough thoroughly. Shape the dough into small balls, flatten them and place on a baking sheet that has been sprinkled with whole wheat flour. Cook in a 375 degree oven for approximately 40 minutes. Cool and refrigerate. These last around 7 days. After 7 days, look for mold.

Liver Treats

Cook liver in water on top of the stove until done (4 minutes at most). Drain, cool and cut into small bite-size pieces. Put them on a lined baking sheet and place in a cool oven (about 200 degrees) for around 2 hours, or until dried out. These are wonderful training treats and are not messy to carry around in your pocket. If you keep them covered in the refrigerator, they last several months.

Kefir

Known as the fountain of youth, kefir contains the richest and most powerful source of enzymes necessary for digestion and absorption. It is a grain food originating in the Caucasus. Because the curds break up easily, thereby releasing enzymes into the digestive system, it is said to be superior to yogurt. It is easier to make than yogurt as no heat process is used. Buy a starter from a health food store.

Carrot Sticks

Scrub carrots thoroughly and rinse under cold water. Cut into strips and put into a plastic bag in the refrigerator. Use these as treats when traveling or at shows. They are refreshing to both dog and handler. They can be used instead of dog biscuits at night.

Other Treats

Any vegetables or fruit, fresh or dried, can be used as treats. Our dogs love lettuce, so when we have salad we save the outer leaves for them. They like cucumbers, radishes and sprouts. Radishes are particularly popular in the winter in our dog family, and we have to be careful that they don't eat too many. If you use treats, make sure they are used in moderation. In training we find raisins to be ideal. They are the right size and they don't take a long time to chew.

Stud Dogs and Brood Bitches

Two weeks prior to breeding, the stud dog needs double the amount of vitamin E. Double up on this in his breakfast. Continue to use this dose during the time he is servicing a female. Add extra eggs to the diet so the dog is receiving them five times a week. Egg yolk contains selenium, which together with vitamin E helps produce sperm.

Your brood bitch will be pregnant for 9 weeks. For the first 6 weeks keep her on a maintenance diet. Over the next 3 weeks gradually increase the food until, at the time of whelping, it is 25 percent more than maintenance. There is a period during pregnancy—around 28 days—when your female will not be hungry. This is normal as the growing puppies push up against the bottom of the stomach, and it lasts around 2 to 3 days.

Add **raspberry leaf tea** to each meal several weeks before delivery. It helps to tone up the uterus, thereby making whelping easier. Put 3 tablespoons of dried raspberry leaves into 2 cups of water. Bring to a boil and simmer for a few moments. Take off the heat and leave overnight. Strain out the leaves, and put the tea into the refrigerator. Use 1 tablespoon per meal for a 50-pound dog. After delivery, halve the amount of raspberry leaf tea, and feed this in each meal for a couple of days. This helps to cleanse the uterus of any debris that may be left.

Your female dog should be exercised well during pregnancy to keep her in shape for whelping. For the last two weeks the exercise should not be too vigorous, and she should be taken to places where she will not be exposed to infections from other dogs.

For 48 hours after delivery, the new mother will be reluctant to leave her puppies. If she has eaten some of the placentas, she won't be very hungry. Her first meal should be a liquid one. Offer some raw milk and honey, or yogurt and honey or kefir and honey to boost her energy. The next meal can be her regular cereal meal, followed by her regular meat meal. Keep the 25 percent increase of food diet. This is a good ratio for her first week of being a mother.

As the puppies grow, their demands for food from her increase until she reaches maximum capacity during the third and fourth weeks. The mother's diet may increase to four times that of maintenance at this time. Few females can eat enough at two meals a day to produce milk to support a litter of fast growing puppies. Our Newfs required four to five feedings a day to keep up with the milk supply of their litters, and the Wirehaired Dachshunds needed six small meals to keep up with the milk production.

The mother should maintain her weight, *plus* produce sufficient milk for her litter *without* the need of supplementation. However, if the stress of feeding puppies is too great, adding the homeopathic remedy Supportasode (1 teaspoon twice a day) can help her cope better. (See Chapter 19 for more information.) If she has a very large litter, weaning may have to start at 21 days.

Weaning Puppies

Puppies from 0 to 28 days old are fed entirely by their mothers. When weaning, we found it easier to take the weight of the entire litter and use it as a guide. For example, if you have six 5-pound puppies, the weight of the litter is 30 pounds. Use the 10-pound chart and multiply by 3 to equal 30 pounds. If the litter weighs 24 pounds, multiply the 10-pound diet by 2.4, and so on.

Make up the food for the entire litter, and then feed each puppy *individually* in a separate bowl. This way all puppies have a chance to eat the same amount of food. In a litter, some puppies eat very quickly, and some slowly, this is normal. Before feeding the puppies, take the mother away from the litter. Let her finish what the puppies leave. As time goes on, her milk supply will dry up naturally. When the puppies are 7 weeks of age, start to decrease the mother's food until it is approximately 10 percent over maintenance. Then reduce her to the normal diet. Increase her exercise to restore her condition and muscle tone.

Weaning Diet for 10 Pounds (Total Litter Weight) of Puppies

Separate the mother dog from the litter.
Feed each puppy in an individual bowl.
Have fresh water available.
After feeding allow the pups outside into the fresh air and sunshine.

28–35 days

8 A.M.	$^1/_2$ cup of raw milk or goats' milk	Put into
	$^1/_2$ teaspoon honey	blender
	$^1/_4$ teaspoon slippery elm powder	and mix.
	Now allow the mother dog to feed her puppies.	
12 noon	1 oz. dry weight baby cereal, oats and barley,	
	mixed and cooked	
	$^1/_2$ cup raw milk	
	50 mg vitamin C	
	Mix up in a blender and serve in individual bowls.	
	Now allow the mother dog to feed her puppies.	

| 4 P.M. | Same as 8 A.M. feeding |
| 8 P.M. | Same as 12 noon feeding; add $1/4$ teaspoon cod liver oil. Before going to bed, allow the mother dog to nurse her puppies. |

If raw cow or goats' milk is not available, use an active, naturally cultured yogurt cut with water, 1 part water to 2 parts yogurt.

36–49 Days

Quantities represent 10 pounds of litter weight, and the increase of solid food. The mother's contribution is decreased from 50 to 25 percent.

| 8 A.M. | $1/2$ eyedropper, Supportasode homeopathic
$2/3$ cup raw milk
$1/3$ teaspoon honey
$1/4$ teaspoon slippery elm powder
1.2 oz. (dry weight) cereal (oats and barley)
50 mg vitamin C
$1/8$ teaspoon Puppy Stress Formula |

Cook cereal, cool and mix with other ingredients. Feed puppies individually, then allow mother dog to nurse pups.

| 12 noon | Same as above, allowing the mother to nurse her pups after feeding. |
| 4 P.M. | 1 teaspoon—increasing to 3.5 oz. over 8–12 days of fresh, raw meat. This represents an increase of around 1 tablespoon each day. Scrape the surface of the meat with a knife, or put it into a blender and chop into tiny pieces.
$1/8$ teaspoon brewers yeast
$1/4$ teaspoon increasing to $2/3$ teaspoon bone meal
$1/2$ teaspoon herbs or greens
$1/16$ teaspoon kelp
$1/2$ teaspoon wheat bran
$1/4$ teaspoon wheat germ
$1/8$ teaspoon cod liver oil
$1/8$ teaspoon Puppy Stress Formula
$1/2$ eyedroppper Supportasode |

Mix together and divide into individual dishes. When pups have finished, allow the mother to feed the puppies.

185

8 P.M.   Same as above, but add $^1/_3$ garlic capsule.

By the time the puppies are $6^1/_2$ weeks of age, they will be on the total diet.

Now the food increases. The puppies are no longer being supplemented by their mother's milk. So if a puppy weighs 10 pounds when it leaves for its new home, the new owner feeds a diet for a 20-pound puppy. This "double" feeding will continue until the puppy is 7 months old.

Stress Associated with Raising Puppies

When puppies are weaned and put on regular commercial food, they experience stress. They are no longer getting the rich diet provided by mother's milk or the complete protection provided by maternal antibodies present in her milk. They also face exposure to vaccines starting around 6 weeks of age. At 7 weeks of age they are usually placed into their new homes and again there is the prospect of a change in diet, visits to the veterinarian and more vaccinations. The stress levels increase. In order to protect puppies from stress-related illnesses, we suggest the following program for those weaned onto commercial dog food.

5–7 weeks $^1/_4$ teaspoon Puppy Stress Mix
            $^1/_2$ eye dropper of Supportasode 2 times a day.
6 weeks   at time of first vaccine, 1 teaspoon Viratox for one
            week.

Supportasode (a homeopathic preparation) supports cell and tissue regeneration. It provides the cell with nutritional factors in metabolically active concentrations, affecting all the organs of the body. If the puppies are raised on commercial dog food, this needs to be continued on a daily basis, increasing to 1 teaspoon daily after 7 weeks, until the puppy is through the vaccination program at approximately 6 months of age. Pups raised on the Natural Diet do not need the Supportasode on a regular basis as their diet compensates for the stress factors of growth and vaccines.

The Viratox is also a homeopathic preparation and it detoxifies any residual toxins from required vaccinations or viral infections. It should be used for one week after any single or combined vaccination whether the pup is raised on commercial food or the natural diet. It can be used with the Supportasode.

It is our suggestion that a breeder should make up a puppy package that includes a bottle of both Supportasode and Viratox, with instructions on how to use them during the critical period up to 6 months of age, when the puppy is placed into his new home, plus a supply of Puppy Stress Formula.

Directly after the puppies are weaned, any food should have some of the Puppy Stress Formula added. If the pups are fed individually, a pinch is sufficient. If you make up the food for the whole litter and then divide it, add $1/8$ teaspoon to each 10-pound batch. This formula contains nutrients that support each organ system and helps to maintain a correctly functioning immune system. This is continued until the puppy is placed on adult food, at which time the regular adult vitamin-mineral mix is substituted for the Puppy Stress Formula.

The stress levels experienced by a puppy in the first 6 months, from growth to entering a new home, inadequate nutrition, as well as the vaccination series, is greater than at any time in life. Managing this time frame carefully helps to produce a dog that as an adult will be more disease resistant and who will have a chance to live a long and healthy life.

Raising Puppies From 7 Weeks

Puppies need to eat double the amount of food for their weight until they are 7 months old. Growing to almost 70 percent of their adult weight during this time, puppies need the correct amount of food. If your puppy weighs 5 pounds, feed a 10-pound diet. This provides the correct number of calories. It is difficult to establish exact amounts as different breeds grow at different rates. The rule of thumb is that a lean puppy is healthier than a fat puppy. Heavy puppies put too much stress on growing bones.

When teething is complete, gradually decrease the quantities fed until the puppy is on the same amount of food as the adult dog and feed three times a day. In a very short time, the puppy will start to leave the third meal, at which time food feedings are cut back to *two a day*. Your dog will stay on two feedings for life. There will be times during the first 18 months of life that the pup goes through growth spurts when you will have to increase the amount of food. If your young dog seems very hungry, increase the food until the dog no longer is able to lick the dish clean, then cut back to the appropriate amount.

Puppies are fed *four times a day* until they are through teething. If your puppy weighs 5 pounds, mix up the breakfast for the 10-pound dog and divide into two meals. Feed one meal at 8 A.M. and the other at 12 noon. Do the same with the meat meal. Mix up the amount for a 10-pound dog and feed half at 4 P.M. and the other half at 8 P.M. If your puppy seems to be hungry before bedtime, you can feed a little cereal, milk and honey. Puppies are not fasted until they are through teething. On the seventh day follow the Day 2 chart.

Traveling With the Diet

We have traveled with several dogs for up to 10 days on the diet with no problems. If you travel in an RV, there is no time limit to using the diet, only the problem of keeping the meat and liver frozen. When we stay in hotels, we make sure the cooler in which the food is stored is kept cold. We load it with fresh ice in the morning and the evening when we return to the room. The apple cider vinegar in the meat meal is a natural preservative, and as long as the meat is kept cold, it will last.

The cereal meal can be prepared ahead of time and frozen in individual meals, with the supplements added separately. Or you can take dry cereal with you and take a small pot that boils water, adding the dry cereal to it before you go to bed and let it stand all night.

Or you can make breakfast bars. If you make the breakfast bars, your dog will need to drink water, since by baking them, most of the moisture is removed and he is not receiving the same amount of water he is used to getting. It is preferable to take your own supply of drinking water, but if that is not possible, use what is available on your trip, and add 2 tablespoons of Willard Water to each bowl so that your dog is not affected by the change.

Breakfast Bars

> 4 cups oats
> 2 cups buckwheat, millet, wheat or barley
> 1 cup boiling water
> 8 tablespoons safflower oil
> 8 tablespoons blackstrap molasses
> 2 tablespoons honey
> 4 medium eggs with shells

Preheat oven to 350 degrees.

Put all the ingredients into a large bowl. Mix with about 1 cup of boiling water. Make a sticky dough. Place into a well-greased baking pan and cook at 350 degrees for 45 minutes. Take out and score into squares. Turn out onto a wire rack to cool.

To determine how much to feed, weigh an individual breakfast bar and compare it to the dry weight of grains on the chart. You can then calculate how many to feed. Vitamin C, B complex, vitamin-mineral mix and the vitamin E are fed separately. We travel with some cans of natural cat food. We place the supplements into the cat food and feed them on a spoon to the dogs.

One easy way to get our finicky dogs to eat when they are traveling is to feed the meat meal in the morning. All the dogs love their meat meal, and if they are going to miss a meal, it will be the cereal meal. We like to start dog show days with dogs that have eaten well and are full of the various vitamins and minerals that will protect their health. We feed their normal breakfasts when we return to the hotel room and when the dogs have had time to rest.

Cravings

If a dog shows a marked preference for certain foods, chances are that your dog needs that food for a balanced diet. We had a dog that craved eggs and cabbage. Two years after these cravings surfaced, she was diagnosed as having a rare blood disease. Her blood would not clot properly. Vitamin K, which is specific for blood clotting, is abundant in eggs and cabbage. She knew before we did what she needed. By observing and listening to our dogs, we can learn what is wrong with them by their preferences for special foods.

Breed Specifics

Reference has been made to the special needs of certain breeds of dogs. German Shepherd Dogs, Labrador Retrievers, Boxers, Newfoundlands and Bull Terriers are among the breeds with which we are most familiar. These are the dogs who require a diet that is more acid based. If your dog is in this category, add an amino acid complex tablet to each morning meal, and on the days that eggs are not used, add 25 mcg selenium and 500 mg L-methionine to maintain constant health. There may be other breeds or individuals that need these adjustments. One indication of these needs is a dog that has dark brown to black discharge in the ears, cystitis or urinary tract infections, poor pigmentation, hair coat and skin eruptions. **Do not use this program without regular veterinary testing.**

Dogs that have problems assimilating their food may have either pancreatic problems or stomach problems. Test the Puppy Stress Formula, which contains many digestive aids, to see if they need it. When you are working with dogs that have specific diseases, repeated blood work is necessary. Some dogs' needs are seasonal, with a greater need for supplements in the winter. Use kinesiology and test frequently. The above amounts are for dogs that weigh 75 to 150 lbs.

Dalmatians, West Highland White Terriers and some Bedlington Terriers represent a special challenge. Since they are unable to deal with high amounts of animal protein in their diets, or cannot eliminate some metals from their systems which are present in food, a diet higher in vegetable protein is probably the best for them. Indeed, some do well on these diets low in meat protein with eggs added. We have been successful with these breeds by adding the amino acid complex tablet in their morning meal, vitamin B complex two times a day and, of course, vitamin C. Many of these tested well for the Puppy Stress Formula. These breeds need careful, continual monitoring by laboratory testing to check their protein levels.

General Information

It is no more expensive to use the Natural Diet than feeding a good-quality dry dog food with supplements. It is dictated by the cost of the meat and liver. Buying meat from the supermarket may not be too expensive if you have a small dog, but if you have several large dogs or a kennel, it can become prohibitive. We found a rendering plant in a city two hours from us that sold meat to dog food companies. We visited the owner of the plant and asked if he dealt in "clean" animals rather than those that were dead, dying or diseased. He told us the plant often had clean animals that had had accidents or had had problems when calving and it was not economical for the farmer to put money into the animal. We asked that if we paid him more than the dog food companies, would he be willing to set aside the clean meat? That was 20 years ago, and today this rendering plant supplies fresh raw, clean meat to many of the northeastern states.

Money can be saved by joining food cooperatives in your area where organic grains can be obtained. Raw honey, blackstrap molasses, wheat germ and herbs can be bought at these cooperatives. We called Walnut Acres in Pennsylvania, where we have bought organic grains for 20 years, and were surprised to find a food cooperative dealing in those grains in a town near to us.

Blackstrap molasses and wheat bran can be bought cheaply from grain feed stores. These items are used in other animal feeds. You will need to take your own containers. Raw cow's milk is hard to find, and in many states it is against the law for farmers to sell unpasturized milk. Call the local 4-H group in your area to find someone who sells raw goat's milk, which is excellent for feeding dogs, indispensable when raising young dogs and great for old dogs. It can be frozen. Take your own containers.

For information on suppliers of the ingredients for this diet, see Chapter 19.

The Natural Diet is not the answer to all problems in dogs, but it offers a quality of life to many dogs who have never had the chance to enjoy good health.

—Chapter 15—

Herbs

Herbs are an integral part of the Natural Diet and are used to stimulate digestion and various organs and glands in the body. They are used medicinally as cleansers and tonics, and they can be used internally as well as externally.

Dogs raised in the country or taken regularly for walks can help themselves to grasses and weeds when they need them. They instinctively choose those that are correct for them to balance their systems. Many people stop their dogs eating grass because they think it makes their dogs sick. Sometimes it does, especially if they eat the coarse couch grass that has serrated edges. Vomiting is the way dogs have of expelling something from their stomachs that is either indigestible or poisonous. The grass encapsulates and binds the foreign object—sometimes only a fluid-type substance, which allows the dog to vomit it up. Do not stop your dogs from eating weeds and grasses, unless they have been chemically treated. They really know what they need.

How to Prepare Herbs

An easy way to use herbs is to make them into a tea (2 tablespoons of fresh or 1 tablespoon dried to a pint of water, boiled and then steeped overnight). Use 1 tablespoon per meal for the 50-pound dog. Keep refrigerated. Chopping up herbs and putting them into food is a popular way of using them. Plants contain cellulose, which is difficult for the dog to break down and utilize. Add some hot water to the herbs and let them steep for a while before feeding. This makes them easier for the dog to digest.

There is a crossover effect with many herbs, which means that combining several herbs works better in many instances than just feeding one herb. The vitamin-mineral mix we use daily, plus the Puppy Stress Formula, contain many herbs, some of which target and stimulate organs and glands in the body, as well as cleansing them.

You will notice on the following list of diseases we have also made reference to vitamins, minerals, amino acids and homeopathics. That is because the combination is needed for that disease state. (See Chapter 18, "At a Glance.").

If your dog is being treated for a specific disease and you are using (for example) soloxine as a thyroid medication, or tiny doses of prednisilone, a common treatment for adrenal gland exhaustion (Addison's disease), it is a good idea to stimulate those individual glands with herbs at the same time they are being medicated. In some cases, the glands can be stimulated enough so that the medication can be reduced or withdrawn completely. Use kinesiology to ascertain which herbs are correct for your dog.

Herbs

Condition	Herbs
Abscesses	burdock, red clover, garlic, dandelion, yellow dock
Addison's disease	Adrenal problems: licorice root, hawthorn and juniper berries, kelp and yucca
Aging	ginseng, barley juice powder, germanium
Allergies—Food	papaya, aloe vera juice, food enzymes
Allergies—Mold	
Pollen	bee pollen, comfrey, alfalfa, chickweed
Anemia	alfalfa, dandelion, chlorophyll, kelp
Appetite	Stimulate: licorice root, ginger root, peppermint, capsicum, chamomile, saw palmetto
	Depress: chickweed, spirulina, l-carnatine
Arthritis	alfalfa, primrose-oil, comfrey, yucca, licorice
Bladder Infection	acidophilus, kyolic garlic, juniper berries, goldenseal (if there is bleeding), uva ursi, corn silk
Breathing Difficulties	lobelia, mullein, yerba santa
Bronchitis	lobelia, pleurisy root, mullein
Bruising	citrus bioflavanoids
Burns	vitamin E, baking soda and olive oil externally; aloe vera juice
Bursitis	comfrey, yucca
Cancer	dandelion, echinacea, pau d'arco, red clover, garlic (burdock, sheep sorrel, rhubarb and elm made into a tea can be helpful)

Colitis	papaya, chamomile, aloe vera, acidophilus
Convulsions and Epilepsy	lobelia, hyssop, black cohosh, passion flower, l-taurine
Cramps in legs	don quai, ginger, butchers broom, vitamin E
Dandruff	dandelion, goldenseal, lecithin, sage, jojoba oil
Dermatitis	comfrey, dandelion, myrrh, pau d'arco, red clover, vitamin B
Diabetes	chromium, goldenseal, juniper berries, uva ursi
Diarrhea	kelp, potassium, slippery elm, charcoal, catnip, mullein, acidophilus
Diuretic	peach, juniper, buckthorn, fennel, parsley
Ears	lobelia, garlic, l-glutamine, echinacea, goldenseal, grapefruit extract (Eco-Vm)
Energy	bee pollen, chlorophyll, kelp, licorice root
Epilepsy	lobelia, passion flower, magnesium, amino acid complex tablet, B complex
Eye Problems	goldenseal, passion flower, vitamin C + zinc.
Eyelids	rosemary or eyebright made up as a tea can be used as an eye wash
Hyperactivity	lobelia, vitamin B, vitamin C, amino acid complex
Hypothyroid	goldenseal, kelp
Incontinence	corn silk
Immune System	echinacea, goldenseal, red clover, acidophilus
Lyme Disease	echinacea, goldenseal, red clover, suma, Chlorophyll, garlic, vitamin C
Motion Sickness	charcoal, ginger, magnesium, B-Complex
Milk Production	To increase: blessed thistle, fennel, red raspberry, marshmallow. To decrease: parsley, kelp, sage
Nervousness	catnip, calcium, magnesium, scullcap, B-Complex, Calm Stress (homeopathic)
Pancreatitis	goldenseal, chromium, vitamin E, calcium, B-Complex, pancreatic enzymes
Parasites, Worms	black walnut, garlic, pumpkin seeds, sage, Paratox (homeopathic), vitamin-mineral mix
Periodontal Disease	goldenseal, white oak bark, vitamins A and C, myrrh

Poison Ivy	vitamin C, aloe vera gel, black walnut, white oak bark, goldenseal, lobelia and rhus tox, a homeopathic made from poison ivy
Ringworm	tea tree oil,* garlic, pau d'arco, apple cider vinegar applied topically
Rocky Mountain Spotted Fever	vitamin C, bentonite clay, Oregon Grape-herbal vitamin-mineral mix
Seizures	lobelia, scullcap, passion flower, magnesium, amino acid complex tablet, B-Complex
Staph Infections	goldenseal, garlic, acidophilus, vitamin A
Stress	B-Complex, vitamin C, magnesium, calcium, catnip, passion flower, valerian root, hops, Calm Stress and ignatia (homeopathics)
Tendonitis	licorice, yucca, lecithin
Tumors	germanium, vitamin C, kelp, lecithin, chickweed, red clover, pau d'arco; Use one of the homeopathic formulas for cleansing the body plus tea listed under Cancer. (See sources chapter 19.)
Thyroid	kelp, Irish moss, vitamin-mineral mix
Viral Infections	garlic, pau d'arco, vitamins A and C, zinc, l-lysine, Viratox (homeopathic)
Wounds	calendula ointment, calendula/hypericum ointment where there is pain, bite wounds
Yeast infections	garlic, vitamins A and C, acidophilus, Pau D'arco; douche with fresh garlic crushed in Willard Water. Acidopilus powder, 2 teaspoons, mixed with water or yogurt, can be used as a douche for 3 days.

Author's Note: *Tea tree oil* can cause convulsions in some dogs if used in a nondiluted form. Areas especially vulnerable are the spine, ears and dosing by mouth. Check with kinesiology if your dog can tolerate this substance, which is found in many natural products—particularly skin care remedies and shampoos.

Systems

Circulation:	yellow dock, omega 3 fatty acids, garlic, capsicum, hawthorn berries
Digestive System—Upper	digestive enzymes, ginger, peppermint, safflowers
Digestive System—Lower	acidophilus capsules to restore intestinal flora, cascara sagrada, psyllium husks, slippery elm bark to promote action of bowels, algin to extract toxins from bowel
Glandular System	Siberian ginseng, black cohosh (for female hormonal system), red clover, yarrow flowers, horsetail, damiana, zinc (for male hormonal system); Adrenals: licorice root; Pancreas: goldenseal, juniper berries, uva ursi, mullein, slippery elm, dandelion; Thyroid: kelp, Irish moss
Nervous System	Stress: B-complex vitamins + choline, vitamin C, calcium, catnip, chamomile, passion flowers, valerian root. Brain: gotu kola. Hops promote sleep and overcomes restlessness.
Immune System	vitamins C, A and E, selenium and zinc; Lymph system: chaparral, burdock root, pau d'arco; General stimulants: echinacea, goldenseal; Use Natural Diet. *Check titers on dogs before getting vaccines. Check heartworm medication.*
Musculoskeletal System	herbal vitamin-mineral mix, bayberry, horsetail, red raspberry leaves, aloe vera, comfrey (do not use this if kidney problems are present), oat straw
Respiratory System	mullein, fenugreek
Urinary System	parsley, uva ursi, juniper berries
Skin and Hair	shampoo that contains jojoba oil or pau d'arco or vitamin E, safflowers, aloe vera, Irish moss or horsetail, plus a good vitamin-mineral mix

Summary

Herbs can be used for many purposes. They are tonics, toners, sedators and energizers and medicines. Have respect for them; they can cure many ailments. If you start to use an herb for a specific complaint, remember to check frequently to see if your dog still needs it. Some medicinal herbs can cause difficulties if they are overused. (For sources, see Chapter 19.)

—Chapter 16—

Homeopathy

Homeopathy was first discovered in 1790 by Dr. Samuel Hahnemann in Germany. A brilliant physician, he was dissatisfied with conventional medicine as it was then practiced and instead became a translator of medical texts. When translating a text by Cullen, a Scottish physician, he disagreed with Cullen's description of how the cinchona bark used to treat malaria acted on the body. Cinchona bark was the effective treatment of the time. In trying to explain the action of the bark Hahnemann took some of it himself, and he produced symptoms of malaria. After a while, the symptoms wore off and he was "normal" again. He tried it again, and reproduced the results.

Thus was born his natural law of "similia similibus curentur," that is, let like be cured by like. He wrote:

> Every medicine which, among the symptoms it can cause in a healthy body, reproduces those most present in a given disease, is capable of curing the disease in the swiftest, most thorough and most enduring fashion.

Hahnemann was a true scientist and over the next 20 years he tested this hypothesis by using close to 70 natural substances on himself, his family and all of his friends, as well as medical school volunteers. Dietary and behavioral controls were exerted with his experiments, and every symptom, however minute, was recorded. A compilation of these symptoms resulted in a book called the *Materia Medica*. It is a documentation of the symptoms each substance (remedy) produced in a healthy person, which was then used to cure the same symptoms in a sick person.

Potencies

Hahnemann discovered, some think by accident, that by diluting his natural remedies they became more and more effective. This is the part of homeopathic medicine that is still being challenged as unscientific. *The more the original substance is diluted, the more powerful it becomes.* Somehow, by what is called "succussion" or banging the substance a specific number of times, the energy of the substance is released, which can then be diluted again, making the original substance more powerful. The substances are succussed either 10 times, called "x" potencies, or 100 times, called "c" potencies. So a 6x potency would be one that is diluted one in ten, six times. Succussion is carried out at each stage and, somehow while making the substance more powerful, also removes the harmful toxins of the original substance. Thus all sorts of poisonous substances are used, anything from deadly snake venom to poisonous plants. Since succussion removes the toxic effects, prescribing the wrong remedy can do no harm.

A Different Approach to Healing

In trying to understand homeopathy, we must change how we think of medicine. Traditional medicine as we know it, uses drugs rather like magic bullets, to target a part of the body where the disease has its hold. If the patient shows signs of liver, kidney or perhaps lung disease, drugs are used to target those specific areas of the body. Homeopathy looks at the whole patient, behavior, appearance, what that patient feels, past illnesses and inherited family diseases plus the symptoms of the disease itself. The homeopathic physician looks up those symptoms in the *Materia Medica*, matching the feelings, appearance and behavior of the patient. When an exact match is found, the homeopathic physician then prescribes a remedy. That remedy enters the body and overpowers the disease, thus releasing the body's natural energies so that the body can heal itself.

Christopher Day, DVM, in his book *The Homeopathic Treatment of Small Animals*, likens homeopathy to the art of judo:

> To apply a force opposite to the aggressor, if the aggressor is strong, will fail, whereas if only one applies a force in the same direction as the aggressor (the art of judo) a very powerful adversary can be defeated with small use of force. This superficially is the strength of homeopathy. (13)

Benefits of Homeopathy

The benefit of homeopathy on our dogs is enormous. *There are no side effects* to worry about. The whole animal, as a unique individual, is taken into consideration when prescribing a remedy: the personality of the dog, the time of the year the symptoms worsen, the time of the day the dog seems uncomfortable, the past illnesses the dog has had, foods, housing and the dog's relationship with the owner. This is called taking the symptoms, developing a drug picture or repetorizing. By supplying the symptoms to a homeopathic veterinarian the owner can, by observation, be part of the healing process. If the homeopathic doctor has chosen the correct remedy and locates the correct drug picture, the disease is cured.

Using conventional medicine with drugs that target a specific organ or disease, palliation or suppression of that disease takes place, not necessarily a cure; the disease may come back. Skin problems are a good example. By the use of antibiotics and steroids, it is fairly easy to suppress the symptoms of itching skin. While the drugs are being used, the dog is comfortable. As soon as the drugs are withdrawn and have worn off, the disease returns, usually worse than it was before. It has not been cured. With the proper use of the correct homeopathic remedy, the disease will not return.

How It Works

How can homeopathic medicine work? If you think of energy you can see quite easily how it is possible for it to work. The dilutions contain the energy of the original product. Some scientists think that the alcohol or water with which the dilutions are made carry memory at an energetic level. They point out that thinking of the energy fields of substances (Einstein's theory of $E = mc^2$) is a possible explanation of how homeopathy works.

Homeopathy, which fell out of favor once antibiotics entered the picture, is enjoying an enormous resurgence worldwide, and in some European countries veterinarians are trained in both homeopathy as well as traditional medicine. In Britain, the royal family is one of homeopathy's greatest proponents. Homeopathic study groups exist in almost every large city in this country, as well as in many small towns.

There are two ways of using homeopathy. Classic homeopathy, where one remedy is used in a high potency to cure a chronic illness, is best left to the expert practitioner because taking the case history and repetorizing is an art in itself, and proficiency takes a lot of study. If high potencies are used without understanding how they work, aggravations of previous illnesses can appear and be frightening and dangerous. *The most appealing aspect of using homeopathy is that when it works, it works, and when it doesn't work, nothing happens.* Made entirely from naturally occurring substances, it has no side effects when used in lower potencies.

As a layperson you can use homeopathy successfully for acute disorders that use the remedies in very low potencies. Following is a list of remedies that cover the most common ailments we see. We keep these on hand in the kennel and take them with us when we travel.

How to Use Homeopathy

Remedies come in different forms. Some are minute pellets, smaller than a pinhead. Some are the size of a pinhead, and some are small tablets. It depends on the manufacturer. Other than the shape and size, they are the same. We prefer the smaller pellets, as they are easy to administer.

Some remedies are in liquid form and come in a bottle with a dropper. These are also easy to use with dogs. By pulling out the flews on the dog's mouth, you can squeeze in a dose. Sometimes you will want to add the remedy to your dog's water bowl. Other remedies are made for external use and come in creams, gels and oils.

When dosing your dog with a remedy, remember you are dealing with the energy of that particular remedy. If you touch the remedy, you are changing the energy. It becomes a mixture of the energy of the remedy, plus your own energy. Read the directions on the bottle, pour the pellets into the hollowed-out cap of the bottle, open your dog's mouth and place the measured remedy onto the back of the tongue. Liquid remedies are used directly from the bottle and dripped from the dropper either onto your dog's tongue or into the flews. All remedies should be housed in a cool, dark place, as they are affected by bright light.

How to Make the Correct Choice

When we were first introduced to homeopathic medicine, we were confused about how to use it. We hadn't yet changed our thinking enough and worried about using the wrong remedy or overdosing, not realizing that with low potencies we would do no harm. This concept took a while to digest. Depending on which book you read, and from whom you learn, there are numerous ways to use homeopathy. We are going to tell you how we use it with our dogs and our families.

When presented with an acute condition—a bee sting, insect bite, poison ivy, a sprain, a pulled muscle and extreme stress—we use one dose of the particular remedy every 5 minutes for 15 minutes, which is *four* doses. We then wait 15 minutes, and if the symptoms are not greatly improved, we use it again. We then wait for half an hour and use it again, then hourly as needed. We use remedies in the potencies from 6x to 30c, and occasionally 200c—rarely higher. Using kinesiology helps us determine which dosage is correct for each situation, and how often to use it.

There are thousands of remedies from which to choose. Listed below are those that we have found most useful. The list is not meant in any way to be complete, but rather as an introduction to get you started. You can make up your own kit. This particular group allows us to deal with most emergency situations and buys time until we can study the situation further.

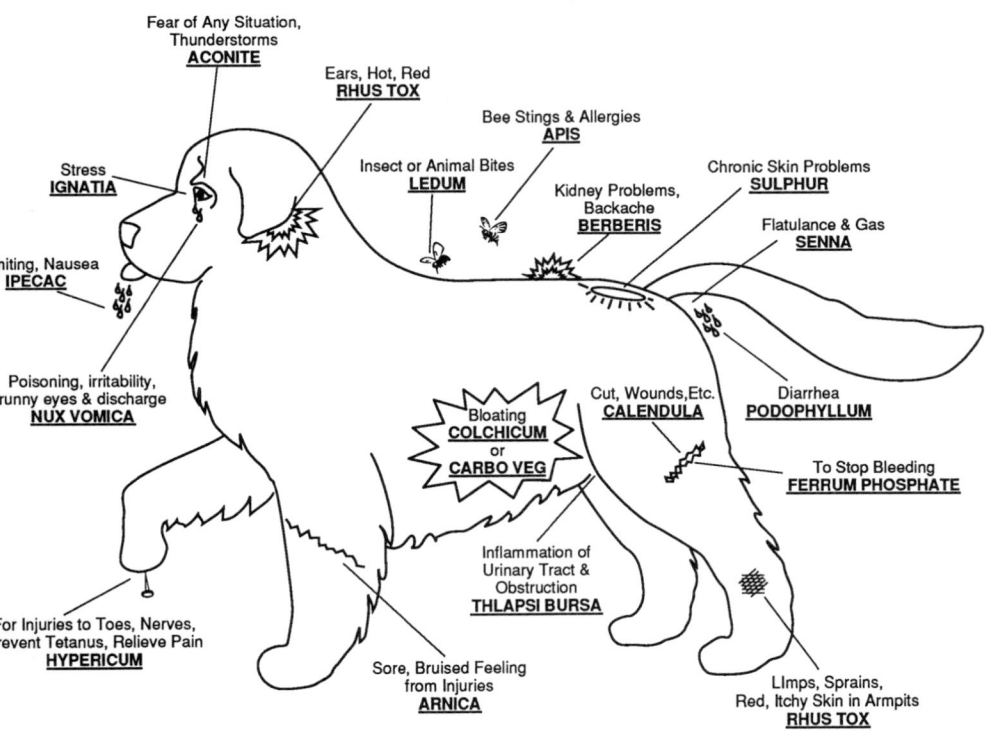

Fear of Any Situation, Thunderstorms
ACONITE

Ears, Hot, Red
RHUS TOX

Bee Stings & Allergies
APIS

Chronic Skin Problems
SULPHUR

Stress
IGNATIA

Insect or Animal Bites
LEDUM

Kidney Problems, Backache
BERBERIS

Flatulance & Gas
SENNA

Vomiting, Nausea
IPECAC

Poisoning, irritability, runny eyes & discharge
NUX VOMICA

Cut, Wounds,Etc.
CALENDULA

Diarrhea
PODOPHYLLUM

Bloating
COLCHICUM
or
CARBO VEG

To Stop Bleeding
FERRUM PHOSPHATE

Inflammation of Urinary Tract & Obstruction
THLAPSI BURSA

For Injuries to Toes, Nerves, Prevent Tetanus, Relieve Pain
HYPERICUM

Sore, Bruised Feeling from Injuries
ARNICA

Limps, Sprains, Red, Itchy Skin in Armpits
RHUS TOX

16-1: The Homeopathic Dog

The remedies are divided into two parts: those remedies we use for physical symptoms and those we use for emotional and behavioral symptoms. Chapter 19 lists places to buy reference books. Do not hesitate to consult a professional if you feel that your dog would benefit from higher doses of a particular remedy.

First-aid kits are available from several sources and come in different potencies.

This drawing can be duplicated and put into your emergency kit, on the refrigerator door, or on the inside of a cupboard door for easy reference in emergencies.

Remedies	Used to Cure
Aconite Napellus	Onset of fever and inflammations. Fear and anxiety. Fear of flying. Ears become red, hot and swollen. Use for fear of thunderstorms or fear of anything.
Aloe Socotrina	Involuntary diarrhea with mucous and gas. Abdomen distended.
Antimonium Tart.	Loose, unproductive cough, respiration difficult and gasping for air.
Ammonium Camb.	Wheezing and labored breathing found in overweight dogs. Nose gets stopped up at night. Nosebleeds. Urinary incontinence on cold nights.
Apis Mellifica	Bee stings, hives. Any swelling that is shiny in appearance, especially joint swelling. Allergic reactions. Can be used for retention of fluids.
Arnica Montana	Use first with injuries. Sore, bruised feeling and any kind of muscle aches. Use after surgery. Fear of being touched. Strong antiseptic properties.
Arsenicum Album	Works on all organs and tissues. Use when there is weakness and exhaustion. Discharges from nose or eyes that cause skin irritation. Wheezing respiration. Scaly or dry skin, especially when it is cold and wet. Great thirst.
Belladonna	Fevers of sudden onset. Heatstroke, convulsions, hot red skin. Acute ear inflammations. Pupils are generally dilated.

Berberis	Inflammation of the kidneys, sore back, very anxious. Urine that drips from male dogs instead of in a stream.
Byronia	Chronic constipation. Dry, hacking cough. Nausea with headache. Yellow-coated tongue. Helps rheumatism or arthritis cases. One of the mastitis remedies.
Calc. Carb.	Pupil dilation, cataracts. Depraved appetite, lymph nodes in throat are swollen. Bone growth abnormalities, umbilical hernia, skin has warts.
Calc. Fluor.	Glandular swellings, mammary growths. Hard swellings. Anal fissures and itching. Backache.
Calc. Phos.	Remedy for the young and growing, especially during teething and puberty. Slowly developing, skinny, weak pups. Poor bone growth. Use during transition times in life.
Calc. Sulph.	Lesions that are slow to heal. Discharges that are thick and yellow.
Calendula	As an oil, lotion or ointment, use externally for open wounds. Stops bleeding when pads are cut. Antiseptic. Internally, natural antibiotic. Helps to relieve pain.
Cantharis	Blood in urine, cystitis, frequent and painful urination. Burns or scalds.
Carbo veg.	Bloated, gassy feeling in stomach with pain.
Caulophyllum	Use before, during or after whelping. Aids in uterine contractions, pushes out the fetus, and pushes out residue left after birth.
Causticum	Chronic cystitis. Flat, rough warts, pains in muscular tissues.
Chamomilla	Irritability in young dog, especially during teething, any toothache. Swollen gums and abscessed teeth. Young dog remedy for diarrhea, colic, swelling of the lymph nodes. Nursing problems with painful mammary glands, false pregnancies.
Chelidonium Maj.	To stimulate the function of a sluggish liver and gallbladder. Yellow, claylike stool.
Cistus canadensis	Throat and neck problems, swollen gums.

Cocculus	Motion sickness. Drooling, vomiting. Difficulty in opening mouth. Acts on central nervous system, sometimes used for epilepsy.
Coffea cruda.	Discomfort after food with a bloated abdomen. Skin is overly sensitive to touch. Insomnia.
Colchincum aut.	Gassy, distended stomach.
Colocynthis	Use for spasmodic colic where the legs are pulled up under the abdomen. Slight swelling of the abdomen, diarrhea with gas. Dog is agitated, grinds teeth and is worse around noise.
Conium	Weakness and trembling, especially in old dogs. Weakness in the hind legs. Helpful in paralysis of rear. Tumors in the mammary glands and lymph glands.
Crataegus	Heart tonic used for chronic heart disease, swelling over whole body, heart murmurs.
Cuprum Metall.	Severe muscle cramps, intestinal colic, convulsions.
Euphrasia	Conjunctivitis, sticky mucus in the eyes. Use in the form of eye drops.
Ferrum Phosphate	To stop bleeding from a wound.
Gelsemium	Fear in general, fear of thunderstorms, fear that leads to urination. Fear in the show ring. Male dogs that get overexcited. Limbs that tremble.
Graphites	Skin that cracks in the folds. Dogs that have smelly skin.
Hepar Sulphuris	Bacterial infections, use when there is pus present, good for hot spots.
Hydrastis	Use for all mucous membranes, gastrointestinal, urinary and respiratory problems.
Hypericum	Nerve damage. Relieves pain, useful in all injuries as well as toe or tail injuries and puncture wounds.
Ignatia	Use for stress, particularly when there is sadness or grief. Loss of a loved one, e.g., mother and puppies separated, or if pet loses owner. Useful for separation anxiety. Dogs that get agitated in showing and break stays.
Ipecacuanna	Vomiting. Nosebleeds, blood in milk of mother dogs.

Kali Bich	Yellow, ropy discharges, gastrointestinal tract, swelling of eyelids.
Kali Carb	Dogs that dislike the cold. Eyelids that stick together in the morning. Yellow discharge from the nose.
Kali Chloricum	Chronic kidney disorders. Bad breath, sore and ulcerated mouth.
Lachesis	Smelly wounds, use when body is toxic with great weakness. Dogs that eat their feet, red in between toes.
Ledum	Puncture wounds, insect bites, after injections. Tetanus nails puncturing feet, poison oak.
Lillium tigrinum	Pyometra in females.
Lycopodium clav.	For dogs that dislike being alone. Works on kidneys, liver, digestive system and respiratory system. Blisters on the tongue. Small, hard stool. Gives confidence.
Lyssin (Hydrophobinum)	Diseases of the nervous system. Used to counteract side effects from the rabies vaccine, which are most often seen up to 30 days after injection. Frothing at the mouth, drooling, snapping in the air, sudden aggression, great weakness, collapse, convulsions and paralysis. Abnormal sexual desire. Worse around running water.
Natrum Carb.	Afraid of thunder. Use in heat exhaustion. Dogs that injure their joints easily especially in summer.
Natrum Sulph.	Use in head injuries. Diarrhea with gas.
Nitric Acid	For warts or any skin lesion that bleeds easily.
Nux Vomica	Digestive system. Upset stomachs. Use for dogs that eat things they should not, sound sensitivity, umbilical hernias. Use when dog is exposed to toxins, externally or internally. Great cleansing remedy.
Phosphorus	Sensitivity to sudden noise, loud bangs, fireworks, thunderstorms. Old dogs, bone degeneration. Food that is vomited back after eating. Hepatitis, pancreatitis and kidney disease. Coughs that seem painful.

	Dogs that seek cold surfaces upon which to sleep when weak. Bleeding from wounds.
Phytolacca	Glands that are swollen and hard. Lymph nodes that are swollen. Swelling in the throat, where the throat is red and there is difficulty swallowing.
Pitric Acid	A male dog remedy. Oversexed dogs, dogs whose penis sticks out. Prostate problems of the old dog.
Platina Metallicum	A female remedy. Oversexed females, those who mount other dogs, disrupted hormonal and heat cycles.
Podophyllum	Primarily a diarrhea remedy where there is gushing, putrid odor and mucus. Watery, greenish feces and sometimes a protusion of the anus. Worse in the morning and in hot weather.
Psorinum	Mange remedy (see also Sulphur). Skin and coat of dog are smelly. Dog is cold and seeks heat.
Pulsatilla	Female remedy, for shyness. Disrupted heats and false pregnancies. Cream-colored discharges. Usually happy dog but gets depressed easily. Used for side effects from measles and Parvo vaccines.
Rhus Tox	Poison ivy. Lameness, rheumatism. Swollen, red and itchy skin. Difficulty in getting up after sleeping.
Ruta	Use for ligament or tendon damage and sprains in general. Use if there are dislocations of joints.
Sanicula	Anal gland problems, or any genital discharges that smell fishy. Fear of being put down after being picked up.
Sarsaparilla	Urinary difficulties and urinary blockages.
Senna	Gas, bloating and flatulence.
Sepia	Female remedy. Mother who rejects puppies. Aggression in females to those they love.
Silicea	Splinters or foreign bodies that lodge in the body. It pushes them out. Shyness or "lacking grit." Brittle nails. Inflammatory conditions. To get abscesses and boils to come to a head and discharge. Brittle bones, some

	epilepsy cases, side effects from any vaccine. Use when there is pus. Skin eruptions on mouth, lips or chin.
Spongia	Congested lungs, coughing without moving, better after eating.
Sulphur	Mange remedy. Use for stubborn, smelly dogs whose skin is dry but red all over. Cleans the system, and works for diarrhea and constipation. Many skin conditions respond to this remedy.
Symphytum	Use with fractures of bones (together with arnica). Injuries to stifle joint. Eye injuries.
Thlaspi Bursa	Inflammation of urinary tract. Often replaces use of catheter in obstructions in dogs and cats. Urine that drips from dog instead of stream.
Thuja Occidentalis	Cauliflower-type warts. Combats adverse reaction to vaccines. (See the following section.)
Urtica urens	Skin remedy, when small red blotches appear. Itching and burning. Mammary glands engorged. To suppress milk use low potency (6x) and to stimulate milk flow use high potency (30c). Use in false pregnancies when milk is present and with bladder problems such as cystitis.
Zincum Metall.	Conjunctivitis, dry eye, convulsions where there is depression.

Detoxifying Side Effects from Vaccines

Thuja Occidentalis is a helpful remedy to counteract the side effects from vaccinations. These may surface anywhere up to 21 days after the vaccine has been administered. We use one dose of Thuja, 12x at bedtime for each vaccine that has been used. For example, if the dog had just received a DA$_2$LPP vaccine, this represents five vaccines, even though they were administered at the same time. The dosage would be given for 5 nights.

Giving Thuja to old dogs gives them a new lease on life. We have had great success with this. Another property of Thuja is that it diminishes and sometimes eliminates cauliflower-shaped warts. Old dogs not only have more energy, but they lose many of those unsightly growths that seem to be common to the aging dog.

Other remedies that are used to counteract the side effect of vaccines (vaccinosis), are Pulsatilla, Lachesis, Silicea and Sulphur. Use kinesiology to determine if your dog needs one of these remedies.

Another effective way to help your dog recover from these side effects is to use Viratox, a homeopathic cleanser. Viratox cleanses the system of the possible residual toxins and side effects from vaccines and clears the system of viral infections. This company makes liquid, easy-to-use products for worming, allergies, detoxification from chemical pollutants associated with long-term feeding of commercial dog food as well as environmental pollutants, cleansers for viral and bacterial attacks, as well as a general system cleanser. The general cleanser contains a combination of homeopathics and is called Theratox. It targets the liver, kidneys, intestines, blood, lymph and immune systems. It tones up the body and is a good Spring cleanser. Available either through your veterinarian or through health practitioners. (See Chapter 19.)

This company also makes a product called Supportasode, which helps cells to regenerate. We have used it for young pups to build up their systems before their first vaccination, and have continued it through the teething period to protect them from the enormous amount of stress they endure during this critical time. They also have produced an equivalent of Rescue Remedy, a combination product that helps to relieve acute stress.

Nosodes

Nosodes are homeopathic remedies made from infected tissues or disease discharges. Today there are nosodes for many of the diseases common in dogs, for example, distemper, parvo and kennel cough. Research continues on how these can be used in a preventative manner and also in actual treatment of the disease states. Short-term clinical trials have been successfully conducted in England on kennel cough. Some veterinarians have programs for giving nosodes instead of vaccinations. Other veterinarians are using them when a disease is diagnosed in an attempt to reverse the disease state.

Bach Flower Remedies

These work primarily on the emotional level and come in liquid form. They can either be added to your dog's water bowl or dropped directly into the mouth:

Rescue Remedy—A composite of 5 remedies:

Star of Bethlehem, for shock

Rock rose, for terror and panic

Impatiens for mental stress and tension
Cherry plum for desperation
Clematis for disorientation

One of the most valuable remedies to have, Rescue Remedy is administered by dropping two drops into the mouth, or rubbing into the gums. Use for shock, trauma, extreme stress, fear and unconsciousness. It brings the animal around almost immediately. Put two drops into some distilled water and pour it onto wounds or cuts. Soak feet several times daily if cut or hurt. It is known to have saved countless lives in emergencies until qualified medical help became available. Our instructors carry it on them every class they teach, and most of us carry it in our cars and emergency kits.

With all the camps, classes and seminars we have given over many years, there have only been two bad dog fights. When they happened, the owners of the dogs were in as bad shape as the dogs. On both occasions, we gave Rescue Remedy first to the owners to get them back under control (the color literally came back into their faces), and then gave it to their dogs. The dogs not only were injured, but they were upset about the condition of their owners. In this situation Rescue Remedy buys you time to make an intelligent assessment of the situation and to act accordingly. Rescue Remedy reduces the panic level of both handler and dog.

Aspen	Inexplicable fear, fear of the unknown
Red chestnut	Anticipatory fear
Cereato	Lack of confidence
Gentian	Dogs that get discouraged easily
Gorse	Hopelessness—giving up
Clematis	Lethargy with no interest in anything
Crabapple	Destructive behavior, eating disorders, obsession; helps in cleansing and healing
Olive	Abused animals that lack strength to get well
Chestnut bud	Dogs that don't learn from experience
Water violet	Dogs that want to be left alone and are happy alone
Impatiens	Lack of patience, act too quickly without thinking; use for pain and tension after accident
Heather	Dogs seeking company, cannot bear to be left alone
Agrimony	Happy dogs that get upset easily when there are arguments or fights; use after injuries for pain

Holly	Jealousy or aggresion to another dog
Larch	Dogs, usually in multi-dog households, that don't try to do their best
Mimulus	Timid, insecure, nervous, anxious, introverted; afraid to use injured limb after it has healed; fear of being alone; fear of pain and of the dark
Sweet chestnut	Overstressed dogs that indulge in self-destructive behavior
Star of Bethlehem	Shock, fright following an accident or trauma
Vervain	For an animal that tries to do too much too soon after surgery or accident

Biochemical Cell Salts

In the mid-nineteenth century, Dr. Wilhelm H. Schuessler, a German physician, discovered that electrolytes or 12 chemical salts were common to all cremated bodies. Electrolytes do not break down, burn or melt. Schuessler devised a system of treatment using these 12 salts.

Schuessler set about finding which body systems were controlled by these 12 salts. He treated diseases of these systems with the tissue salts. Subsequent scientific tests showed that these tissue salts do indeed exist in the body and are essential to health.

The tissue salts are prepared in much the same way as homeopathic remedies and are taken in similar doses. They are used as symptom relievers to rebalance the body. Since Schuessler's time, more trace elements have been identified and modern-day practitioners use these in their practice. What follows is a brief description of each of the 12 original salts and their use in people. We have used these for many years in combination form, mostly as a prophylactic for dogs with weak immune systems.

Calc Fluor.	Maintains elasticity of tissues. Good for bad circulation, varicose veins, hemorrhoids, tooth enamel.
Calc Phos.	Essential to the formation of bones, teeth and gastric juices. Good for indigestion, chilblains and teething.
Calc Sulph.	Purifies the blood. Good for acne, pimples, sores and wounds that are slow to heal and catarrh.
Ferr Phos.	Essential to the oxygenation of the blood. Good for coughs, colds, fevers, congestion and inflammation.

Kali Mur.	Keeps the blood in good condition. Good for coughs, colds, bronchitis, tonsillitis and measles.
Kali Phos.	Nutrient essential to nerves. Good for stress, worry, headaches, nervous indigestion and nervous headaches.
Kali Sulph.	Oxygenates tissue cells. Good for skin complaints, catarrh, loss of hair, poor nails and stuffiness.
Mag Phos.	The nerve stabilizer. Good for cramp, neuralgia, sharp pains, sciatica, spasms, hiccups and females experiencing pain when in season.
Nat Mur.	Distributor of water. Good for loss of taste or smell, tears, constipation, drowsiness, muscular weakness.
Nat Phos.	Acid neutralizer. Good for acidity of blood, gastric problems, heartburn, rheumatism, back pain, fibrositis.
Nat Sulph.	Eliminator of excess water. Good for liver problems, nausea, influenza, conditions made worse during humid weather.
Silic Oxide	SILICA Conditioner, cleanser and stimulator. Good for brittle nails, bones, dull hair, bad cases of body odor and boils.

Combination Remedies: These remedies can be bought together in a combination of all 12 salts or in groups. Found in many supermarkets and drug stores, they are listed by letter for certain problems, for example, Combination F for backache and allied pain, Combination R for stomach upset and so on. Since all the salts work together, I prefer to use the combination remedies for the dogs.

Summary

There is a temptation, when first learning about and then using homeopathy, to abandon traditional medicine. Once you start to read about the possibilities of its use and its enormous scope in treatment, you feel as if it is the absolute answer to everything that you encounter with your dog. *Don't succumb to this temptation.* It takes many, many years to become proficient at using homeopathy properly. The ideal is to find a veterinarian trained in both traditional as well as homeopathic medicine who will use the best treatment for the situation presented. There may be something happening to your dog that you have missed. There is no substitute for a good diagnostic work up.

If the homeopathic treatment is not working, and your dog does not improve in a few days, go to your veterinarian. Resist the temptation of jumping from one remedy to another.

This chapter recommends the use of homeopathy in acute (sudden) disease states. Classical homeopathy, where one remedy is prescribed to cure all the symptoms, is an art, and takes many years of study. There are many veterinarians who are trained this way, and their names can be found by writing to the society listed in Chapter 19.

Homeopathy is powerful when you find the correct remedy to match the problem, as illustrated by the following story: Obedience class was almost over when I heard Stu yell from the other side of the room. He was clutching his eye. He had been stung by a bee on the right bottom eyelid. He was in agony. After pulling out the stinger, I went to my emergency first-aid kit and took out Apis 12x. I gave him a dose and repeated it every 5 minutes for five doses. In half an hour, there was no swelling, no pain, and in fact you couldn't see that he had been bitten at all. Stu was able to drive home. I called the next day to see if there had been any bruising. He had forgotten all about being bitten and was feeling fine. When homeopathic remedies work, they work!

The Healing Crisis

Using homeopathy to treat acute problems, that is, those of sudden onset, with the low potencies we have suggested usually avoids a healing crisis. This is a phenomenon that is also described as an aggravation. It is the appearance of the original symptoms in an aggravated form. If you were dealing with hot spots, for instance, you could use the remedy Hepar Sulph. If used in a potency too high, it is possible that the hot spots would get bigger, or more could break out over the body. In other words, using the incorrect potency makes the existing symptoms worse. What this tells you is that you have picked the correct remedy, but the dosage is too strong. If you had used a 200c potency, you would drop down to a 30c. While alarming, it does not harm the animal, and the symptoms only last 48 hours. Allow the aggravation to pass, then use the same remedy in a lower potency. Mishandling of an aggravation by the use of drugs can suppress the disease and make it more difficult to treat. That is why using high potencies is best left to a trained homeopathist.

Chapter 17

Other Alternative Therapies

In the alternative medicine field there are many modalities that can be used in adjunct with more traditional therapies. Some are therapies and others are diagnostic tools. We have supplied in the bibliography books for further study by the reader. What follows is a synopsis of the more common alternative therapies now being practiced.

Chiropractic

This is a method of treatment based on the theory that disease is caused by interference with nerve function. By manipulating the spine and the joints of the body, normal nerve function can be reestablished and the body is able to heal itself.

The following information comes from Sue Ann Lesser, DVM, who is a senior instructor for the American Veterinary Chiropractic Association.

Veterinary chiropractic in the dog is relatively new. It excels in the treatment of biomechanical problems, thus minimizing, if not eliminating, objectionable gait patterns due to misalignments. Veterinary chiropractic can be used in conjunction with traditional veterinary medicine in the treatment of organic disorders.

Members of the American Veterinary Chiropractic Association (AVCA) are currently reviewing the human chiropractic literature as well as evaluating contemporary clinical studies in dogs in order to develop a complete canine chart. The development of the human chart was based originally on research done with animals.

Without delving into neurophysiological chiropractic theory, which is beyond the scope of this book, it is important to note that spinal misalignments can create disorders within the internal organs of the dog. Interruptions in the nervous system can occur and disorders of the internal organs through reflex neurologic pathways can create subluxations of the spine. Because of the difficulty of ascertaining which disorder came first, that of the internal organ or that of the spine, the AVCA recommends that the whole dog be adjusted so that balance is achieved between the sympathetic (thoracic-lumbar) and parasympathetic (cranial-sacral) nervous systems, both of which affect the function of the internal organs of the dog.

It is this balancing of the autonomic nervous system that achieves the optimal result when treating canine patients with internal (visceral) disorders.

Relieving musculoskeletal pain by correcting misalignments contributes to the dog's whole body function. It can be argued from a physiologic standpoint that pain is responsible for incorrect or irregular neurologic reflexes that contribute to both spinal subluxation and visceral disorders. To paraphrase a popular advertisement, "It's all connected." This principle is critical to remember when correlating spinal subluxations with visceral disorders.

The following relationships between organic diseases and spinal subluxations can be made. The reader is advised that the diseases listed below may also have causes beyond simple chiropractic subluxations, and **that the dog should be examined by a traditional veterinarian prior to referral to a veterinary chiropractor.** A veterinary chiropractor will refer patients back to the primary care traditional veterinarian when certain diseases (e.g., Lyme disease, hypothyroidism and cystitis) are suspected from the chiropractic exam.

Cervical subluxations (especially of the atlas, occiput and axis) can be related to various behavioral abnormalities: the slow learner, the hyperactive dog, the dog with attention deficit, blurred vision—especially in certain types of fear-biters, sound sensitivity, recurrent ear infections, certain varieties of seizures and olfactory disorders.

Mid- and lower cervical subluxations can be related to motion sickness, certain anxiety states, lick granulomas and hypothyroidism. Subluxations in the thoracic region between the shoulder blades can be related to hypothyroidism, heart problems (especially mitral valve insufficiencies in older dogs) and liver disorders.

In the horse, subluxations in the area of the withers are related to lung problems, including allergic bronchitis, chronic obstructive pulmonary disease and both inflammatory and infectious diseases of the respiratory tract. There is no reason to suspect that a similar situation does not also exist in the dog, but this has yet to be definitively demonstrated.

Thoraco-lumbar junction **subluxations** are the most common in the dog and can be related to both cystitis and diarrhea. **Caudal lumbar subluxations** combined with sacral rotations are related to acute onset incontinence and constipation. Thoraco-lumbar and cervical subluxations can also be manifested as incontinence. Back pain from **athletic overindulgence** can also create incontinence. The chiropractic diagnosis

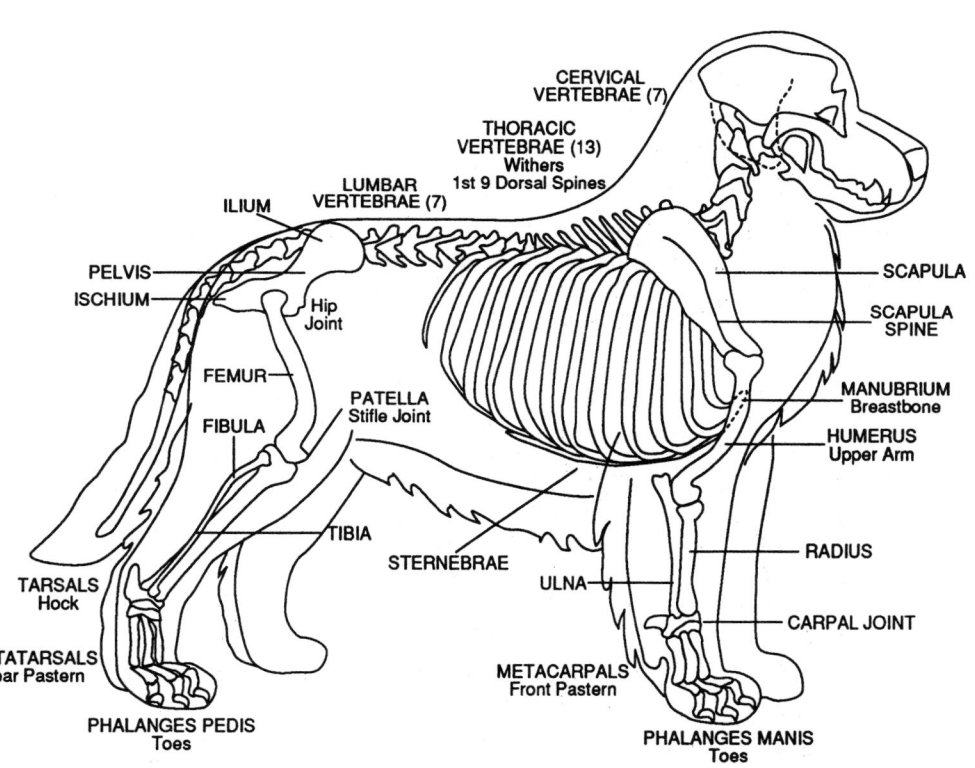

17-1: Comparative Skeletal Diagram

CERVICAL
VERTEBRAE (7)

THORACIC
VERTEBRAE (13)
Withers
1st 9 Dorsal Spines

LUMBAR
VERTEBRAE (7)

ILIUM

PELVIS

ISCHIUM

Hip
Joint

FEMUR

FIBULA

PATELLA
Stifle Joint

TIBIA

TARSALS
Hock

METATARSALS
Rear Pastern

PHALANGES PEDIS
Toes

STERNEBRAE

ULNA

METACARPALS
Front Pastern

PHALANGES MANIS
Toes

SCAPULA

SCAPULA
SPINE

MANUBRIUM
Breastbone

HUMERUS
Upper Arm

RADIUS

CARPAL JOINT

of **hypothyroidism** depends on a number of subluxations found simultaneously; the condition is then confirmed by a laboratory analysis.

The subluxation complex is profoundly affected by exercise, environmental conditions (ice, snow, slippery floors etc.), emotional stresses (kenneling, etc.) and nutrition. Dogs fed properly do not exhibit the spinal abnormalities of dogs whose nutritional needs are not met. A proper nutritional plane will improve the dog's chiropractic picture, as demonstrated elsewhere in this book.

Although every dog is an individual, certain patient histories and current physical findings are consistent for the new canine chiropractic patient. Dogs that have one or more of the following symptoms or experiences should ideally be examined by an experienced, qualified veterinary chiropractor. Most dogs with a combination of these histories and physical signs have required adjustment. Other medical conditions can contribute to the physical signs listed. **Veterinary chiropractic is an addition to, not a replacement for, traditional veterinary care.**

History

1. Hit by a car.
2. Playing, then becoming suddenly lame. Lameness usually improves with minimal traditional treatment but dog is never "quite right" afterward.
3. "Body slamming"—patient is sideswiped by another dog while playing and gets rolled.
4. Fell off the porch, deck, downstairs etc.
5. Lost balance while running and hit wall, tree, door, etc.
6. Any dog working in Obedience, Agility, Schutzhund, etc.
7. All German Shepherd Dogs over 4 years of age.
8. Dogs that play Frisbee.
9. Decreasing performance—especially show dogs that show inconsistent behavior and are not doing as well as they used to in either Conformation or Obedience.
10. Dogs that have been put under general anesthesia.
11. Dogs that cannot jump on couch, bed etc., or won't go up and down stairs.
12. Poor leash manners—number one cause of cervical subluxations.

Physical Findings

1. Personality change, not as active or happy. May start biting, or look like they have a headache. Dogs that have faces that continuously look anxious.
2. A tail that does not wag symmetrically.
3. Stiff back, does not roll, or rolls and stops at one point.

4. Lumpy/bumpy feeling through the spine, especially near back of the rib cage.
5. Head tilt, or dog has problems in turning head in one direction.
6. Scuffs one foot when gaiting.
7. "Baby with wet diapers" look—gait in rear stilted.
8. Lack of symmetry limb to limb—catches or rattles through shoulder or hock.
9. Tail clamped to body or under body. Tail held straight out, not relaxed.
10. Dog wiggles skin on back or shakes when a particular point is touched.
11. Hip dysplasia: While chiropractic cannot cure the truly dysplastic dog, it can make the dog more comfortable and balanced.
12. Esthetics: Instead of seeing the whole dog, the eye is drawn to one part of the dog (back, pelvis, head, neck etc.). Correct dogs have a certain presence about them, a sort of glow. If you have difficulty determining if the dog being examined is gaiting properly or not, have the animal chiropractically examined.

When our dogs are at their showing and training peak, they go for adjustments every month to counteract the stresses of travel and work—especially jumping. Dogs that are regularly adjusted this way have longer show careers than those dogs who are not worked on chiropractically.

Behavior problems that involve aggression or those that do not fit the norm should always be checked out by a competent veterinary chiropractor before any decision is made on how to treat the dog.

Further information on veterinary chiropractic as well as certified individuals can be obtained from the American Veterinary Chiropractic Association, P.O. Box 249, Port Byron, IL 61275 (309) 523-3995.

Iridology

This is another tool to use in diagnosing health. Based on the concept that the eyes mirror the health of the body, it was first discovered by Ignatz von Peczeley. As a young man he kept a pet owl. The owl broke a leg and correspondingly, von Peczeley noticed a "hole" in the iris of both the owl's eyes. When the leg healed, the "holes" disappeared. Von Peczeley charted all of his patients thereafter, recording the correlation between the spots in the eyes and the diseases presented. Iridology is practiced widely in Europe today and many medical doctors are trained in this accurate diagnostic approach.

View the eye as a clock, each eye being a mirror image of the other. (When left or right is mentioned, it refers to the dog's left or right, not

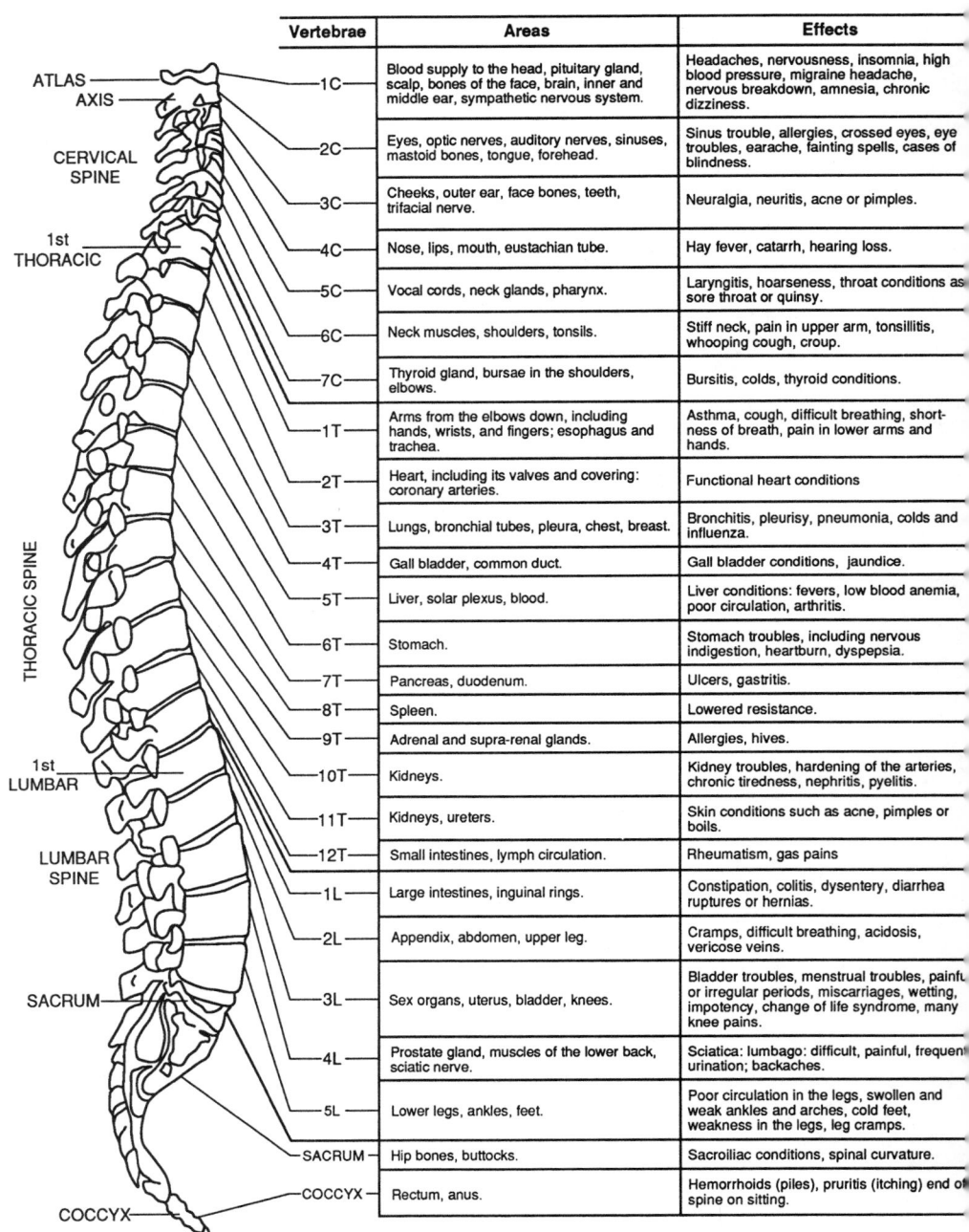

Vertebrae	Areas	Effects
1C	Blood supply to the head, pituitary gland, scalp, bones of the face, brain, inner and middle ear, sympathetic nervous system.	Headaches, nervousness, insomnia, high blood pressure, migraine headache, nervous breakdown, amnesia, chronic dizziness.
2C	Eyes, optic nerves, auditory nerves, sinuses, mastoid bones, tongue, forehead.	Sinus trouble, allergies, crossed eyes, eye troubles, earache, fainting spells, cases of blindness.
3C	Cheeks, outer ear, face bones, teeth, trifacial nerve.	Neuralgia, neuritis, acne or pimples.
4C	Nose, lips, mouth, eustachian tube.	Hay fever, catarrh, hearing loss.
5C	Vocal cords, neck glands, pharynx.	Laryngitis, hoarseness, throat conditions as sore throat or quinsy.
6C	Neck muscles, shoulders, tonsils.	Stiff neck, pain in upper arm, tonsillitis, whooping cough, croup.
7C	Thyroid gland, bursae in the shoulders, elbows.	Bursitis, colds, thyroid conditions.
1T	Arms from the elbows down, including hands, wrists, and fingers; esophagus and trachea.	Asthma, cough, difficult breathing, shortness of breath, pain in lower arms and hands.
2T	Heart, including its valves and covering; coronary arteries.	Functional heart conditions
3T	Lungs, bronchial tubes, pleura, chest, breast.	Bronchitis, pleurisy, pneumonia, colds and influenza.
4T	Gall bladder, common duct.	Gall bladder conditions, jaundice.
5T	Liver, solar plexus, blood.	Liver conditions: fevers, low blood anemia, poor circulation, arthritis.
6T	Stomach.	Stomach troubles, including nervous indigestion, heartburn, dyspepsia.
7T	Pancreas, duodenum.	Ulcers, gastritis.
8T	Spleen.	Lowered resistance.
9T	Adrenal and supra-renal glands.	Allergies, hives.
10T	Kidneys.	Kidney troubles, hardening of the arteries, chronic tiredness, nephritis, pyelitis.
11T	Kidneys, ureters.	Skin conditions such as acne, pimples or boils.
12T	Small intestines, lymph circulation.	Rheumatism, gas pains
1L	Large intestines, inguinal rings.	Constipation, colitis, dysentery, diarrhea ruptures or hernias.
2L	Appendix, abdomen, upper leg.	Cramps, difficult breathing, acidosis, vericose veins.
3L	Sex organs, uterus, bladder, knees.	Bladder troubles, menstrual troubles, painful or irregular periods, miscarriages, wetting, impotency, change of life syndrome, many knee pains.
4L	Prostate gland, muscles of the lower back, sciatic nerve.	Sciatica: lumbago: difficult, painful, frequent urination; backaches.
5L	Lower legs, ankles, feet.	Poor circulation in the legs, swollen and weak ankles and arches, cold feet, weakness in the legs, leg cramps.
SACRUM	Hip bones, buttocks.	Sacroiliac conditions, spinal curvature.
COCCYX	Rectum, anus.	Hemorrhoids (piles), pruritis (itching) end of spine on sitting.

17-2: Chart of Effects of Spinal Misalignments (Human)

218

yours.) Not all diseases show up in both eyes. The eye needs to be observed in strong sunlight or with a flashlight. If a flashlight is used, do not leave it on the eye for more than 10 seconds before removing it.

Think of the eye as a tunnel to the body, with the outside rim of the iris representing the skin and the innermost part of the iris next to the pupil, as internal organs such as the stomach and intestines. Any discolorations or markings mean something to an iridologist, who can predict diseases up to two years prior to clinical manifestation. Abnormalities also reveal inherited diseases. For example, if you have a dog whose mother had heart disease, you may notice a black spot or hole between the 2 and 3 o'clock positions on your dog's left eye. This does not necessarily mean that your dog has heart disease. What it is more likely to mean is that there is an inherited *tendency* toward weakness in the heart.

Iridology can be an invaluable tool for breeders because it can indicate possible genetic disorders in breeding animals. A simple understanding of iridology shows the breeder *not* to double up on breed-specific problems. Why, for example, double up on a dog with inherited heart weakness if you have a choice of another dog that does not carry that weakness?

When we were breeding Newfoundlands, stock was routinely selected for dark eyes. It was thought that dark brown, almost black eyes denoted good overall pigmentation. Understanding iridology taught us that aside from genetically dark brown eyes, there are eyes that *appear* dark brown because the body is toxic. The difference is that a healthy dog can bring into a breeding program genes for good pigmentation versus an unhealthy dog, who does not possess these genes.

Genetically dark brown eyes of a healthy dog have a sparkle and shine to them. The whites of the eyes are clear with no bleeding out of the rim of the iris. The color of the iris, while being dark brown, is clear of markings. Toxic brown eyes, on the other hand, look as if there is a film of darkness over them; the eyes have many black markings on the iris, and the outside of the iris bleeds into the white of the eye. This "bleeding" effect is a sign of toxins in the system and can be associated with chronic skin problems. These eyes appear dull and without life.

One amusing side effect that we had when studying this subject was with our Labrador, Bean. When we got Bean he was quite unhealthy and it took us several years to get him to the state of health that we felt was acceptable. As a young puppy, he had the most beautiful dark, almost black eyes. As the healing progressed, his eyes got lighter and lighter, until today, at age 7, he has light brown eyes with many black specks in them, which represent all the inherited health difficulties.

Light

Light plays an important part in the health, growth, reproduction and behavior of animals. Dogs housed in an area that has improper light have been observed with chronic skin disease, an inability to reproduce, strange and neurotic behaviors and improper growth in young dogs. There may be a direct correlation between the rise in dental decay in dogs and the use of improper light.

Light controls the survival mechanisms of most species of animals. Young animals almost universally are brought into the world in the spring. This is when there is enough food for the young to eat. It would be non-adaptive behavior to have young in the fall or winter, when it is often impossible to forage for food. Animals instinctively know by the quality of light in their environment, what time of the year it is. *They must know this if the species is to survive.* If light is controlled, or is of inferior quality, it gives false information to the animal's brain, triggering inappropriate behavior.

What is improper light? Regular bulbs that are used in lighting fixtures and fluorescent cool white lights are found in hospitals, offices, homes and kennels. Many articles have been written about the effect of light on behavior of animals. One that caught our eye was from the *Journal of Optometry*, June 1979. This article talked about effects of light on rats' breeding behaviors. Male rats raised under normal fluorescent lighting had to be taken away from the females before they gave birth, due to the males' tendency to eat the babies as they were born. Under full spectrum lighting, the male rat showed good parental instincts and helped to take care of the young.

Other experiments were done on fish, where it is normal to keep different species apart because of fighting and fin nipping. Under full spectrum lights, it was possible to keep the fish together with no fighting displayed.

Experiments were conducted on mice divided into two groups. One group was exposed to daylight and others were exposed to pink fluorescent lights. These experiments were run by John Ott, head of the Environmental Health and Light Research Institute in Florida, who is the foremost authority on the effect of light on health. In six months, mice under the pink lights had lost their tails! In another experiment, spontaneous tumors arose on those mice continually exposed to fluorescent light.

A brand of full spectrum lighting that is easy to obtain is called Vita Lite. See Chapter 19 for more information.

Full spectrum lighting with an extra amount of blue (kiva lights) decreases bacteria and inhibits the spread of disease in an area where a lot of dogs are housed. These lights are used in supermarkets to keep bacteria from growing on exposed meat and fish. They have been used to promote healing in hospitals. If put above counters and sinks, the light penetrates the water, which becomes softer.

Color and Light

Many experiments have been conducted on the effect of color and light. People who wear tinted contact lenses or sunglasses have shown a marked decrease in muscle strength when natural light was not allowed to penetrate the eyes. Moods of tennis players and baseball players have been monitored by changing the color of the visors they wear to protect their eyes from the sun. Athletes who already showed temperamental behavior had their sunglasses, visors and uniform colors changed. Hyperaggressive, helmet-throwing athletes then become calm, relaxed and confident when the proper colors were used.

How does this information help us with our dogs? Dogs need to have time in their day when they are outside getting daylight. Even if they are in the shade of a tree, they are still getting adequate light. In bad weather and during long hard winters they are denied that light. Using full spectrum lighting in a kennel, house or veterinary hospital will yield a more calm, relaxed and healthier animal. Sick animals will heal faster and breeding cycles will become normal.

If you are decorating a kennel, choose blue as your primary color as it is the most calming color, green for good overall health and white, which is neutral. Stay away from red, bright pink, orange and yellow, which can create aggression and sickness from prolonged exposure.

Dr. Parcell's Food Cleansing

Hazel Parcell, Ph.D., D.C., N.D., has created a system for cleansing food of pesticides, fungi, parasites, bacteria and heavy metals. This has been valuable when working with natural food diets.

When a small amount of chlorine bleach is added to a large amount of water and raw foods are soaked in the mixture, the bleach acts like a magnet to toxins. Dr. Parcell maintains that there are many advantages to using this system. Fruits and vegetables last much longer, and wilted vegetables return to their normal crispness and the flavor is enhanced. Most of the toxins used in the production of that food are removed. This is particularly important for apples and grapes, for example, which are sprayed at least 15 times before they reach the marketplace.

Using the System

Sort the vegetables and fruits into different piles. Eggs and meat should be separated. Use $1/2$ teaspoon of Clorox bleach to 1 gallon of water. Fruits and vegetables are soaked for 10 minutes, then rinsed. Fill up the sink and

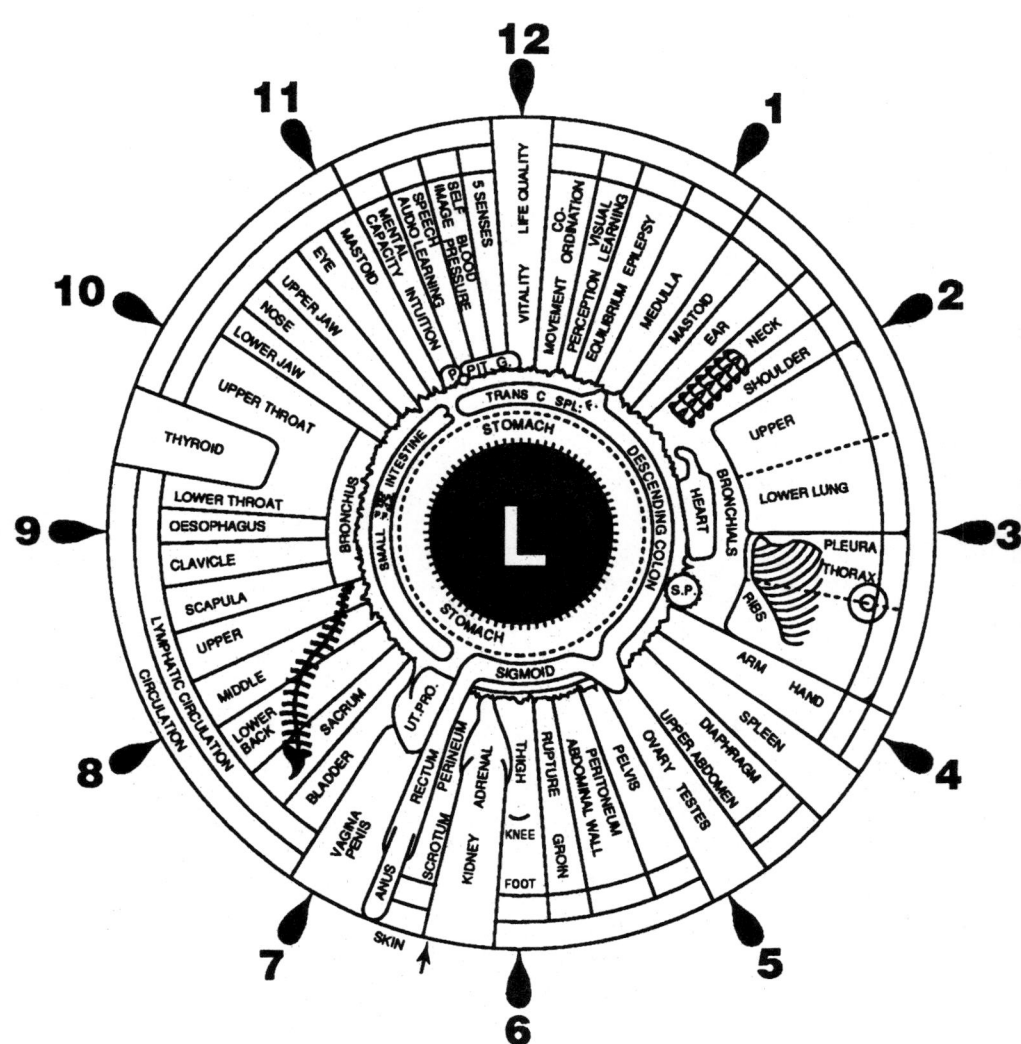

The Iris Map, Left Eye
(looking at another person's left eye)

17-3a: Iridology Chart

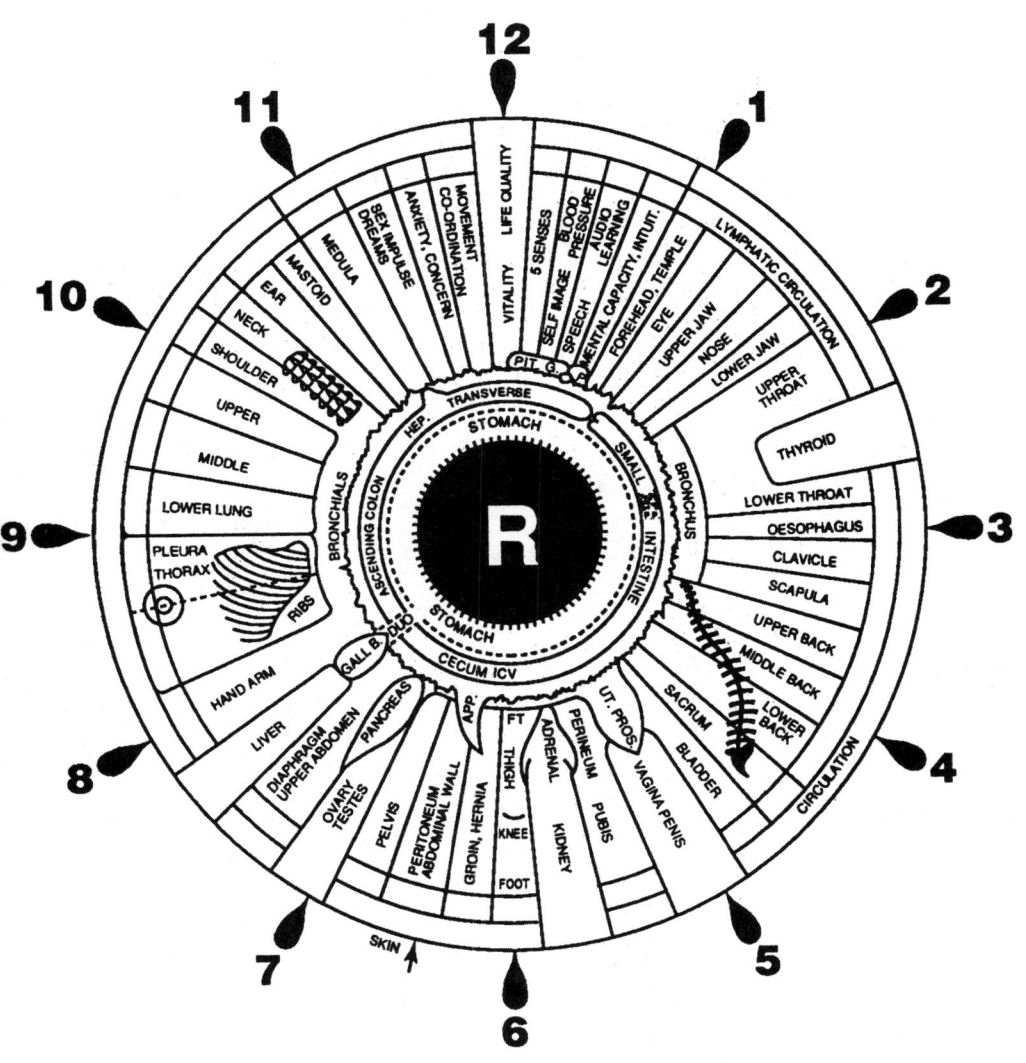

The Iris Map, Right Eye
(looking at another person's right eye)

17-3b: Iridology Chart

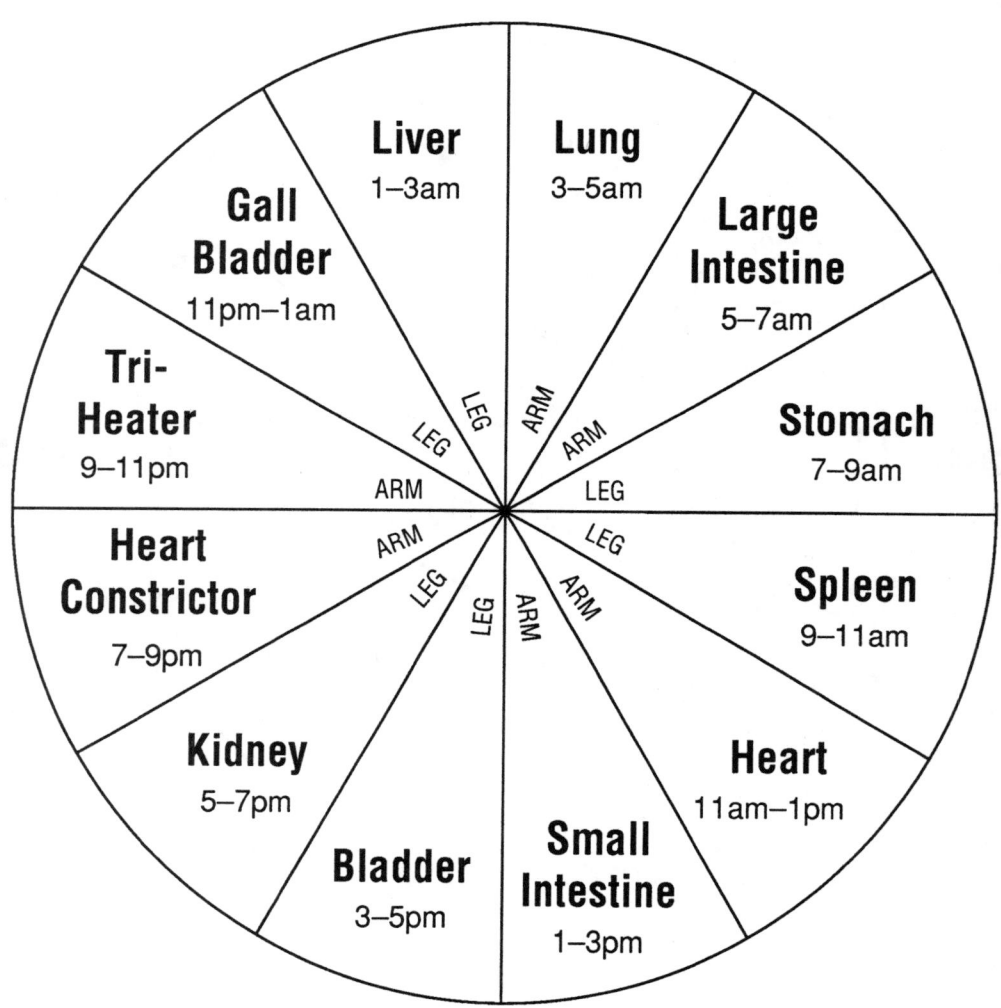

17-4: General Circulation Energy

soak again in fresh water for 10 minutes. Drain and store. Eggs should be soaked in the bleach bath for 30 minutes and then rinsed as above, and meat should be soaked for 10 to 15 minutes for 2 to 5 pounds of meat, then rinsed as above.

We have successfully used this cleansing system for years. Indeed, the fruit and vegetables last twice as long and retain their crispness. When we are lazy, there is a noticeable difference in the length of time the food lasts.

Chronobiology

This is a theory of time and rhythm. Chronobiology studies the interaction of time among the nervous, hormonal and metabolic systems in the body. It means that at any given time of the day, the energy of the body in certain systems is either ebbing or flowing. If these times can be determined, then using medication targeted at certain organs would be more effective. It also means that false/negative responses may be recorded if diagnostic procedures are carried out at the wrong time of the day. This concept has been effectively used in diagnosing heartworm.

When diagnostic work is being done on a dog, draw blood and do other diagnostic testing when the energy is in that organ (see chart on previous page). For example, if you want to make an accurate kidney diagnosis, have your veterinarian draw blood between 5 and 7 P.M. in the evening. If kidney medication is indicated, it would make sense to give it to your dog at that time. Stanford University is doing a lot of work on people using the concepts of chronobiology; however, more work needs to be done with animals.

Aggression
AT A GLANCE

CAUSES & SYMPTOMS

NEARLY ALWAYS ASSOCIATED WITH LIVER PROBLEMS WHEN AGGRESSION IS DIRECTED TOWARDS PEOPLE, ANIMALS OR UNPROVOKED. SEEN MOSTLY FROM MARCH-JUNE.
AGGRESSION FROM FEAR IS RELATED TO KIDNEY PROBLEMS, MORE OFTER SEEN IN WINTER FROM LATE DECEMBER TO EARLY MARCH, BUT CAN BE ANY TIME OF YEAR.
DOG IS TOXIC IN BOTH INSTANCES.
THIS CAN BE CAUSED THROUGH IMPROPER DIET, PLUS OVER-VACCINATION.

BITING OR SNAPPING AT PEOPLE, OTHER ANIMALS OR RANDOMLY.
POOR VISION, INFLAMED EARS, ALLERGIC REACTIONS TO ENVIRONMENT OR TO RABIES VACCINE.
CERVICAL, THORACIC OR LUMBAR VERTEBRAE OUT OF ALIGNMENT, CAUSING PAIN.
POSSIBLE THYROID OR ADRENAL GLAND INVOLVEMENT.
AGGRESSION CAN BE CAUSED FROM MISHANDLING AND A MISUNDERSTANDING OF DOG BEHAVIOR.

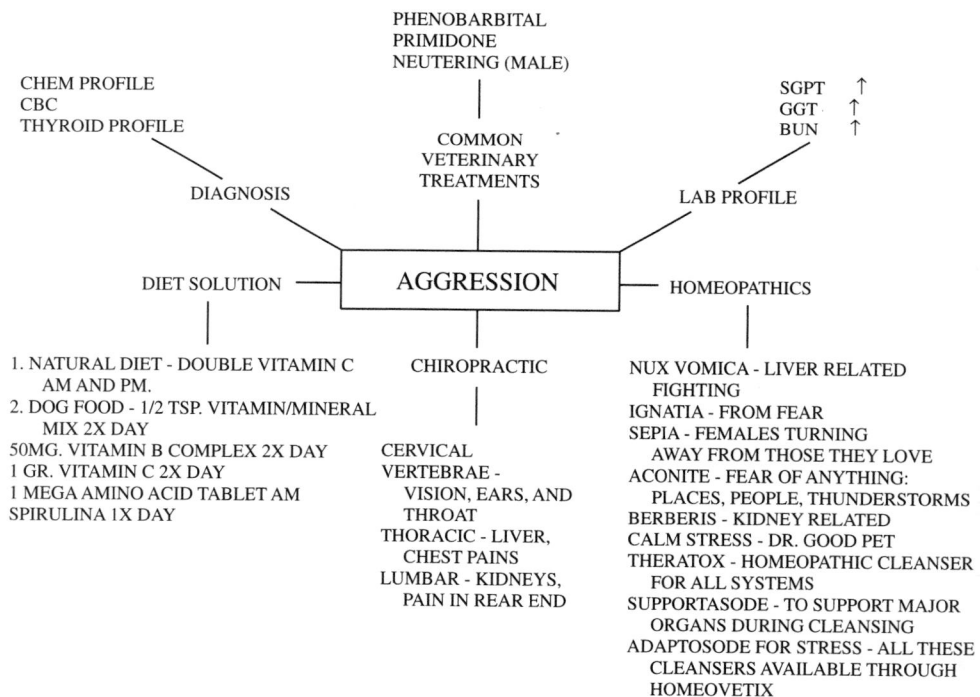

PHENOBARBITAL
PRIMIDONE
NEUTERING (MALE)

CHEM PROFILE
CBC
THYROID PROFILE

COMMON
VETERINARY
TREATMENTS

SGPT ↑
GGT ↑
BUN ↑

DIAGNOSIS

LAB PROFILE

DIET SOLUTION —

AGGRESSION

— HOMEOPATHICS

1. NATURAL DIET - DOUBLE VITAMIN C AM AND PM.
2. DOG FOOD - 1/2 TSP. VITAMIN/MINERAL MIX 2X DAY
50MG. VITAMIN B COMPLEX 2X DAY
1 GR. VITAMIN C 2X DAY
1 MEGA AMINO ACID TABLET AM
SPIRULINA 1X DAY

CHIROPRACTIC

CERVICAL
VERTEBRAE -
VISION, EARS, AND
THROAT
THORACIC - LIVER,
CHEST PAINS
LUMBAR - KIDNEYS,
PAIN IN REAR END

NUX VOMICA - LIVER RELATED FIGHTING
IGNATIA - FROM FEAR
SEPIA - FEMALES TURNING AWAY FROM THOSE THEY LOVE
ACONITE - FEAR OF ANYTHING: PLACES, PEOPLE, THUNDERSTORMS
BERBERIS - KIDNEY RELATED
CALM STRESS - DR. GOOD PET
THERATOX - HOMEOPATHIC CLEANSER FOR ALL SYSTEMS
SUPPORTASODE - TO SUPPORT MAJOR ORGANS DURING CLEANSING
ADAPTOSODE FOR STRESS - ALL THESE CLEANSERS AVAILABLE THROUGH HOMEOVETIX

Chapter 18

At a Glance

The following charts are intended as an easy reference guide to certain diseases or conditions. Your dog may express only one or two of the symptoms listed.

Each chart is divided into sections for symptoms, possible causes, diet, homeopathy, chiropractic, laboratory profiles and drugs for that disease state. The suggestions on treatment are the most commonly used to cure these states. For further information we refer the reader back to the chapters covering each individual subject. The suggestions in each column should be checked by using kinesiology, to ascertain which is the correct treatment for your dog.

We have used the Natural Diet in many instances because we have had excellent results. It provides the greatest latitude in tailoring a diet to the individual dog. This is labeled (1). Supplementation to the correctly tested dog food, where applicable, is labeled (2). The amounts suggested are for a 50-pound dog and should be calculated for different weights. Some common herbal treatments are also listed.

The laboratory profile column indicates what tests should be done with a dog exhibiting certain symptoms. It also pinpoints the changes expected with that disease state and helps to eliminate other diseases, too. It confirms the diagnoses done by physical examination that will determine what tests are necessary.

Homeopathics are listed that cover the widest possible symptom etiology. You will need to use kinesiology to ascertain which remedy is correct for your dog.

Common drugs or treatments are listed for each disease. If the disease shows that there are several approaches that can be taken, then by using kinesiology, check to see which is the correct one for your dog.

In many instances, regular chiropractic adjustments have produced wonderful results.

Many disease states relate to an improperly functioning thyroid gland. When in doubt, have your veterinarian run the appropriate tests.

Allergies—Acute
AT A GLANCE

<u>CAUSES & SYMPTOMS</u>

STRESS FROM INCORRECT DIET
DEFICIENCIES IN DIET OF VITAMINS,
MINERALS AND PROPER PROTEIN
ENVIRONMENTAL POLLUTANTS -
   POLLENS, GARDEN OR
   HOUSEHOLD SPRAYS
FLEA, TICK, SPIDER OR INSECT BITES
   (VENOMS)
DRUG REACTIONS
VACCINES
ANAPHYLAXIS
THYROID OR ADRENAL GLAND
   INVOLVEMENT

* GENERALIZED HIVES
* FACIAL SWELLING
* RAPID TO DIFFICULT BREATHING
* SHOCK
  DIARRHEA
  SLUGGISHNESS
  IRRITABILITY

* THESE ARE EMERGENCY SITUATIONS

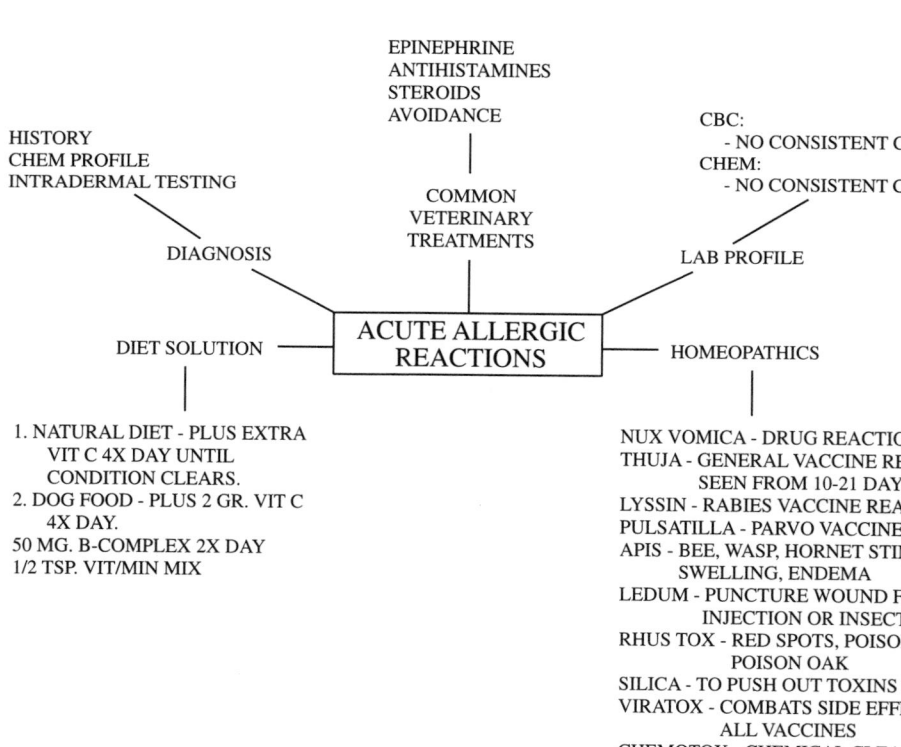

EPINEPHRINE
ANTIHISTAMINES
STEROIDS
AVOIDANCE

HISTORY
CHEM PROFILE
INTRADERMAL TESTING

CBC:
  - NO CONSISTENT CHANGES
CHEM:
  - NO CONSISTENT CHANGES

COMMON
VETERINARY
TREATMENTS

DIAGNOSIS

LAB PROFILE

DIET SOLUTION — ACUTE ALLERGIC REACTIONS — HOMEOPATHICS

1. NATURAL DIET - PLUS EXTRA
   VIT C 4X DAY UNTIL
   CONDITION CLEARS.
2. DOG FOOD - PLUS 2 GR. VIT C
   4X DAY.
50 MG. B-COMPLEX 2X DAY
1/2 TSP. VIT/MIN MIX

NUX VOMICA - DRUG REACTION
THUJA - GENERAL VACCINE REACTION
   SEEN FROM 10-21 DAYS AFTER
LYSSIN - RABIES VACCINE REACTION
PULSATILLA - PARVO VACCINE REACTION
APIS - BEE, WASP, HORNET STING, SHINY
   SWELLING, ENDEMA
LEDUM - PUNCTURE WOUND FROM
   INJECTION OR INSECT BITE
RHUS TOX - RED SPOTS, POISON IVY,
   POISON OAK
SILICA - TO PUSH OUT TOXINS FROM BODY
VIRATOX - COMBATS SIDE EFFECTS FROM
   ALL VACCINES
CHEMOTOX - CHEMICAL CLEANSING
   BUILD UP FROM FOOD OR
   POLLUTANTS
THERATOX - GENERAL SYSTEMS CLEANSE
ADAPTOSODE - GENERALIZED STRESS TO
   SYSTEM
CALM STRESS
RESCUE REMEDY - SHOCK

Allergies—Chronic
AT A GLANCE

CAUSES & SYMPTOMS

FOOD - ALLERGY TO
   INGREDIENTS
DEFICIENCIES IN ANIMAL
   PROTEIN, VITAMINS AND
   MINERALS
DIET TOO ALKALINE
METABOLIC AND GENETICALLY
   INHERITED DISEASES
ENVIRONMENTAL CAUSES

RED, DISCHARGING EYES
INFLAMED, ITCHING EARS
INFLAMED, ITCHING SKIN
SEBORRHEA
DERMATITIS
PROBLEMS WITH BONES, TENDONS,
   LIGAMENTS

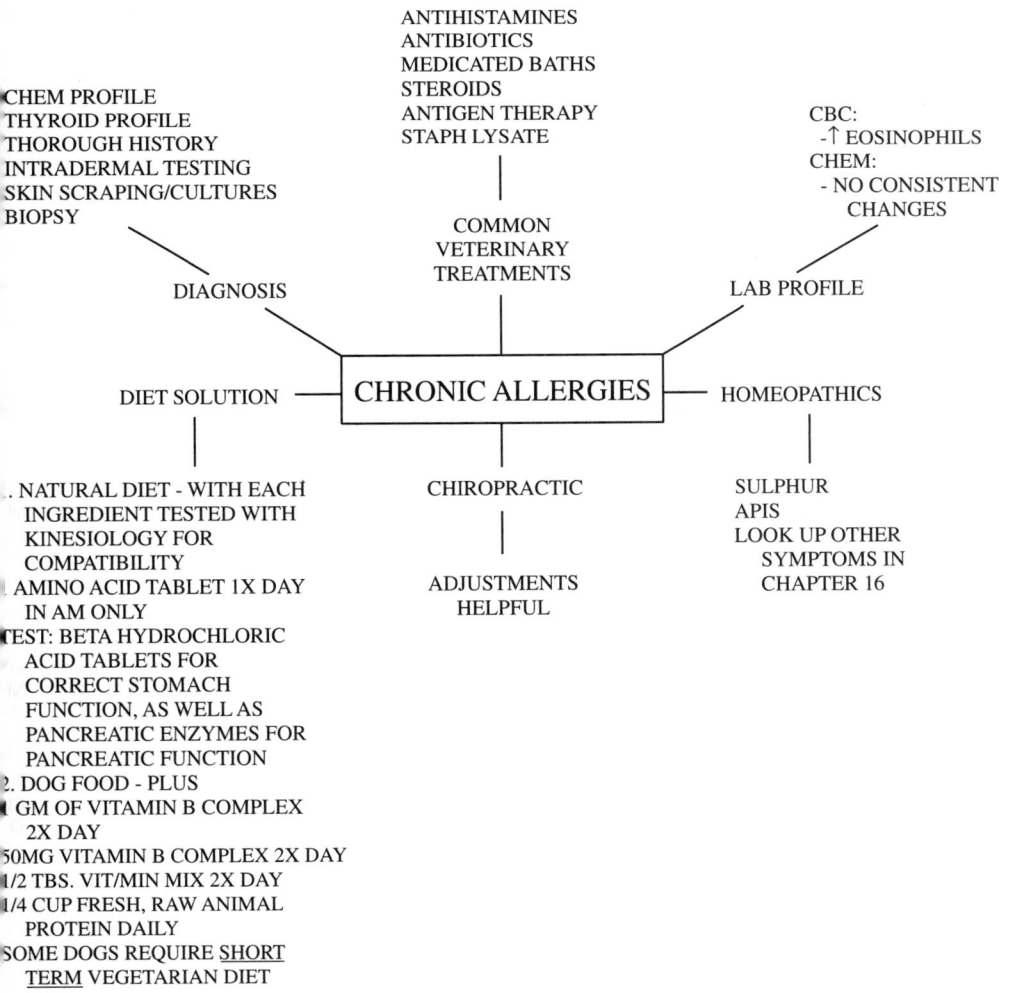

ANTIHISTAMINES
ANTIBIOTICS
MEDICATED BATHS
STEROIDS
ANTIGEN THERAPY
STAPH LYSATE

COMMON
VETERINARY
TREATMENTS

CHEM PROFILE
THYROID PROFILE
THOROUGH HISTORY
INTRADERMAL TESTING
SKIN SCRAPING/CULTURES
BIOPSY

DIAGNOSIS

CBC:
-↑ EOSINOPHILS
CHEM:
- NO CONSISTENT
   CHANGES

LAB PROFILE

CHRONIC ALLERGIES

DIET SOLUTION

HOMEOPATHICS

CHIROPRACTIC

ADJUSTMENTS
HELPFUL

SULPHUR
APIS
LOOK UP OTHER
   SYMPTOMS IN
   CHAPTER 16

1. NATURAL DIET - WITH EACH
   INGREDIENT TESTED WITH
   KINESIOLOGY FOR
   COMPATIBILITY
AMINO ACID TABLET 1X DAY
   IN AM ONLY
TEST: BETA HYDROCHLORIC
   ACID TABLETS FOR
   CORRECT STOMACH
   FUNCTION, AS WELL AS
   PANCREATIC ENZYMES FOR
   PANCREATIC FUNCTION
2. DOG FOOD - PLUS
GM OF VITAMIN B COMPLEX
   2X DAY
50MG VITAMIN B COMPLEX 2X DAY
1/2 TBS. VIT/MIN MIX 2X DAY
1/4 CUP FRESH, RAW ANIMAL
   PROTEIN DAILY
SOME DOGS REQUIRE <u>SHORT</u>
   <u>TERM</u> VEGETARIAN DIET

Bloat
AT A GLANCE

CAUSES & SYMPTOMS

INHERITED TENDENCY IN SOME
  BREEDS
STRESS FROM IMPROPER DIET
  AND MANAGEMENT
DIET TOO ALKALINE
STOMACH ACID TOO WEAK
FOOD STAYS TOO LONG IN
  STOMACH
THYROID MALFUNCTION
VACCINE RELATED

GASTRIC DILATION WITH VOLVULUS
DOG'S ABDOMEN IS HARD & DISTENDED
  (WITH GAS)
ESPECIALLY NOTICEABLE ON LEFT SIDE
DOG MAY DROOL & DRY HEAVE, VOMIT
HEAD USUALLY LEVEL WITH OR LOWER
  FROM BACKLINE
SHOCK CAN ENSUE RAPIDLY
GET TO VETERINARIAN IMMEDIATELY
THIS IS AN EMERGENCY

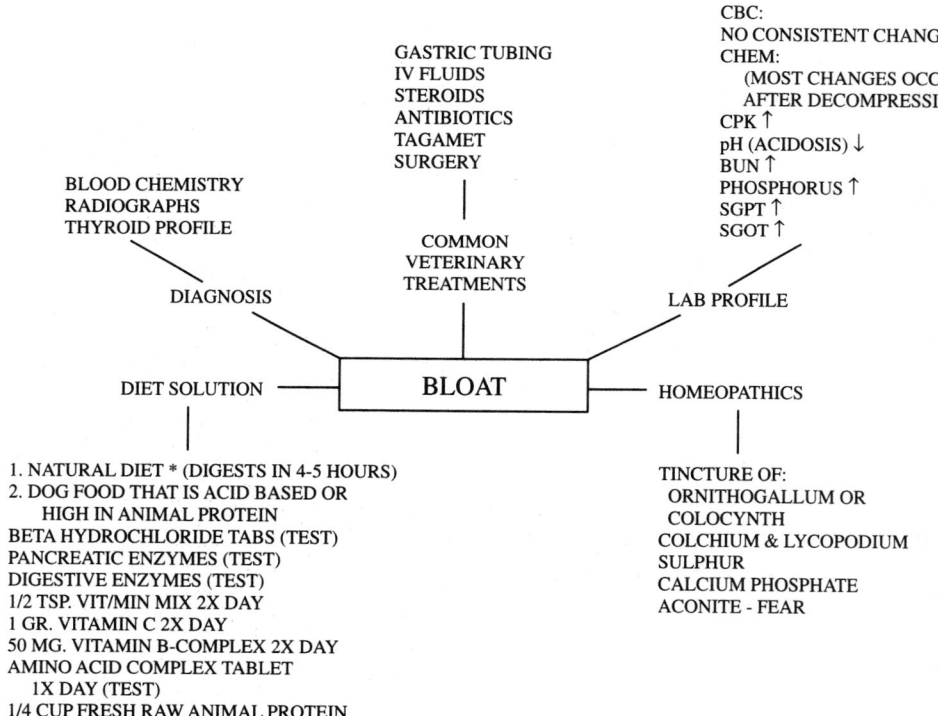

BLOOD CHEMISTRY
RADIOGRAPHS
THYROID PROFILE

DIAGNOSIS

GASTRIC TUBING
IV FLUIDS
STEROIDS
ANTIBIOTICS
TAGAMET
SURGERY

COMMON
VETERINARY
TREATMENTS

CBC:
NO CONSISTENT CHANGE
CHEM:
  (MOST CHANGES OCCUR
  AFTER DECOMPRESSION
CPK ↑
pH (ACIDOSIS) ↓
BUN ↑
PHOSPHORUS ↑
SGPT ↑
SGOT ↑

LAB PROFILE

DIET SOLUTION — **BLOAT** — HOMEOPATHICS

1. NATURAL DIET * (DIGESTS IN 4-5 HOURS)
2. DOG FOOD THAT IS ACID BASED OR
  HIGH IN ANIMAL PROTEIN
BETA HYDROCHLORIDE TABS (TEST)
PANCREATIC ENZYMES (TEST)
DIGESTIVE ENZYMES (TEST)
1/2 TSP. VIT/MIN MIX 2X DAY
1 GR. VITAMIN C 2X DAY
50 MG. VITAMIN B-COMPLEX 2X DAY
AMINO ACID COMPLEX TABLET
  1X DAY (TEST)
1/4 CUP FRESH RAW ANIMAL PROTEIN
MOISTEN BEFORE FEEDING

TINCTURE OF:
  ORNITHOGALLUM OR
  COLOCYNTH
COLCHIUM & LYCOPODIUM
SULPHUR
CALCIUM PHOSPHATE
ACONITE - FEAR

* NATURAL DIET CONTAINS RAW FOODS FULL OF DIGESTIVE ENZYMES. BLOAT IS ALMOST UNHEARD OF
WHEN FEEDING A BALANCED NATURAL DIET. DIET MUST BE KEPT ON ACIDIC SIDE FOR THESE DOGS.
GRAINS OF CHOICE: OATS AND WHEAT.

Cystitis
AT A GLANCE

CAUSES & SYMPTOMS

DIET IS TOO ALKALINE
HAPPENS MORE OFTEN IN WINTER

FREQUENT URINATION OFTEN
WITH STRAINING
ONLY A FEW DROPS AT A TIME
ACCIDENTS IN HOUSE
BLOODY URINE

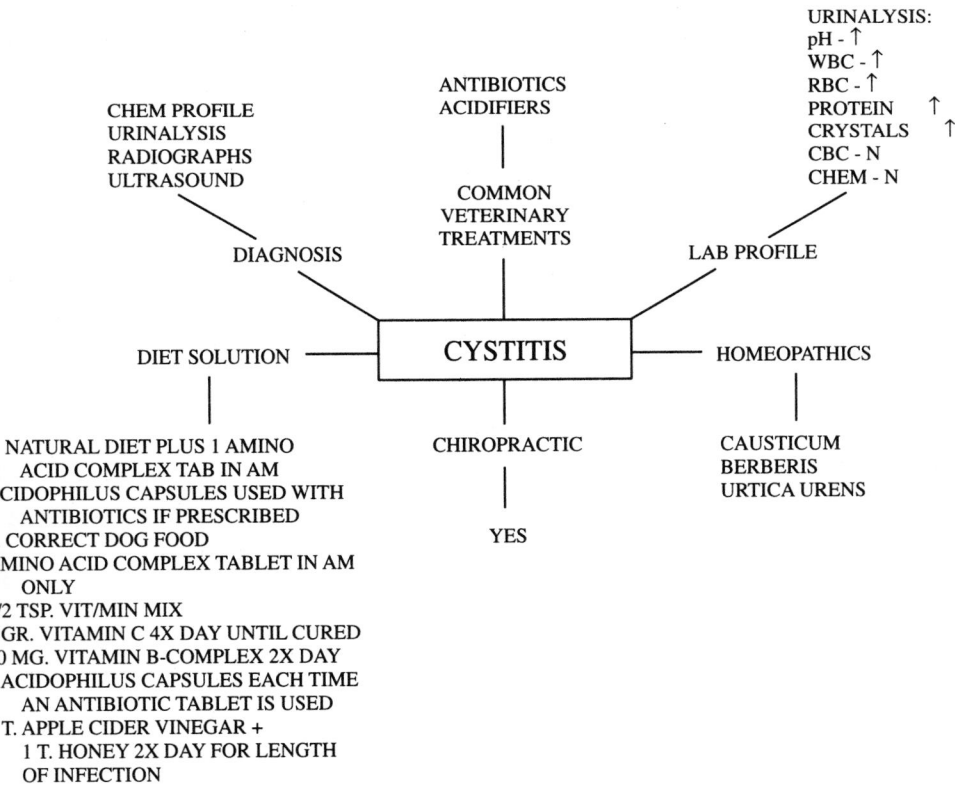

URINALYSIS:
pH - ↑
WBC - ↑
RBC - ↑
PROTEIN ↑
CRYSTALS ↑
CBC - N
CHEM - N

CHEM PROFILE
URINALYSIS
RADIOGRAPHS
ULTRASOUND

ANTIBIOTICS
ACIDIFIERS

COMMON
VETERINARY
TREATMENTS

DIAGNOSIS

LAB PROFILE

DIET SOLUTION — CYSTITIS — HOMEOPATHICS

CHIROPRACTIC

CAUSTICUM
BERBERIS
URTICA URENS

1. NATURAL DIET PLUS 1 AMINO
ACID COMPLEX TAB IN AM
ACIDOPHILUS CAPSULES USED WITH
ANTIBIOTICS IF PRESCRIBED
2. CORRECT DOG FOOD
AMINO ACID COMPLEX TABLET IN AM
ONLY
1/2 TSP. VIT/MIN MIX
1 GR. VITAMIN C 4X DAY UNTIL CURED
50 MG. VITAMIN B-COMPLEX 2X DAY
2 ACIDOPHILUS CAPSULES EACH TIME
AN ANTIBIOTIC TABLET IS USED
1 T. APPLE CIDER VINEGAR +
1 T. HONEY 2X DAY FOR LENGTH
OF INFECTION

YES

Diarrhea
AT A GLANCE

CAUSES & SYMPTOMS

INFECTION
STRESS
ADVERSE REACTION TO DRUGS OR VACCINES
FOOD ALLERGY - OLD MOLDY, RANCID FOOD
INABILITY TO DIGEST TYPE OF FOOD FED
EATING TOO MUCH FRUIT, OR GARBAGE ETC.
WORMS
POISONING
NEED TO DIFFERENTIATE BETWEEN
   SMALL BOWEL & LARGE BOWEL DISEASE

STOOLS THAT ARE VERY WATERY OR BLOOD
   OR UNFORMED OVER SEVERAL DAYS.
STOOLS THAT SMELL SUDDENLY DIFFERENT
   "BAD"
CONTINUOUS STOOLS
STOOLS THAT ARE YELLOW OR GREEN OR TH
   CONTAIN DISCHARGES
WITH ELEVATED TEMPERATURE, GET TO
VETERINARIAN IMMEDIATELY

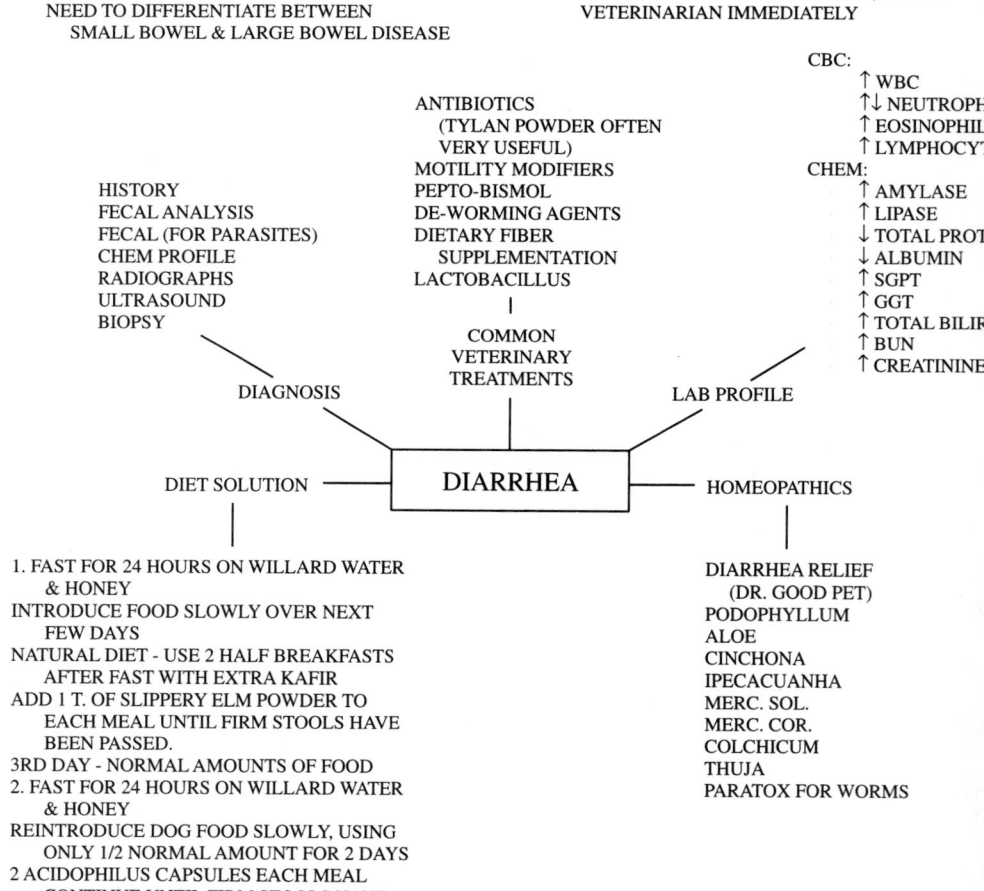

HISTORY
FECAL ANALYSIS
FECAL (FOR PARASITES)
CHEM PROFILE
RADIOGRAPHS
ULTRASOUND
BIOPSY

ANTIBIOTICS
   (TYLAN POWDER OFTEN
   VERY USEFUL)
MOTILITY MODIFIERS
PEPTO-BISMOL
DE-WORMING AGENTS
DIETARY FIBER
   SUPPLEMENTATION
LACTOBACILLUS

CBC:
   ↑ WBC
   ↑↓ NEUTROPH
   ↑ EOSINOPHIL
   ↑ LYMPHOCYT
CHEM:
   ↑ AMYLASE
   ↑ LIPASE
   ↓ TOTAL PROT
   ↓ ALBUMIN
   ↑ SGPT
   ↑ GGT
   ↑ TOTAL BILIR
   ↑ BUN
   ↑ CREATININE

COMMON
VETERINARY
TREATMENTS

DIAGNOSIS

LAB PROFILE

DIET SOLUTION — **DIARRHEA** — HOMEOPATHICS

1. FAST FOR 24 HOURS ON WILLARD WATER
   & HONEY
INTRODUCE FOOD SLOWLY OVER NEXT
   FEW DAYS
NATURAL DIET - USE 2 HALF BREAKFASTS
   AFTER FAST WITH EXTRA KAFIR
ADD 1 T. OF SLIPPERY ELM POWDER TO
   EACH MEAL UNTIL FIRM STOOLS HAVE
   BEEN PASSED.
3RD DAY - NORMAL AMOUNTS OF FOOD
2. FAST FOR 24 HOURS ON WILLARD WATER
   & HONEY
REINTRODUCE DOG FOOD SLOWLY, USING
   ONLY 1/2 NORMAL AMOUNT FOR 2 DAYS
2 ACIDOPHILUS CAPSULES EACH MEAL
   CONTINUE UNTIL FIRM STOOLS HAVE
   BEEN PASSED
1/2 CUP YOGURT OR KEFIR MIXED WITH
   EACH MEAL
1 GR. VITAMIN C 2X DAY
50 MG. VITAMIN B-COMPLEX 2X DAY
1/2 TSP. VIT/MIN MIX
2 T. WHEAT BRAN AT EACH MEAL UNTIL
   FIRM STOOLS HAVE PASSED

DIARRHEA RELIEF
   (DR. GOOD PET)
PODOPHYLLUM
ALOE
CINCHONA
IPECACUANHA
MERC. SOL.
MERC. COR.
COLCHICUM
THUJA
PARATOX FOR WORMS

Digestive Problems
AT A GLANCE

CAUSES & SYMPTOMS

PANCREATIC INSUFFICIENCY (EPI)
MALDIGESTION/MALABSORPTION
NEOPLASIA
INCORRECT DIET
ALLERGY TO INGREDIENTS IN DIET
STRESS
INHERITED METABOLIC DISORDERS
DRUGS
VACCINES

WEIGHT LOSS
POOR QUALITY STOOLS
LOSS OF STAMINA
ABDOMINAL DISCOMFORT
INCREASED INTESTINAL STRESS
PERIODIC TO FREQUENT VOMITING

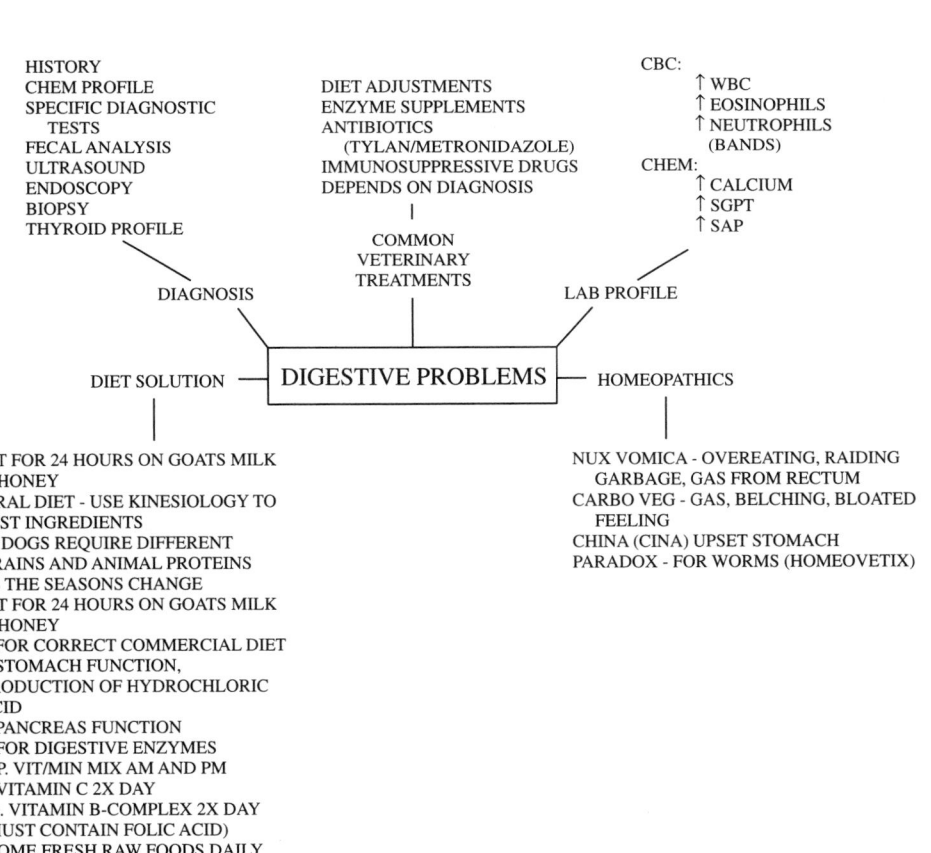

DIAGNOSIS

HISTORY
CHEM PROFILE
SPECIFIC DIAGNOSTIC
   TESTS
FECAL ANALYSIS
ULTRASOUND
ENDOSCOPY
BIOPSY
THYROID PROFILE

COMMON VETERINARY TREATMENTS

DIET ADJUSTMENTS
ENZYME SUPPLEMENTS
ANTIBIOTICS
   (TYLAN/METRONIDAZOLE)
IMMUNOSUPPRESSIVE DRUGS
DEPENDS ON DIAGNOSIS

LAB PROFILE

CBC:
↑ WBC
↑ EOSINOPHILS
↑ NEUTROPHILS
   (BANDS)
CHEM:
↑ CALCIUM
↑ SGPT
↑ SAP

DIGESTIVE PROBLEMS

DIET SOLUTION

1. FAST FOR 24 HOURS ON GOATS MILK
   & HONEY
NATURAL DIET - USE KINESIOLOGY TO
   TEST INGREDIENTS
SOME DOGS REQUIRE DIFFERENT
   GRAINS AND ANIMAL PROTEINS
   AS THE SEASONS CHANGE
2. FAST FOR 24 HOURS ON GOATS MILK
   & HONEY
TEST FOR CORRECT COMMERCIAL DIET
TEST STOMACH FUNCTION,
   PRODUCTION OF HYDROCHLORIC
   ACID
TEST PANCREAS FUNCTION
TEST FOR DIGESTIVE ENZYMES
1/2 TSP. VIT/MIN MIX AM AND PM
1 GR. VITAMIN C 2X DAY
50 MG. VITAMIN B-COMPLEX 2X DAY
   (MUST CONTAIN FOLIC ACID)
USE SOME FRESH RAW FOODS DAILY

HOMEOPATHICS

NUX VOMICA - OVEREATING, RAIDING
   GARBAGE, GAS FROM RECTUM
CARBO VEG - GAS, BELCHING, BLOATED
   FEELING
CHINA (CINA) UPSET STOMACH
PARADOX - FOR WORMS (HOMEOVETIX)

Ears
AT A GLANCE

CAUSES & SYMPTOMS

ALLERGIES TO FOOD OR ENVIRONMENT
ADRENAL OR THYROID GLAND
  MALFUNCTION
KIDNEY PROBLEMS (VERY COMMON)
DIET TOO ALKALINE
BODY STRESSED IN HEAT AND HIGH
  HUMIDITY
EAR MITES
YEAST INFECTIONS
SOMETHING CAUGHT IN THE EAR
CERVICAL AND LUMBAR VERTEBRAE
  OUT OF ALIGNMENT

DISCHARGE FROM EAR CANAL
DRY SCALY FLAPS
INFLAMED EAR FLAPS/CANALS
PAIN
HEAD TILT
ODOR
SHAKING OF HEAD
SCRATCHING WITH BACK FEET IN EARS
  AND GROANING
BLACK DISCHARGE, KIDNEY RELATED
  OR MITES
GINGER OR BROWN DISCHARGE
  EXTENDING ON TO EAR FLAPS,
  YEAST OR FUNGUS

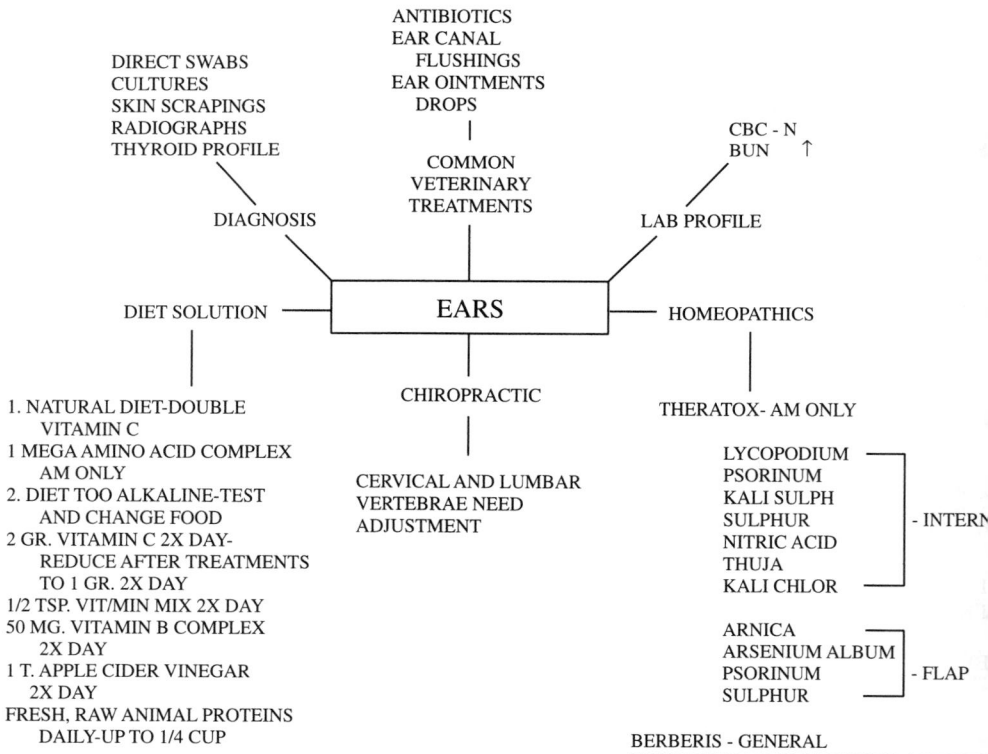

DIRECT SWABS
CULTURES
SKIN SCRAPINGS
RADIOGRAPHS
THYROID PROFILE

ANTIBIOTICS
EAR CANAL
  FLUSHINGS
EAR OINTMENTS
DROPS

CBC - N
BUN ↑

COMMON
VETERINARY
TREATMENTS

DIAGNOSIS

LAB PROFILE

DIET SOLUTION —

EARS

— HOMEOPATHICS

CHIROPRACTIC

THERATOX- AM ONLY

1. NATURAL DIET-DOUBLE
  VITAMIN C
1 MEGA AMINO ACID COMPLEX
  AM ONLY
2. DIET TOO ALKALINE-TEST
  AND CHANGE FOOD
2 GR. VITAMIN C 2X DAY-
  REDUCE AFTER TREATMENTS
  TO 1 GR. 2X DAY
1/2 TSP. VIT/MIN MIX 2X DAY
50 MG. VITAMIN B COMPLEX
  2X DAY
1 T. APPLE CIDER VINEGAR
  2X DAY
FRESH, RAW ANIMAL PROTEINS
  DAILY-UP TO 1/4 CUP

CERVICAL AND LUMBAR
VERTEBRAE NEED
ADJUSTMENT

LYCOPODIUM
PSORINUM
KALI SULPH
SULPHUR   - INTERN
NITRIC ACID
THUJA
KALI CHLOR

ARNICA
ARSENIUM ALBUM
PSORINUM   - FLAP
SULPHUR

BERBERIS - GENERAL
VERBASCUM AND CALENDULA TINCTU
  USED AS DROPS

*USE APPLE CIDER VINEGAR AND WATER AS EAR WASH IF EARS ARE NOT INFLAMED TO KEEP
ENVIRONMENT ACIDIC

Epilepsy

AT A GLANCE

CAUSES & SYMPTOMS

GENETIC METABOLIC DEFICIENCIES
DEFICIENCIES IN AMINO ACIDS,
   MAGNESIUM, MANGANESE
"PETIT MAL" SEIZURES
"GRAND MAL" SEIZURES
SEIZURES CAN VARY FROM STAR GAZING
   TO SEVERE GRAND MAL (EPILEPTICUS)

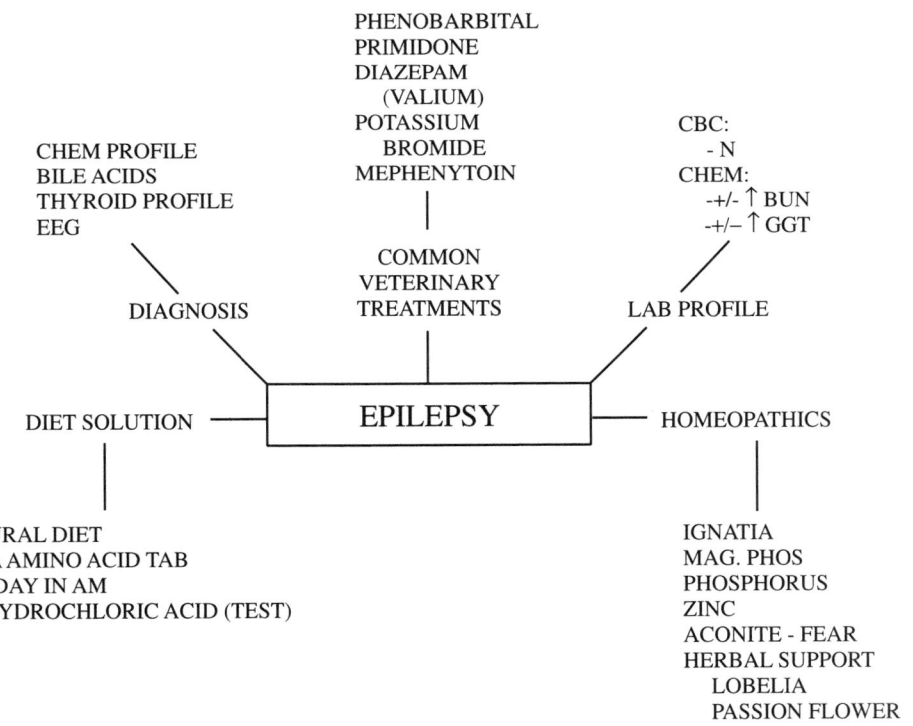

PHENOBARBITAL
PRIMIDONE
DIAZEPAM
(VALIUM)
POTASSIUM
BROMIDE
MEPHENYTOIN

COMMON
VETERINARY
TREATMENTS

CHEM PROFILE
BILE ACIDS
THYROID PROFILE
EEG

DIAGNOSIS

CBC:
- N
CHEM:
-+/- ↑ BUN
-+/- ↑ GGT

LAB PROFILE

DIET SOLUTION — EPILEPSY — HOMEOPATHICS

1. NATURAL DIET
1 MEGA AMINO ACID TAB
  1X DAY IN AM
BETA HYDROCHLORIC ACID (TEST)

IGNATIA
MAG. PHOS
PHOSPHORUS
ZINC
ACONITE - FEAR
HERBAL SUPPORT
  LOBELIA
  PASSION FLOWER

Eye Problems—Acute
AT A GLANCE

TRAUMA
LIVER PROBLEMS
BACTERIAL/VIRAL INFECTIONS
CAUSTIC IRRITATION
ACUTE ALLERGIC REACTIONS

BLINKING (BLEPHAROSPASM)
TEARING EXCESSIVELY
CLOUDY CORNEA
RED OR PUS WITHIN EYE

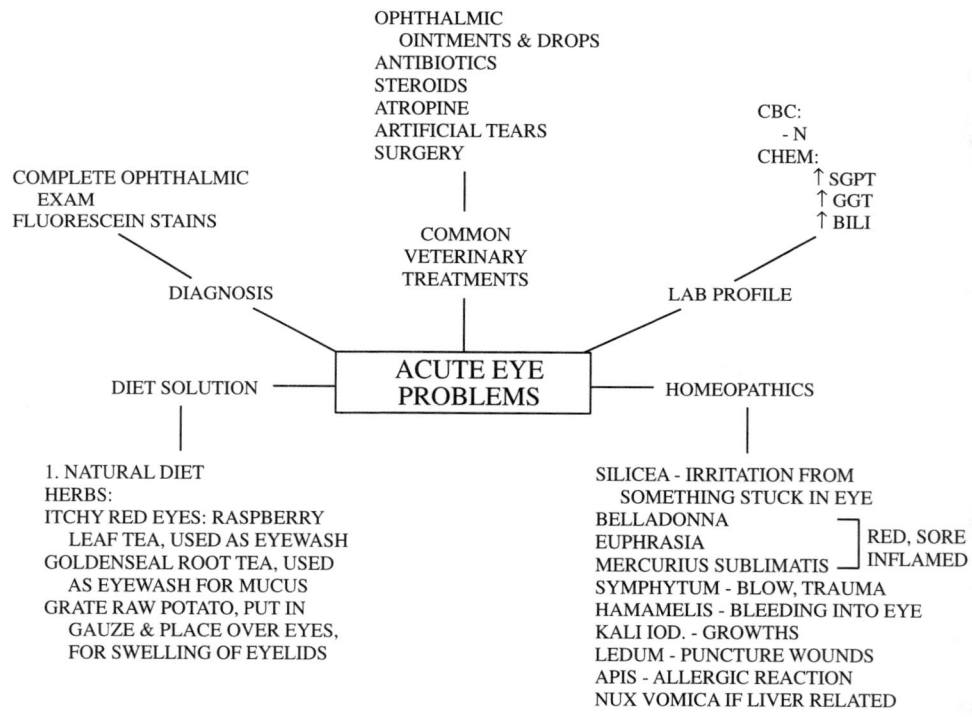

OPHTHALMIC
 OINTMENTS & DROPS
ANTIBIOTICS
STEROIDS
ATROPINE
ARTIFICIAL TEARS
SURGERY

CBC:
 - N
CHEM:
 ↑ SGPT
 ↑ GGT
 ↑ BILI

COMPLETE OPHTHALMIC
 EXAM
FLUORESCEIN STAINS

COMMON
VETERINARY
TREATMENTS

DIAGNOSIS

LAB PROFILE

ACUTE EYE
PROBLEMS

DIET SOLUTION

HOMEOPATHICS

1. NATURAL DIET
HERBS:
ITCHY RED EYES: RASPBERRY
 LEAF TEA, USED AS EYEWASH
GOLDENSEAL ROOT TEA, USED
 AS EYEWASH FOR MUCUS
GRATE RAW POTATO, PUT IN
 GAUZE & PLACE OVER EYES,
 FOR SWELLING OF EYELIDS

SILICEA - IRRITATION FROM
 SOMETHING STUCK IN EYE
BELLADONNA
EUPHRASIA   ⎤ RED, SORE
MERCURIUS SUBLIMATIS ⎦ INFLAMED
SYMPHYTUM - BLOW, TRAUMA
HAMAMELIS - BLEEDING INTO EYE
KALI IOD. - GROWTHS
LEDUM - PUNCTURE WOUNDS
APIS - ALLERGIC REACTION
NUX VOMICA IF LIVER RELATED

236

Eye Problems—Chronic
AT A GLANCE

CAUSES & SYMPTOMS

MANY EYE PROBLEMS CAN BE
  GENETIC
IMPROPER SHAPE OF EYE IN SOME
  BREEDS (NOT OVAL)
GENETIC LIVER DISEASE
TOXIC LIVER
ALLERGIES TO DOG FOOD OR
  ENVIRONMENT
POSSIBLE THYROID PROBLEMS

DRY EYES (KERATITIS SICCA)
ENTROPION/ECTROPION
EXTRA & DISPLACED EYELASHES
RETINAL PROBLEMS
BLOCKED DIFFICULTIES
CHRONIC ALLERGIES

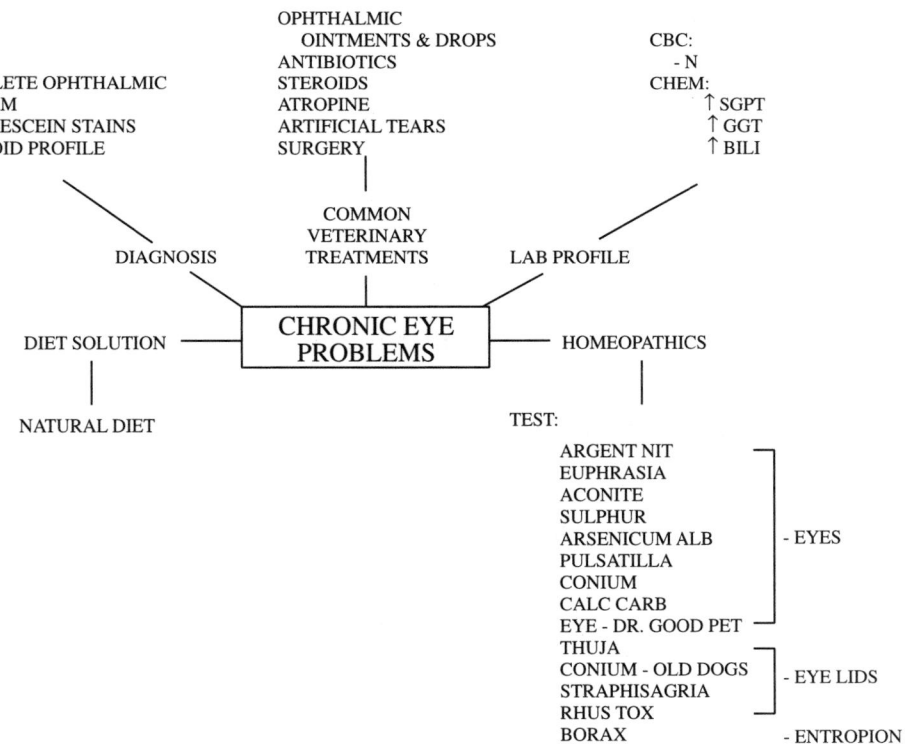

OPHTHALMIC
  OINTMENTS & DROPS
ANTIBIOTICS
STEROIDS
ATROPINE
ARTIFICIAL TEARS
SURGERY

CBC:
  - N
CHEM:
  ↑ SGPT
  ↑ GGT
  ↑ BILI

COMPLETE OPHTHALMIC
  EXAM
FLUORESCEIN STAINS
THYROID PROFILE

DIAGNOSIS

COMMON
VETERINARY
TREATMENTS

LAB PROFILE

DIET SOLUTION — CHRONIC EYE PROBLEMS — HOMEOPATHICS

NATURAL DIET

TEST:

ARGENT NIT
EUPHRASIA
ACONITE
SULPHUR
ARSENICUM ALB
PULSATILLA
CONIUM
CALC CARB
EYE - DR. GOOD PET

- EYES

THUJA
CONIUM - OLD DOGS
STRAPHISAGRIA
RHUS TOX
BORAX

- EYE LIDS

- ENTROPION

Heat Stroke
AT A GLANCE

CAUSES & SYMPTOMS

BEING LEFT IN A CAR WITHOUT ADEQUATE
   VENTILATION ON HOT DAYS
DOGS WORKING IN TEMPERATURES ABOVE
   90° F WITHOUT ADEQUATE REST
   OR PLACE TO COOL DOWN
INADEQUATE WATER
DOGS HOUSED IN AREAS WITHOUT
   ADEQUATE SHADE
EXTREME STRESS

HIGH FEVER > 108° F
PANTING/INCREASED HEARTRATE
SHOCK TO COMATOSE
BLOODY DIARRHEA
PINPOINT HEMORRHAGES ON MEMBRA
EMERGENCY STEPS:
   PUT ICE UNDER ARMS & LEGS
   ALCOHOL WRAPS ON FEET
   IMMERSE IN COLD WATER
   SEEK VETERINARY HELP IMMEDIATE

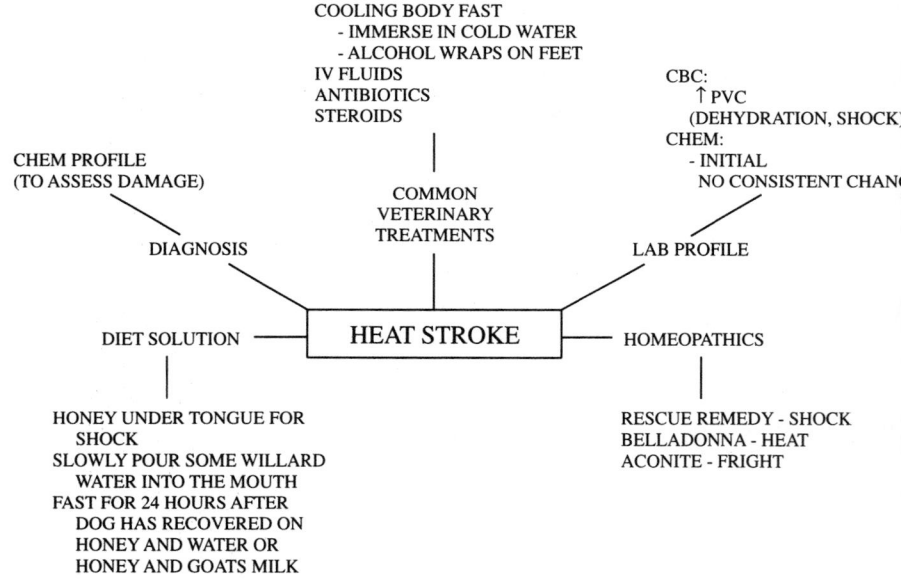

COOLING BODY FAST
  - IMMERSE IN COLD WATER
  - ALCOHOL WRAPS ON FEET
IV FLUIDS
ANTIBIOTICS
STEROIDS

CBC:
  ↑ PVC
  (DEHYDRATION, SHOCK)
CHEM:
  - INITIAL
    NO CONSISTENT CHANG

CHEM PROFILE
(TO ASSESS DAMAGE)

COMMON
VETERINARY
TREATMENTS

DIAGNOSIS

LAB PROFILE

DIET SOLUTION — **HEAT STROKE** — HOMEOPATHICS

HONEY UNDER TONGUE FOR
  SHOCK
SLOWLY POUR SOME WILLARD
  WATER INTO THE MOUTH
FAST FOR 24 HOURS AFTER
  DOG HAS RECOVERED ON
  HONEY AND WATER OR
  HONEY AND GOATS MILK

RESCUE REMEDY - SHOCK
BELLADONNA - HEAT
ACONITE - FRIGHT

Hyperadrenocorticism
AT A GLANCE

CAUSES & SYMPTOMS

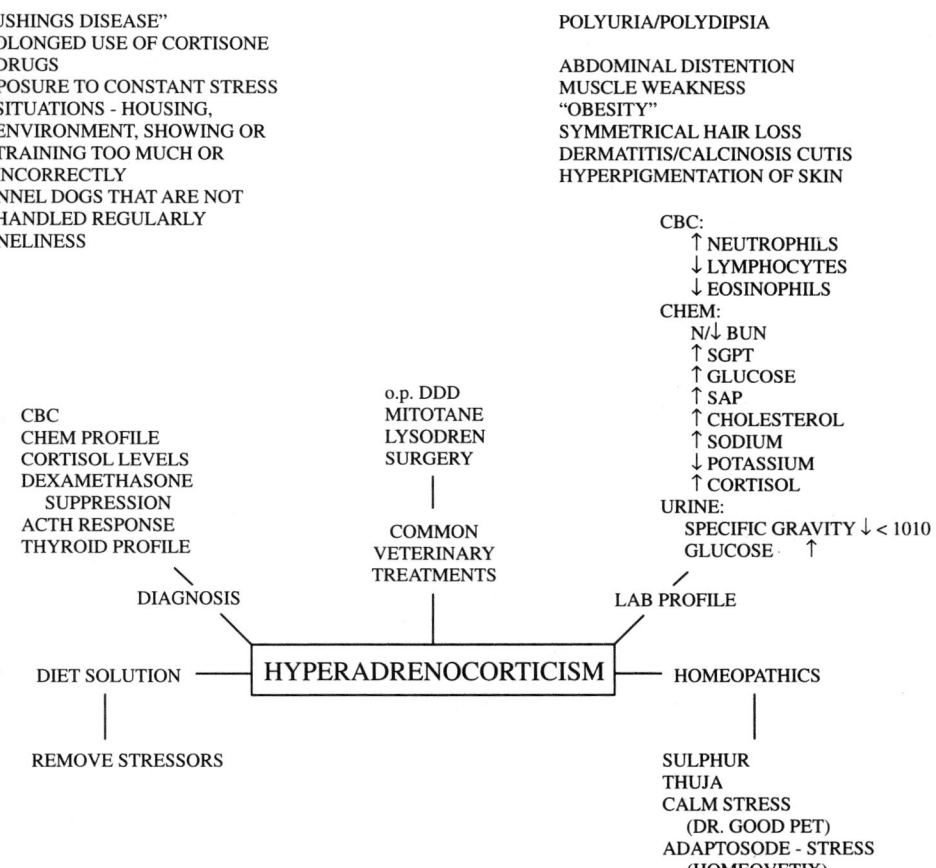

USHINGS DISEASE"
ROLONGED USE OF CORTISONE
 DRUGS
XPOSURE TO CONSTANT STRESS
 SITUATIONS - HOUSING,
 ENVIRONMENT, SHOWING OR
 TRAINING TOO MUCH OR
 INCORRECTLY
:NNEL DOGS THAT ARE NOT
 HANDLED REGULARLY
)NELINESS

POLYURIA/POLYDIPSIA

ABDOMINAL DISTENTION
MUSCLE WEAKNESS
"OBESITY"
SYMMETRICAL HAIR LOSS
DERMATITIS/CALCINOSIS CUTIS
HYPERPIGMENTATION OF SKIN

CBC:
 ↑ NEUTROPHILS
 ↓ LYMPHOCYTES
 ↓ EOSINOPHILS
CHEM:
 N/↓ BUN
 ↑ SGPT
 ↑ GLUCOSE
 ↑ SAP
 ↑ CHOLESTEROL
 ↑ SODIUM
 ↓ POTASSIUM
 ↑ CORTISOL
URINE:
 SPECIFIC GRAVITY ↓ < 1010
 GLUCOSE   ↑

CBC
CHEM PROFILE
CORTISOL LEVELS
DEXAMETHASONE
 SUPPRESSION
ACTH RESPONSE
THYROID PROFILE

o.p. DDD
MITOTANE
LYSODREN
SURGERY

COMMON
VETERINARY
TREATMENTS

DIAGNOSIS

LAB PROFILE

DIET SOLUTION — **HYPERADRENOCORTICISM** — HOMEOPATHICS

REMOVE STRESSORS

SULPHUR
THUJA
CALM STRESS
 (DR. GOOD PET)
ADAPTOSODE - STRESS
 (HOMEOVETIX)

Hypoadrenocorticism
AT A GLANCE

<u>CAUSES & SYMPTOMS</u>

"ADDISONS DISEASE"
THYROID MALFUNCTION
ALLERGY TO DOG FOOD
DIET LACKING IN POTASSIUM
   OR DOG DEPLETED OF
   POTASSIUM
EXCESS SALT IN DIET
DRINKING TOO MUCH
CHLORINATED WATER
LACK OF VITAMIN B AND/OR C IN
   DIET
LACK OF AMINO ACIDS IN DIET
OVER VACCINATION

DEPRESSION
WEIGHT LOSS
CHRONIC EAR INFECTIONS
EXCESSIVE THIRST
LOSS OF HAIR

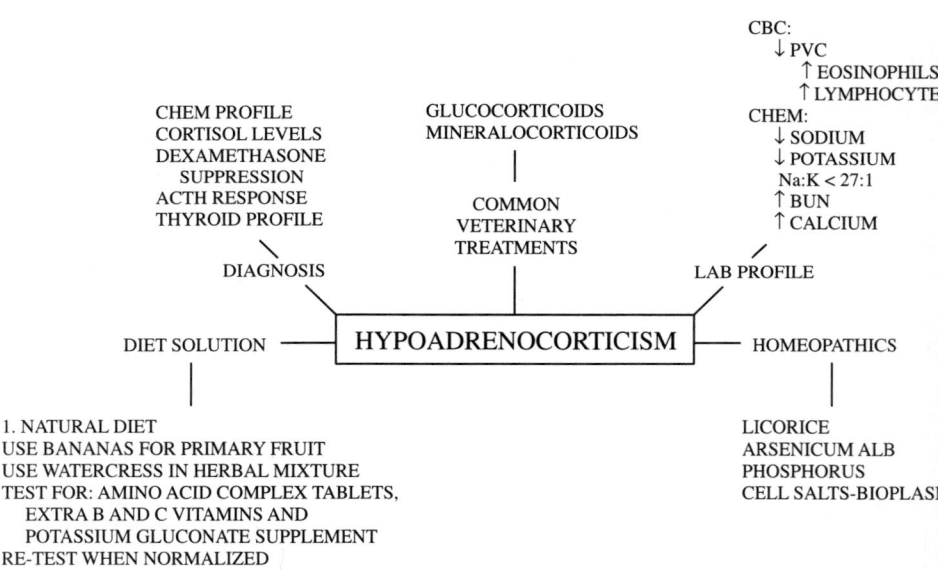

CBC:
   ↓ PVC
     ↑ EOSINOPHILS
     ↑ LYMPHOCYTE

CHEM PROFILE
CORTISOL LEVELS
DEXAMETHASONE
   SUPPRESSION
ACTH RESPONSE
THYROID PROFILE

GLUCOCORTICOIDS
MINERALOCORTICOIDS

CHEM:
   ↓ SODIUM
   ↓ POTASSIUM
   Na:K < 27:1
   ↑ BUN
   ↑ CALCIUM

COMMON
VETERINARY
TREATMENTS

DIAGNOSIS

LAB PROFILE

DIET SOLUTION — **HYPOADRENOCORTICISM** — HOMEOPATHICS

1. NATURAL DIET
USE BANANAS FOR PRIMARY FRUIT
USE WATERCRESS IN HERBAL MIXTURE
TEST FOR: AMINO ACID COMPLEX TABLETS,
   EXTRA B AND C VITAMINS AND
   POTASSIUM GLUCONATE SUPPLEMENT
RE-TEST WHEN NORMALIZED

LICORICE
ARSENICUM ALB
PHOSPHORUS
CELL SALTS-BIOPLASM

Hyperthyroid
AT A GLANCE

<u>CAUSES & SYMPTOMS</u>

GENETIC   TUMOR ON GLAND
DEFICIENCY OF   IMMUNE RELATED
   AMINO ACIDS
DEFICIENCY OF
   VITAMINS C & B

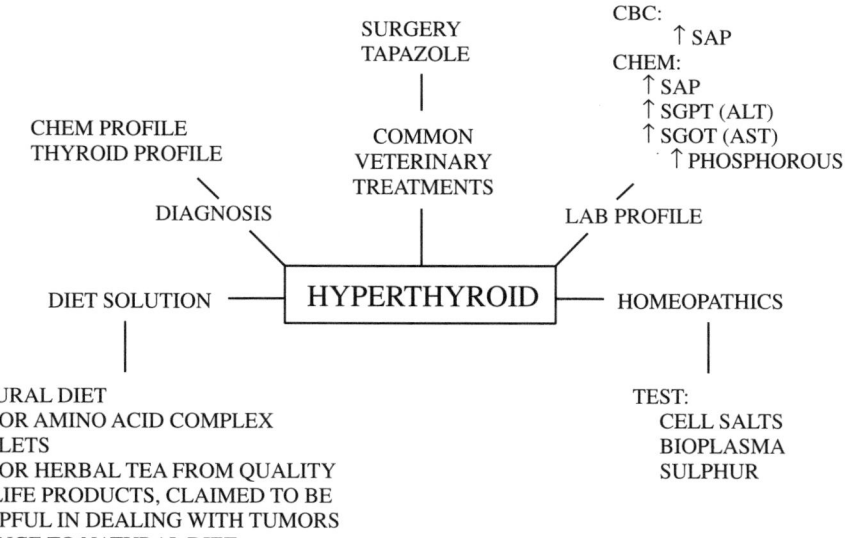

SURGERY
TAPAZOLE

CBC:
   ↑ SAP
CHEM:
   ↑ SAP
   ↑ SGPT (ALT)
   ↑ SGOT (AST)
   ↑ PHOSPHOROUS

CHEM PROFILE
THYROID PROFILE

COMMON
VETERINARY
TREATMENTS

DIAGNOSIS   LAB PROFILE

DIET SOLUTION ———— **HYPERTHYROID** —— HOMEOPATHICS

1. NATURAL DIET
TEST FOR AMINO ACID COMPLEX
   TABLETS
TEST FOR HERBAL TEA FROM QUALITY
   OF LIFE PRODUCTS, CLAIMED TO BE
   HELPFUL IN DEALING WITH TUMORS
2. CHANGE TO NATURAL DIET

TEST:
   CELL SALTS
   BIOPLASMA
   SULPHUR

Hypothyroid
AT A GLANCE

CAUSES & SYMPTOMS

MALFUNCTION OF THYROID GLAND
CAN BE A GENETIC PREDISPOSITION
DEFICIENCY IN DOG FOOD OF
    AMINO ACIDS, VITAMINS B AND C,
    MINERALS, IODINE
OVER-VACCINATION OF YOUNG
    DOGS
AUTO IMMUNE PROBLEMS *
NEUTERING

LETHARGY
MENTAL DULLNESS
WEIGHT GAIN
SKIN PROBLEMS
REPRODUCTIVE DISORDERS
BEHAVIOR PROBLEMS

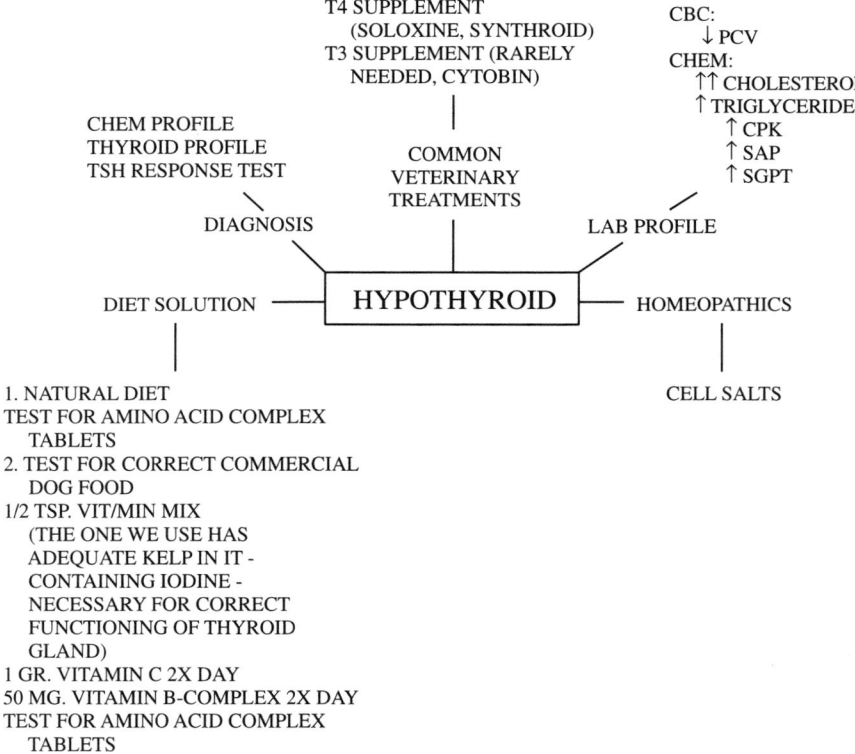

T4 SUPPLEMENT
(SOLOXINE, SYNTHROID)
T3 SUPPLEMENT (RARELY
NEEDED, CYTOBIN)

CBC:
  ↓ PCV
CHEM:
  ↑↑ CHOLESTEROL
  ↑ TRIGLYCERIDES
  ↑ CPK
  ↑ SAP
  ↑ SGPT

CHEM PROFILE
THYROID PROFILE
TSH RESPONSE TEST

COMMON
VETERINARY
TREATMENTS

DIAGNOSIS

LAB PROFILE

DIET SOLUTION —— HYPOTHYROID —— HOMEOPATHICS

1. NATURAL DIET
TEST FOR AMINO ACID COMPLEX
    TABLETS
2. TEST FOR CORRECT COMMERCIAL
    DOG FOOD
1/2 TSP. VIT/MIN MIX
    (THE ONE WE USE HAS
    ADEQUATE KELP IN IT -
    CONTAINING IODINE -
    NECESSARY FOR CORRECT
    FUNCTIONING OF THYROID
    GLAND)
1 GR. VITAMIN C 2X DAY
50 MG. VITAMIN B-COMPLEX 2X DAY
TEST FOR AMINO ACID COMPLEX
    TABLETS

CELL SALTS

* DOGS THAT HAVE AUTO IMMUNE PROBLEMS NEED TO HAVE THEIR TITERS CHECKED YEARLY
BEFORE ROUTINELY USING VACCINE BOOSTERS.

Skin
AT A GLANCE

CAUSES & SYMPTOMS

ALLERGIES IN GENERAL
THYROID OR ADRENAL
   GLAND MALFUNCTION
INFLAMMATION
TRAUMA
LACK OF FAT IN DIET
STRESS
DIET TOO ALKALINE OR
   DEFICIENT IN NUTRIENTS
CAN BE GENETIC

INFLAMMATION
RED SPLOTCHES
ITCHY, SMELLY, SCALY, DRY
PUSTULES
THINNING COAT
HOT SPOTS
TRAUMA

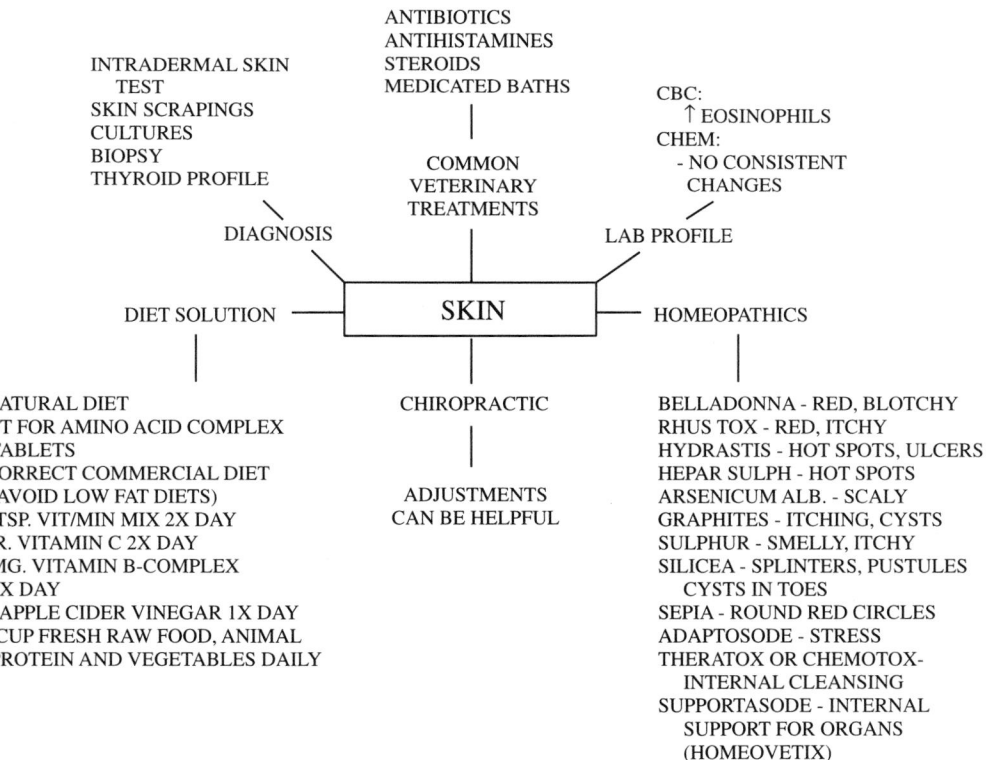

INTRADERMAL SKIN
   TEST
SKIN SCRAPINGS
CULTURES
BIOPSY
THYROID PROFILE

ANTIBIOTICS
ANTIHISTAMINES
STEROIDS
MEDICATED BATHS

CBC:
  ↑ EOSINOPHILS
CHEM:
  - NO CONSISTENT
   CHANGES

DIAGNOSIS

COMMON
VETERINARY
TREATMENTS

LAB PROFILE

DIET SOLUTION ———

SKIN

——— HOMEOPATHICS

NATURAL DIET
ST FOR AMINO ACID COMPLEX
TABLETS
CORRECT COMMERCIAL DIET
  (AVOID LOW FAT DIETS)
TSP. VIT/MIN MIX 2X DAY
R. VITAMIN C 2X DAY
MG. VITAMIN B-COMPLEX
  2X DAY
. APPLE CIDER VINEGAR 1X DAY
CUP FRESH RAW FOOD, ANIMAL
  PROTEIN AND VEGETABLES DAILY

CHIROPRACTIC

ADJUSTMENTS
CAN BE HELPFUL

BELLADONNA - RED, BLOTCHY
RHUS TOX - RED, ITCHY
HYDRASTIS - HOT SPOTS, ULCERS
HEPAR SULPH - HOT SPOTS
ARSENICUM ALB. - SCALY
GRAPHITES - ITCHING, CYSTS
SULPHUR - SMELLY, ITCHY
SILICEA - SPLINTERS, PUSTULES
  CYSTS IN TOES
SEPIA - ROUND RED CIRCLES
ADAPTOSODE - STRESS
THERATOX OR CHEMOTOX-
  INTERNAL CLEANSING
SUPPORTASODE - INTERNAL
  SUPPORT FOR ORGANS
  (HOMEOVETIX)

* BATHE DOG IN MILD HERBAL SHAMPOO, RINSE THOROUGHLY AND THEN RINSE AGAIN WITH
APPLE CIDER VINEGAR AND WATER. SPONGE ON AND LET DOG DRIP DRY.

Timidity
AT A GLANCE

KIDNEY PROBLEMS
THYROID OR ADRENAL GLAND
  MALFUNCTION
CAN BE ALLERGIC REACTION TO
  IMPROPER DIET, OR DIET
  WITHOUT ADEQUATE
  SUPPLEMENTATION
INABILITY TO ABSORB CALCIUM
  AND MAGNESIUM
UNDIAGNOSED PAIN

SHYNESS
ANXIETY
NOT EATING
BEHAVIOR PROBLEMS

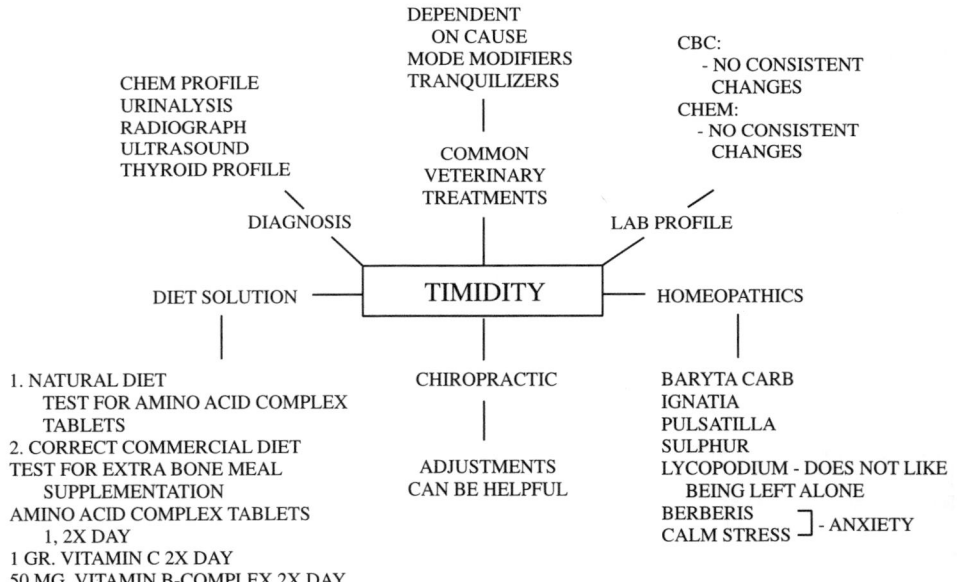

DEPENDENT
ON CAUSE
MODE MODIFIERS
TRANQUILIZERS

CBC:
  - NO CONSISTENT
    CHANGES
CHEM:
  - NO CONSISTENT
    CHANGES

CHEM PROFILE
URINALYSIS
RADIOGRAPH
ULTRASOUND
THYROID PROFILE

COMMON
VETERINARY
TREATMENTS

DIAGNOSIS

LAB PROFILE

DIET SOLUTION — | TIMIDITY | — HOMEOPATHICS

1. NATURAL DIET
   TEST FOR AMINO ACID COMPLEX
   TABLETS
2. CORRECT COMMERCIAL DIET
TEST FOR EXTRA BONE MEAL
   SUPPLEMENTATION
AMINO ACID COMPLEX TABLETS
   1, 2X DAY
1 GR. VITAMIN C 2X DAY
50 MG. VITAMIN B-COMPLEX 2X DAY
   (FOR APPETITE)
1/2 VIT/MIN MIX 2X DAY

CHIROPRACTIC

ADJUSTMENTS
CAN BE HELPFUL

BARYTA CARB
IGNATIA
PULSATILLA
SULPHUR
LYCOPODIUM - DOES NOT LIKE
   BEING LEFT ALONE
BERBERIS
CALM STRESS] - ANXIETY

Trauma
AT A GLANCE

ACCIDENTS
ANAPHYLACTIC REACTIONS

THIS IS AN EMERGENCY

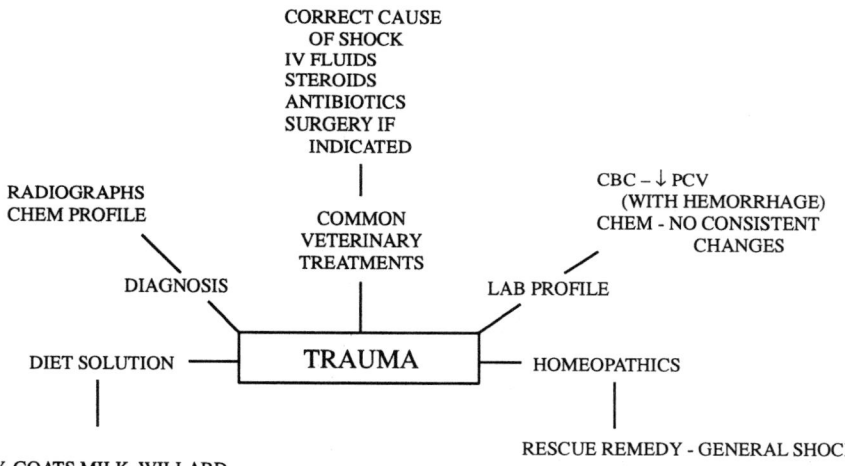

CORRECT CAUSE
OF SHOCK
IV FLUIDS
STEROIDS
ANTIBIOTICS
SURGERY IF
INDICATED

RADIOGRAPHS
CHEM PROFILE

CBC – ↓ PCV
(WITH HEMORRHAGE)
CHEM - NO CONSISTENT
CHANGES

COMMON
VETERINARY
TREATMENTS

DIAGNOSIS

LAB PROFILE

DIET SOLUTION — **TRAUMA** — HOMEOPATHICS

FAST
HONEY, GOATS MILK, WILLARD
WATER FOR 1 MEAL
1/2 REGULAR MEAL 2nd MEAL
3rd MEAL RETURN TO NORMAL
MEGA AMINO ACID COMPLEX
DURING RECOVERY 1X DAY
IN AM

RESCUE REMEDY - GENERAL SHOCK

Weak Hindquarters
AT A GLANCE

CAUSES & SYMPTOMS

GENETIC
POOR DIET
ACCUMULATION OF TOXINS
DEFICIENCIES AND ALLERGIES
INJURY
OVER-VACCINATION OF OLDER
   DOGS. DO TITERS BEFORE
   ROUTINELY VACCINATING
   DOGS OVER 5.

HIP DYSPLASIA
SPINAL MYELOPATHY
INTRAVERTEBRAL DISC DISEASE
LAMENESS

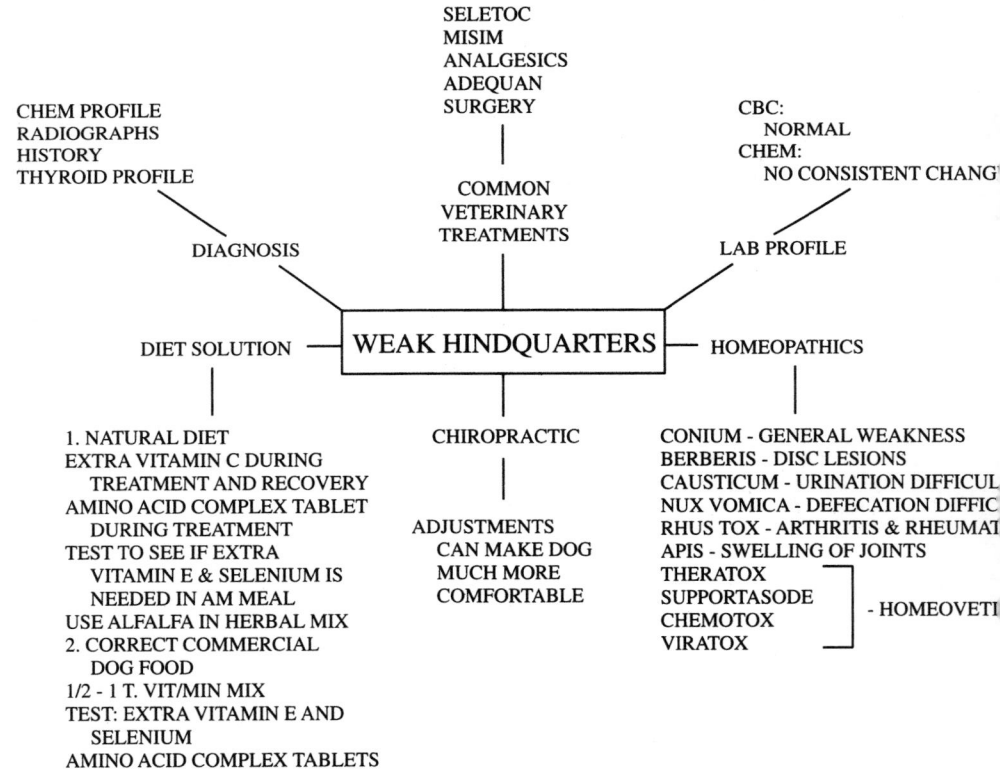

SELETOC
MISIM
ANALGESICS
ADEQUAN
SURGERY

CHEM PROFILE
RADIOGRAPHS
HISTORY
THYROID PROFILE

COMMON
VETERINARY
TREATMENTS

CBC:
   NORMAL
CHEM:
   NO CONSISTENT CHANG

DIAGNOSIS

LAB PROFILE

DIET SOLUTION — **WEAK HINDQUARTERS** — HOMEOPATHICS

1. NATURAL DIET
EXTRA VITAMIN C DURING
   TREATMENT AND RECOVERY
AMINO ACID COMPLEX TABLET
   DURING TREATMENT
TEST TO SEE IF EXTRA
   VITAMIN E & SELENIUM IS
   NEEDED IN AM MEAL
USE ALFALFA IN HERBAL MIX
2. CORRECT COMMERCIAL
   DOG FOOD
1/2 - 1 T. VIT/MIN MIX
TEST: EXTRA VITAMIN E AND
   SELENIUM
AMINO ACID COMPLEX TABLETS
VITAMIN C AND B-COMPLEX
ALFALFA AND COD LIVER OIL

CHIROPRACTIC

ADJUSTMENTS
CAN MAKE DOG
MUCH MORE
COMFORTABLE

CONIUM - GENERAL WEAKNESS
BERBERIS - DISC LESIONS
CAUSTICUM - URINATION DIFFICUL
NUX VOMICA - DEFECATION DIFFIC
RHUS TOX - ARTHRITIS & RHEUMAT
APIS - SWELLING OF JOINTS
THERATOX
SUPPORTASODE
CHEMOTOX   - HOMEOVETI
VIRATOX

—Chapter 19—

Sources

Some excellent products are now on the market to supplement dog food or to make your own food. We have used the sources for products listed below over time and have conducted our testing both by laboratory work and kinesiology on these products. Each of the products has been used for a very specific reason. In some instances, companies have worked with us to make what we needed available. Although other products can be substituted, we cannot guarantee those results.

Vitamins, Minerals and Amino Acids

Nature's Most
P.O. Box 721
Middletown, CT 06457
(800) 234-2112

vitamins, minerals, dried liver, amino acid complex, kyolic garlic pancreatic enzymes

Bronson Pharmaceuticals
1945 Craig Road,
P.O. Box 46903
St. Louis, MO 63146-6903
(800) 235-3200

vitamins and some minerals, deodorized garlic

L & H Vitamins
37-10 Crescent Street
Long Island City, NY 11101
(800) 221-1152

hydrochloric acid tablets (Synergy plus); Willard Water; homeopathic eye drops (Similasan); Bach flower remedies

This company wholesales products from many well-known vitamin and mineral houses.

Vitamin and Mineral Mixes

Quality of Life Products
Hartley Associates
373 Chestnut St.
Middlenburg, PA 17844
717-966-9280
(800) 206-1861

Puppy Stress Formula; adult vitamin-mineral mix; respiratory formula for working and older dogs; stiffness formula for older or injured dogs; coat and skin formula

The Quality of Life products are the ones on which we have run the majority of our laboratory work. The vitamin-mineral mixes contain herbs that not only stimulate the major organ systems but also cleanse them. They contain enzymes for digestion and herbs that cleanse the intestinal tract, making it an environment in which worms do not like to live. The Puppy Stress Formula is similar, but its ingredients support the thymus gland and the whole digestive tract. It contains amino acids plus special herbs to boost the immune system of young puppies so they are protected during the first critical months of life. This unique product was made at our request. We are using it successfully for older and debilitated dogs. We recommend these products.

Organically Grown Grains and Ingredients for the Natural Diet

Walnut Acres
Penns Creek, PA 17862
(800) 433-3998

organic grains, kelp, NBC 600 yeast powder (brewers yeast), raw wheat germ

Herbs

Blessed Herbs
109 Barre Plains Road
Oakham, MA 01068
(508) 882-3839

Organically grown herbs

These are among the freshest we have found. They can be obtained in 1-pound bags.

Bone Meal, Di Calcium Phosphate and Cod Liver Oil

UPCO
3705 Pear Street
Box 969
St. Joseph, MO 64502
(816) 233-8800

cod liver oil is called Codivet

Natural Pet Products

Morrill's New Directions
P.O. Box 30
Orient, ME 04471
(800) 368-5057

Vitamins, Minerals, Amino Acids, Quality of Life products, Homeopathics, Willard Water, natural shampoos, natural dog foods, environmentally safe cleansers and many of the books used in our research; write or call for a catalog.

Homeopathics

Standard Homeopathics
P.O. Box 61067
Los Angeles, CA 90061
(800) 624-9659

Combination remedies sold in supermarkets under the name of Hyland

Luyties Pharmacal Co.
4200 Laclede Avenue
St. Louis, MO 63108
(800) 325-8080

Remedies, books, cell salts, emergency kits, natural remedies, some herbs, combination vitamins and minerals

Homeovetix
P.O. Box 8243
Naples, FL 33941
(800) 851-5444
(800) 964-7177

Homeopathic cleansers and detoxifiers made especially for animals, allergy control, natural detox from worms, vaccinations, chemicals in dog food, Supportasode, Viratox, etc.

Available only through veterinarians or health professionals. Call for catalog and list of distributors. Used in our research projects.

Boiron-Borneman
1208 Amosland Road
P.O. Box 54
Norwood, PA 19074
(800) 258-8823

Single remedies, emergency kits

Books

Direct Book Services
8 Summercreek Place
P.O. Box 3073
Wenatchee, WA 98807
(800) 776-2665

Write for catalog

Homeopathic Educational Services
2124 Kittredge Street
Berkeley, CA 94704
(800) 359-9051

Books, tapes, remedies, computer software, kits and more; write or call for catalog

Woodland Health Books
P.O. Box 1422
Provo, UT 84603
(801) 785-8100

Write for catalog

Redwing Book Company
44 Linden Street
Brookline, MA 02146
(617) 738-4664

A good source for old, out-of-print as well as health books; write for catalog

B. Jain Publishers Overseas
1920 Chuna Mandi, Street 10th
Post Box 5775
Paharganj, New Delhi 110055 India.
Fax: 91-11-7510471

Carries many expensive homeopathic and medical texts that are printed on thin paper and are much cheaper to buy; remedy kits; write for catalog

Lights

Kiva Lights (Full sprectrum plus blue)

These lights keep down the bacterial count in the environment. Place over counters and sinks. Excellent for use in kennels, veterinary hospitals etc.

Kimo International Vitalized Association Inc.
912 Broadway, NE
Albuquerque, NM 87102

Full Spectrum Lights

Use anywhere dogs are housed, also in kitchen, offices etc. Can be found at most good lighting stores.

ph Strips

Available through drugstores or your veterinarian.

Associations

Write for practitioners in your area.

American Holistic Veterinary Medical Association
2214 Old Emmorton Road
Bel Air, MD 21015
(410) 569-0795

Directory of practicing veterinarians who offer holistic services

This association puts out an excellent magazine that anyone can buy. Membership is open to everyone. Write the association for more details.

American Veterinary Chiropractic Association
P.O. Box 249
Port Byron, IL 61275
(309) 523-3995

Write for directory of practitioners in the United States

Homeopathic Educational Services
Dana Ullman, President
2124 Kittredge Street
Berkeley, CA 94704
(800) 359-9051

Remedies, books, tapes, computer software, kits and more; write or call for catalog

National Center for Homeopathy
6231 Leesburg Pike, Suite 506
Falls Church, VA 22044

Directory of practitioners

National Iridology Research Association
P.O. Box 33637
Seattle, WA 98133
(206) 365-5980

Other Food Sources

Many ingredients for the Natural Diet are available through health food stores. The meat and liver can be bought through the supermarket. If you are looking for a place to buy meat in bulk, check local rendering plants to see if they will sell you *clean* meat directly. Most of these plants supply dog food companies and often have carcasses of animals that are not contaminated. If you can get several people together to buy meat in bulk, many of these companies will be willing to work with you. Chicken can be bought in bulk directly from restaurant supply companies.

There are some states where organic meat can be bought. Check your health food store for more information.

— Bibliography —

Airola, Pavo. *How to Get Well*. Sherwood, OR: Health Plus Publishers, 1974.

Balch, James F., and Phyllis A. Balch. *Prescription for Nutritional Healing*. Garden City Park, N.Y.: Avery Publishing, 1993.

Belfield, Wendell O., and Martin Zucker. *How to Have a Healthier Dog*. Garden City, N.Y. : Doubleday & Co. Inc., 1981.

Birchard, Stephen J. *Saunders Manual of Small Animal Practice*. Philadelphia: W. B. Saunders Co., 1993.

Burrows, C. *The Compendium Collection Gastroenterology in Practice*. Trenton N.J.: Veterinary Learning Systems, 1993.

Cargill, J., and S. Thorpe-Vargas. "Feed that Dog," Parts IV–VI. *Dog World*, 78, no. 10–12 (1994): 28–31, 36–42.

Chaitow, Leon. *Thorson's Guide to Amino Acids*. London: Harper Collins, 1991.

Cimino, J. A., S. Jhangiani, and E. Schwartz. "Riboflavin Metabolism." *Proceedings of the Society for Experimental Biology and Medicine*, issue no. 184. (1987): 151–153.

Collins, Donald R. *The Collins Guide to Dog Nutrition*. New York: Howell Book House, 1972.

Day, Christopher. *The Homeopathic Treatment of Small Animals*. Saffron Walden, England: C.W. Daniel Co. Ltd., 1990.

Diamond, John. *Your Body Doesn't Lie*. New York: Harper and Row, 1979.

Dodds, W.J. "Autoimmune Thyroid Disease." *Dog World*, 77 no. 4 (1992): 36–40.

———. "Genetic, Environmental and Nutritional Influences on Autoimmune Disease States." Holistic Study Group Seminar, June 3–4, 1994. Vandekamp Center, Cleveland, New York.

———. "The Immune System." *Dog World* (March 1995): 26–31.

———. "Vaccine Safety and Efficacy Revisited." *Veterinary Forum*, May, 1993: 68–71.

Dodds, W.J. and S. Donoghue. "Interactions of Clinical Nutrition with Genetics." Chapter 8. *The Waltham Book of Clinical Nutrition of the Dog and Cat*. Oxford: Pergamon Press, Ltd., 1994.

Ettinger, Stephen. *Diseases of the Dog and Cat*. Vol. 11 of *Textbook of Veterinary Internal Medicine*. 2d ed. Philadelphia: W.B. Saunders Co., 1983, 1381–82.

Evans, Howard E., and George C. Christensen. *Miller's Anatomy of the Dog*. Philadelphia: W. B. Saunders Co., 1979.

Feldman, Edward C., and Richard W. Nelson. *Canine and Feline Endocrinology and Reproduction*. Philadelphia: W. B. Saunders Co., 1979.

Fiengold, Ben. *Why Your Child Is Hyperactive*. New York: Random House, 1974.

Gerber, Richard. *Vibrational Medicine: New Choices of Healing Ourselves.* Santa Fe, NM: Bear and Company, 1988.

Haas, Elson. *Staying Healthy with Nutrition.* Berkeley, CA: Celestial Arts, 1992.

Hall, Dorothy. *Iridology: How the Eyes Reveal Your Health and Your Personality.* New Canaan, CT: Keats Publishing, 1981.

Hills Pet Products. *Hills Atlas of Veterinary Clinical Anatomy.* Lenexa, KS: Veterinary Medicine Publishing Co., 1989.

Jarvis, D.C. *Folk Medicine.* New York: Fawcett Books, 1988.

Jones, Brent D. *Canine and Feline Gastroenterology.* Philadelphia: W. B. Saunders Co., 1986.

Kirk, Robert W. *Kirk's Current Veterinary Therapy X1 - 205.* Philadelphia: W.B. Saunders Co., 1989.

Lepore, Donald. *The Ultimate Healing System.* Woodland, UT: Woodland Books, 1988.

Levy, Juliette de Bairacli. *Common Herbs for Natural Health.* New York: Schocken Books, 1974.

———. *The Complete Herbal Book for the Dog and Cat.* 6th ed. Winchester, MA: Faber & Faber, Ltd., 1991.

Macleod, G. *A Veterinary Materia Medica and Clinical Repertory with a Materia Medica of the Nosodes.* Saffron Walden, England: C.W. Daniel Co. Ltd., 1983.

Mindell, Earl. *Earl Mindell's Vitamin Bible.* New York: Warner Books, 1981.

Nutrient Requirement of Dogs. Rev. ed. Washington, DC: National Academy Press, 1985.

Ott, John N. *Health & Light: The Effects of Natural and Artificial Light on Man and Other Living Things.* Greenwich, CT: Devin-Adair Publishers, 1973.

Parry, Bruce W. *The Veterinary Clinic of North America-Clinical Pathology.* Part 1, Vol. 19.4. Philadelphia: W. B. Saunders Co., 1989.

———. *The Veterinary Clinic of North America-Clinical Pathology.* Part II, Vol. 19.5. Philadelphia: W. B. Saunders Co., 1989.

Plechner, Alfred, and Martin Zucker. *Pet Allergies: Remedies for an Epidemic.* Inglewood, CA: Very Healthy Enterprises, 1986.

60 Minutes CBS Nov. 23, 1980. Harry Reasoner.

Slatter, D. *Textbook of Small Animal Surgery.* 2nd ed. Vol 1. Philadelphia: W. B. Saunders Co., 1993.

Soditcoff, Charles, and Paul W. Pratt. *Laboratory Profiles of Small Animal Diseases.* American Publications, 1981.

Tizard, Ian. "Risks Associated with the Use of Live Vaccines." *Journal of American Veterinary Medical Association,* 196, no. 11 (1990): 1851–1858.

———. *Veterinary Immunology: An Introduction.* 4th ed. Philadelphia: W.B. Saunders Co., 1992, p. 498.

Williams, Sue Rodwell. *Nutrition Diet Therapy,* 6th ed. St. Louis: C.V. Mosby, 1989.

—Appendix I—

Amino Acids in Dogs

Essential (EAA)

arginine
histidine
isoleucine
leucine
lysine
methionine
phenylalanine
threonine
tryptophan
valine

Nonessential (NEAA)

alanine
asparagine
aspartic acid
carnitine
citroline
cysteine
gaba
glutamic acid
glutamine
glycine
hydroxyproline
ornithine
proline
serine
taurine
tyrosine

Arginine
ESSENTIAL AMINO ACID

EAA

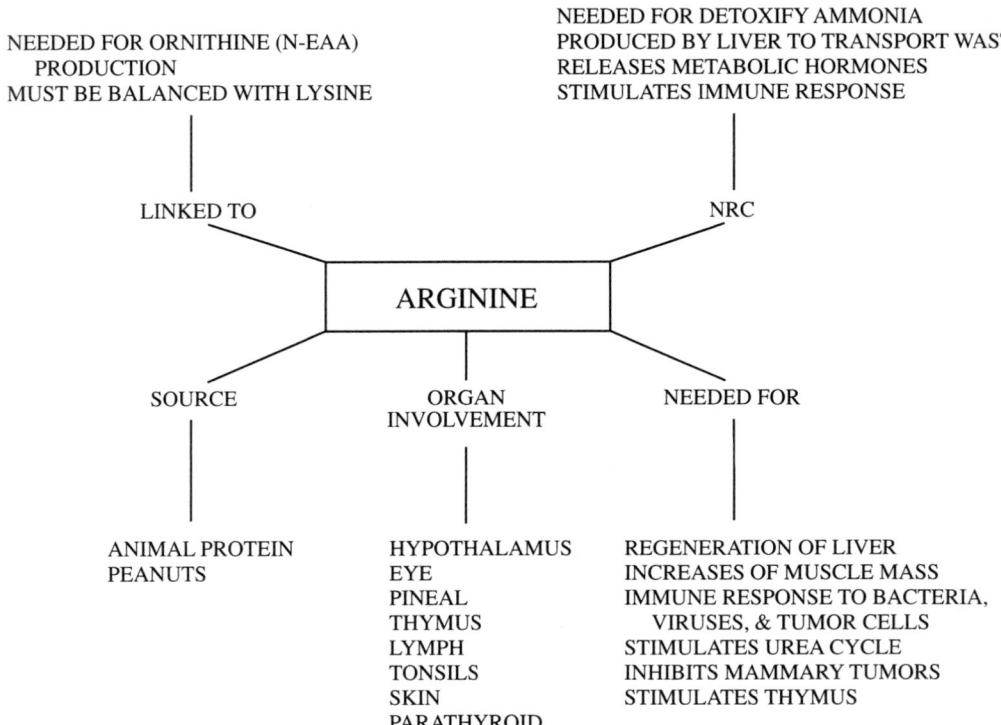

NEEDED FOR ORNITHINE (N-EAA)
PRODUCTION
MUST BE BALANCED WITH LYSINE

NEEDED FOR DETOXIFY AMMONIA
PRODUCED BY LIVER TO TRANSPORT WAST▮
RELEASES METABOLIC HORMONES
STIMULATES IMMUNE RESPONSE

LINKED TO

NRC

ARGININE

SOURCE

ORGAN
INVOLVEMENT

NEEDED FOR

ANIMAL PROTEIN
PEANUTS

HYPOTHALAMUS
EYE
PINEAL
THYMUS
LYMPH
TONSILS
SKIN
PARATHYROID

REGENERATION OF LIVER
INCREASES OF MUSCLE MASS
IMMUNE RESPONSE TO BACTERIA,
    VIRUSES, & TUMOR CELLS
STIMULATES UREA CYCLE
INHIBITS MAMMARY TUMORS
STIMULATES THYMUS

Histidine

EAA

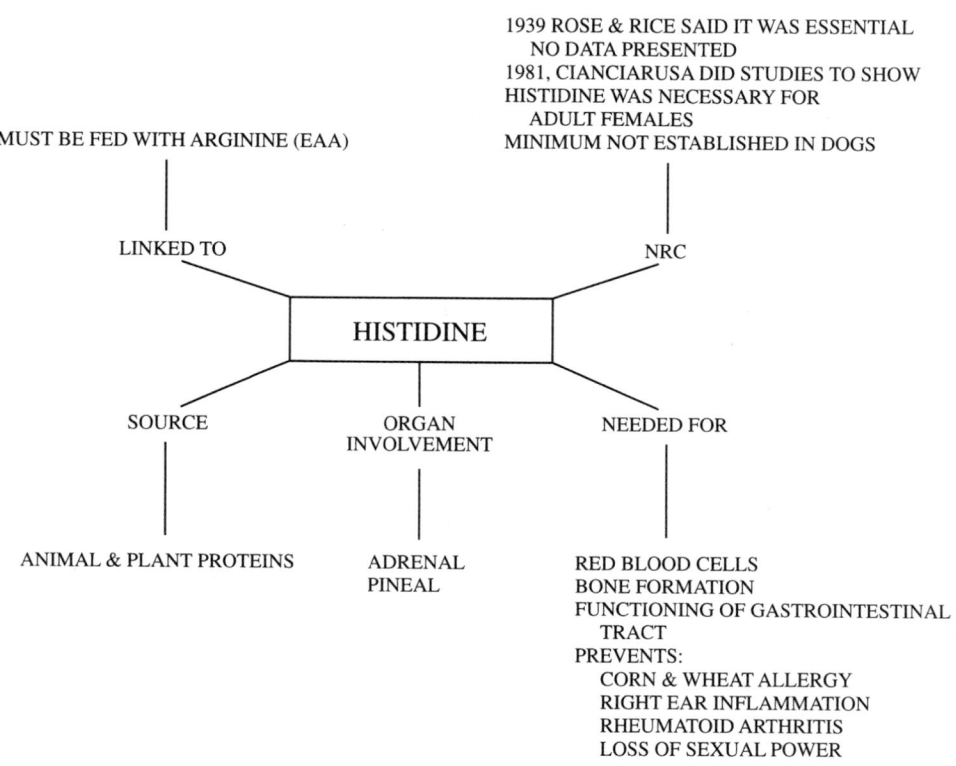

1939 ROSE & RICE SAID IT WAS ESSENTIAL
   NO DATA PRESENTED
1981, CIANCIARUSA DID STUDIES TO SHOW
HISTIDINE WAS NECESSARY FOR
   ADULT FEMALES
MINIMUM NOT ESTABLISHED IN DOGS

MUST BE FED WITH ARGININE (EAA)

LINKED TO

NRC

HISTIDINE

SOURCE

ORGAN
INVOLVEMENT

NEEDED FOR

ANIMAL & PLANT PROTEINS

ADRENAL
PINEAL

RED BLOOD CELLS
BONE FORMATION
FUNCTIONING OF GASTROINTESTINAL
   TRACT
PREVENTS:
   CORN & WHEAT ALLERGY
   RIGHT EAR INFLAMMATION
   RHEUMATOID ARTHRITIS
   LOSS OF SEXUAL POWER

Isoleucine

EAA

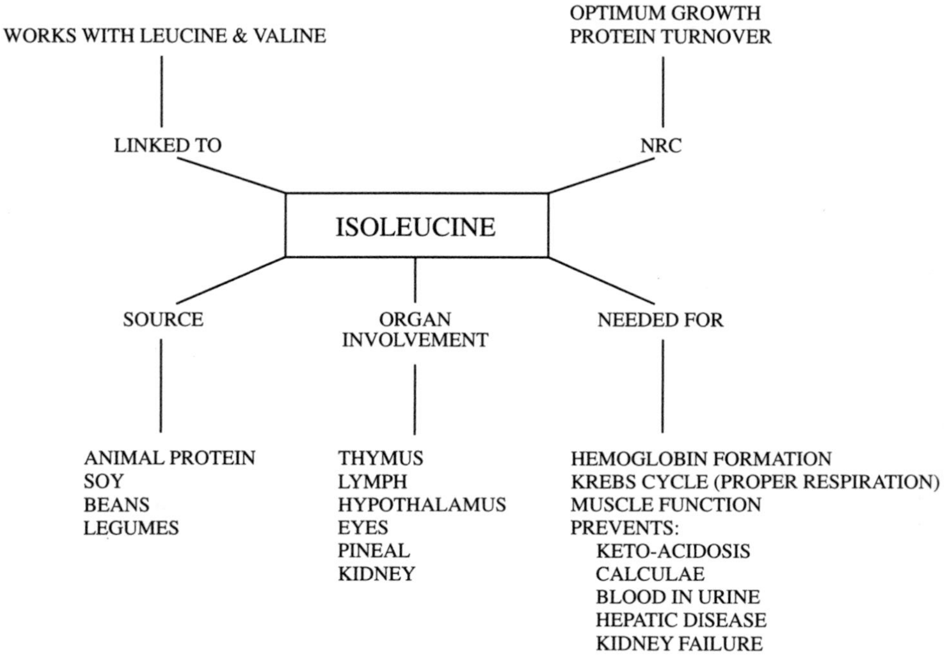

WORKS WITH LEUCINE & VALINE

OPTIMUM GROWTH
PROTEIN TURNOVER

LINKED TO

NRC

ISOLEUCINE

SOURCE

ORGAN
INVOLVEMENT

NEEDED FOR

ANIMAL PROTEIN
SOY
BEANS
LEGUMES

THYMUS
LYMPH
HYPOTHALAMUS
EYES
PINEAL
KIDNEY

HEMOGLOBIN FORMATION
KREBS CYCLE (PROPER RESPIRATION)
MUSCLE FUNCTION
PREVENTS:
    KETO-ACIDOSIS
    CALCULAE
    BLOOD IN URINE
    HEPATIC DISEASE
    KIDNEY FAILURE

Leucine

EAA

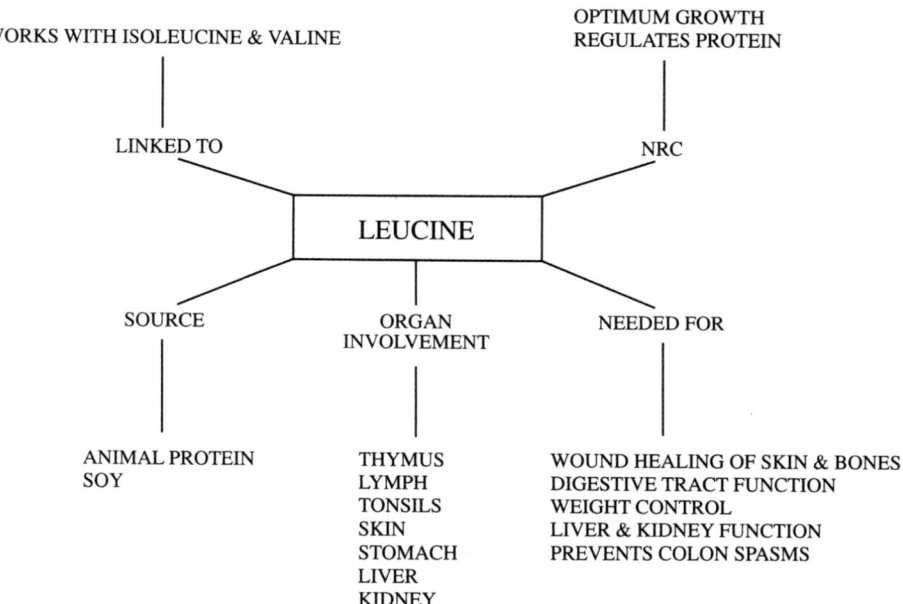

WORKS WITH ISOLEUCINE & VALINE

OPTIMUM GROWTH
REGULATES PROTEIN

LINKED TO

NRC

LEUCINE

SOURCE

ORGAN
INVOLVEMENT

NEEDED FOR

ANIMAL PROTEIN
SOY

THYMUS
LYMPH
TONSILS
SKIN
STOMACH
LIVER
KIDNEY

WOUND HEALING OF SKIN & BONES
DIGESTIVE TRACT FUNCTION
WEIGHT CONTROL
LIVER & KIDNEY FUNCTION
PREVENTS COLON SPASMS

Lysine

EAA

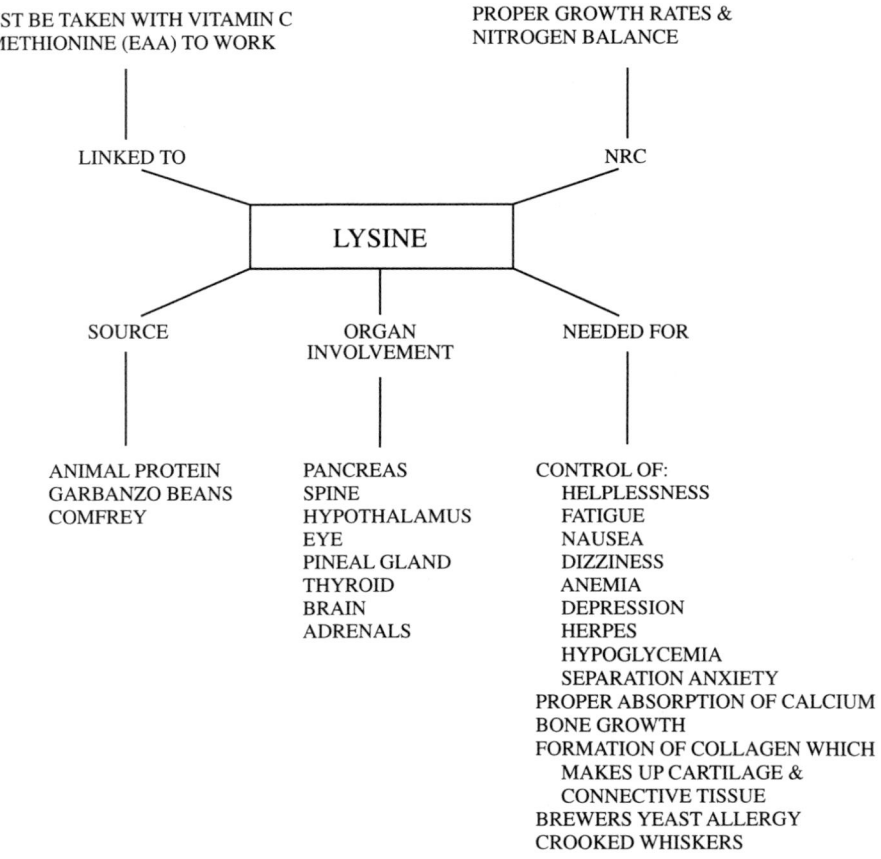

MUST BE TAKEN WITH VITAMIN C
& METHIONINE (EAA) TO WORK

PROPER GROWTH RATES &
NITROGEN BALANCE

LINKED TO

NRC

LYSINE

SOURCE

ORGAN
INVOLVEMENT

NEEDED FOR

ANIMAL PROTEIN
GARBANZO BEANS
COMFREY

PANCREAS
SPINE
HYPOTHALAMUS
EYE
PINEAL GLAND
THYROID
BRAIN
ADRENALS

CONTROL OF:
  HELPLESSNESS
  FATIGUE
  NAUSEA
  DIZZINESS
  ANEMIA
  DEPRESSION
  HERPES
  HYPOGLYCEMIA
  SEPARATION ANXIETY
PROPER ABSORPTION OF CALCIUM
BONE GROWTH
FORMATION OF COLLAGEN WHICH
  MAKES UP CARTILAGE &
  CONNECTIVE TISSUE
BREWERS YEAST ALLERGY
CROOKED WHISKERS

Methionine

EAA

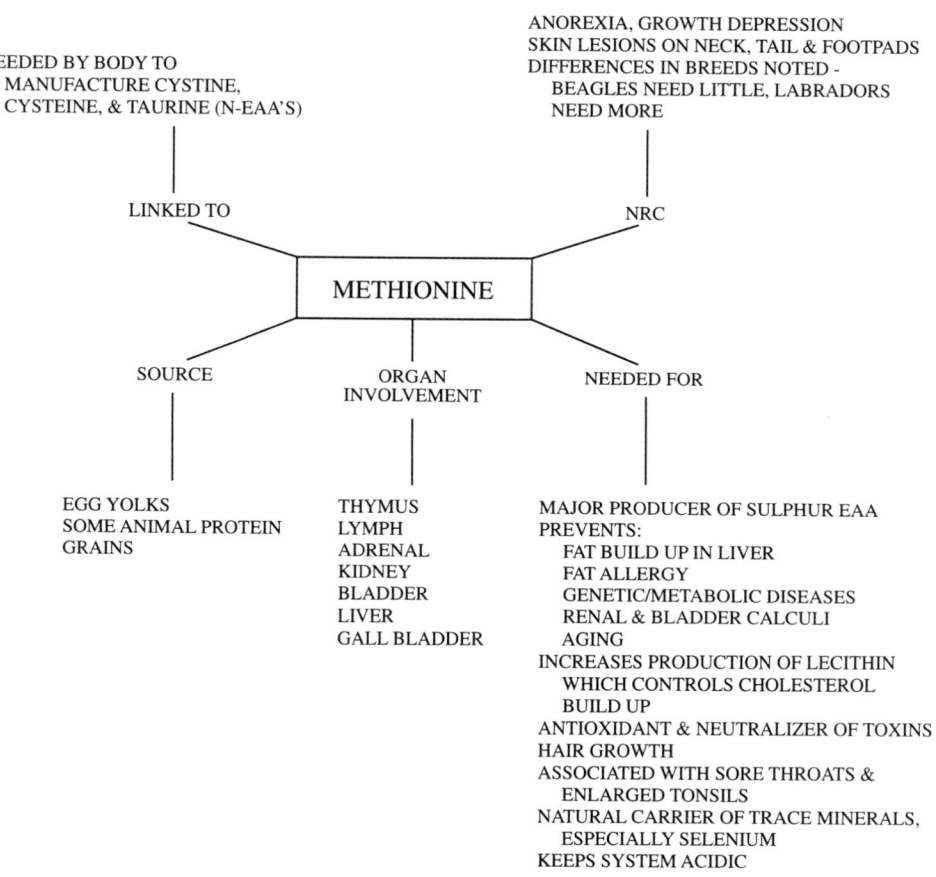

NEEDED BY BODY TO
   MANUFACTURE CYSTINE,
   CYSTEINE, & TAURINE (N-EAA'S)

ANOREXIA, GROWTH DEPRESSION
SKIN LESIONS ON NECK, TAIL & FOOTPADS
DIFFERENCES IN BREEDS NOTED -
   BEAGLES NEED LITTLE, LABRADORS
   NEED MORE

LINKED TO

NRC

METHIONINE

SOURCE

ORGAN
INVOLVEMENT

NEEDED FOR

EGG YOLKS
SOME ANIMAL PROTEIN
GRAINS

THYMUS
LYMPH
ADRENAL
KIDNEY
BLADDER
LIVER
GALL BLADDER

MAJOR PRODUCER OF SULPHUR EAA
PREVENTS:
   FAT BUILD UP IN LIVER
   FAT ALLERGY
   GENETIC/METABOLIC DISEASES
   RENAL & BLADDER CALCULI
   AGING
INCREASES PRODUCTION OF LECITHIN
   WHICH CONTROLS CHOLESTEROL
   BUILD UP
ANTIOXIDANT & NEUTRALIZER OF TOXINS
HAIR GROWTH
ASSOCIATED WITH SORE THROATS &
   ENLARGED TONSILS
NATURAL CARRIER OF TRACE MINERALS,
   ESPECIALLY SELENIUM
KEEPS SYSTEM ACIDIC

DO NOT SUPPLEMENT WITH THIS
ALONE IF LIVER DISEASE IS PRESENT.

Phenylalanine
EAA

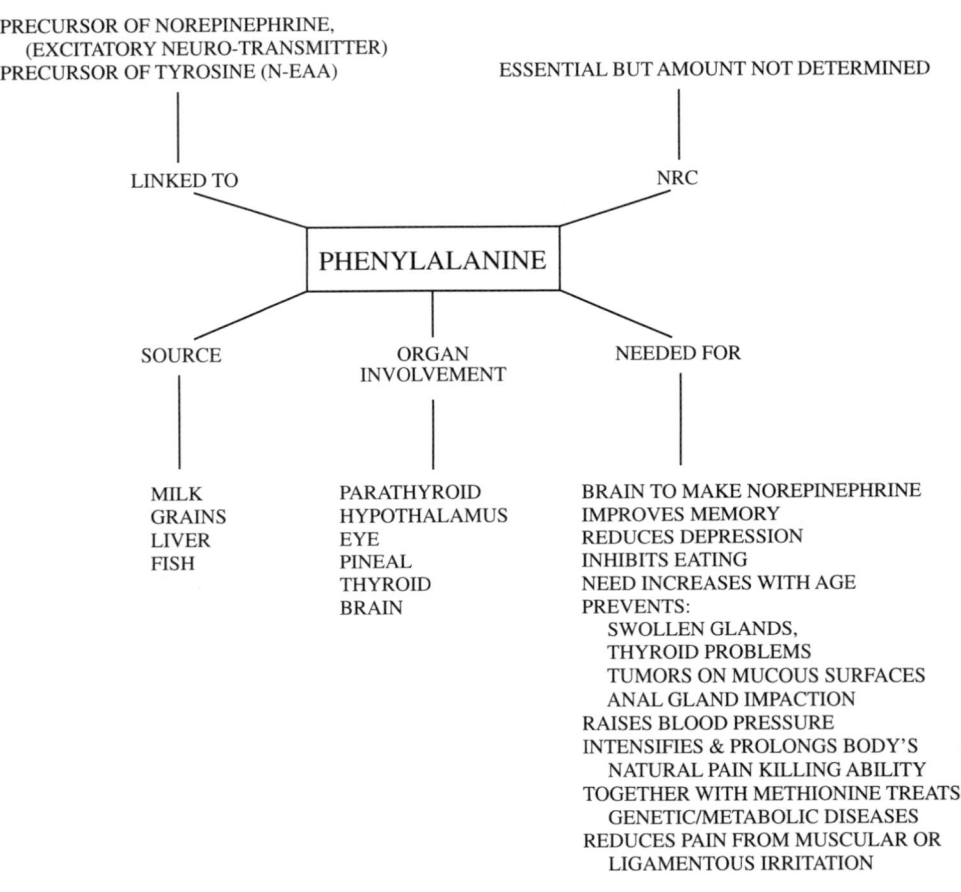

PRECURSOR OF NOREPINEPHRINE,
   (EXCITATORY NEURO-TRANSMITTER)
PRECURSOR OF TYROSINE (N-EAA)

ESSENTIAL BUT AMOUNT NOT DETERMINED

LINKED TO

NRC

PHENYLALANINE

SOURCE

ORGAN
INVOLVEMENT

NEEDED FOR

MILK
GRAINS
LIVER
FISH

PARATHYROID
HYPOTHALAMUS
EYE
PINEAL
THYROID
BRAIN

BRAIN TO MAKE NOREPINEPHRINE
IMPROVES MEMORY
REDUCES DEPRESSION
INHIBITS EATING
NEED INCREASES WITH AGE
PREVENTS:
   SWOLLEN GLANDS,
   THYROID PROBLEMS
   TUMORS ON MUCOUS SURFACES
   ANAL GLAND IMPACTION
RAISES BLOOD PRESSURE
INTENSIFIES & PROLONGS BODY'S
   NATURAL PAIN KILLING ABILITY
TOGETHER WITH METHIONINE TREATS
   GENETIC/METABOLIC DISEASES
REDUCES PAIN FROM MUSCULAR OR
   LIGAMENTOUS IRRITATION

Threonine

EAA

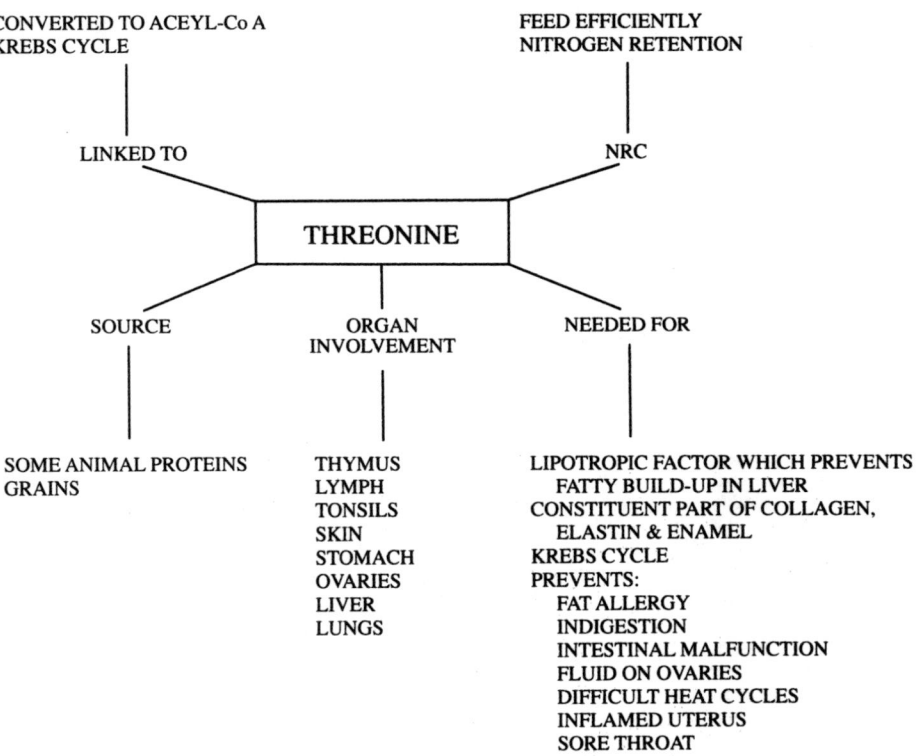

CONVERTED TO ACEYL-Co A
KREBS CYCLE

FEED EFFICIENTLY
NITROGEN RETENTION

LINKED TO

NRC

THREONINE

SOURCE

ORGAN
INVOLVEMENT

NEEDED FOR

SOME ANIMAL PROTEINS
GRAINS

THYMUS
LYMPH
TONSILS
SKIN
STOMACH
OVARIES
LIVER
LUNGS

LIPOTROPIC FACTOR WHICH PREVENTS
    FATTY BUILD-UP IN LIVER
CONSTITUENT PART OF COLLAGEN,
    ELASTIN & ENAMEL
KREBS CYCLE
PREVENTS:
    FAT ALLERGY
    INDIGESTION
    INTESTINAL MALFUNCTION
    FLUID ON OVARIES
    DIFFICULT HEAT CYCLES
    INFLAMED UTERUS
    SORE THROAT

Tryptophan

EAA

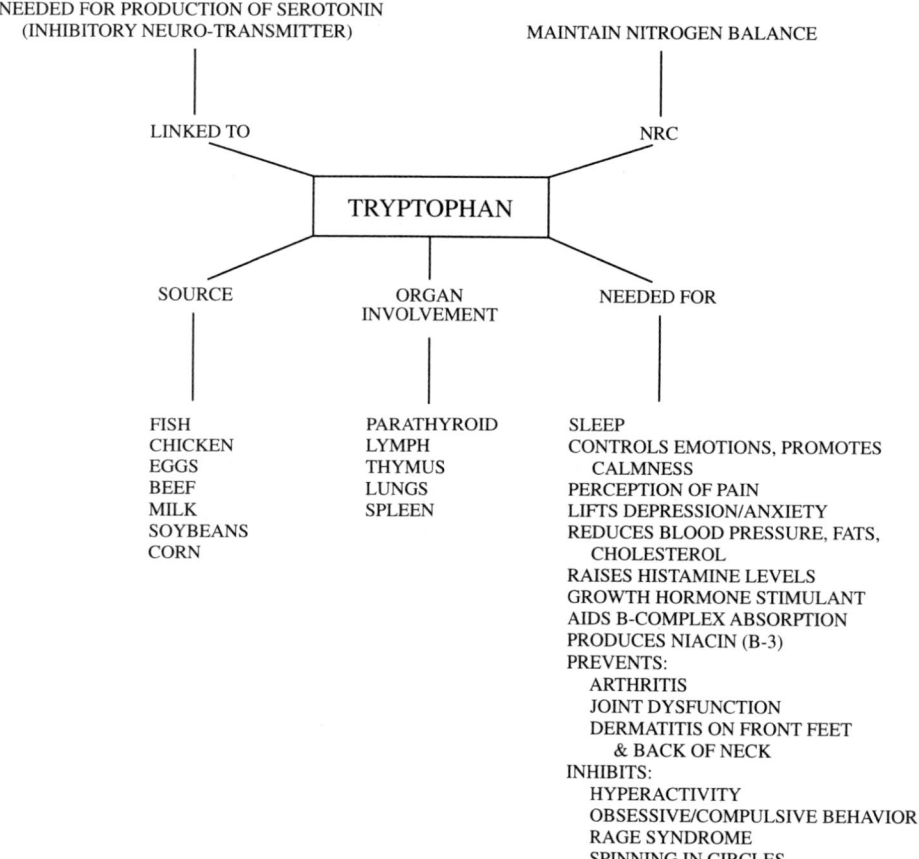

NEEDED FOR PRODUCTION OF SEROTONIN
(INHIBITORY NEURO-TRANSMITTER)

MAINTAIN NITROGEN BALANCE

LINKED TO

NRC

TRYPTOPHAN

SOURCE

ORGAN
INVOLVEMENT

NEEDED FOR

FISH
CHICKEN
EGGS
BEEF
MILK
SOYBEANS
CORN

PARATHYROID
LYMPH
THYMUS
LUNGS
SPLEEN

SLEEP
CONTROLS EMOTIONS, PROMOTES
   CALMNESS
PERCEPTION OF PAIN
LIFTS DEPRESSION/ANXIETY
REDUCES BLOOD PRESSURE, FATS,
   CHOLESTEROL
RAISES HISTAMINE LEVELS
GROWTH HORMONE STIMULANT
AIDS B-COMPLEX ABSORPTION
PRODUCES NIACIN (B-3)
PREVENTS:
   ARTHRITIS
   JOINT DYSFUNCTION
   DERMATITIS ON FRONT FEET
     & BACK OF NECK
INHIBITS:
   HYPERACTIVITY
   OBSESSIVE/COMPULSIVE BEHAVIOR
   RAGE SYNDROME
   SPINNING IN CIRCLES

Valine

EAA

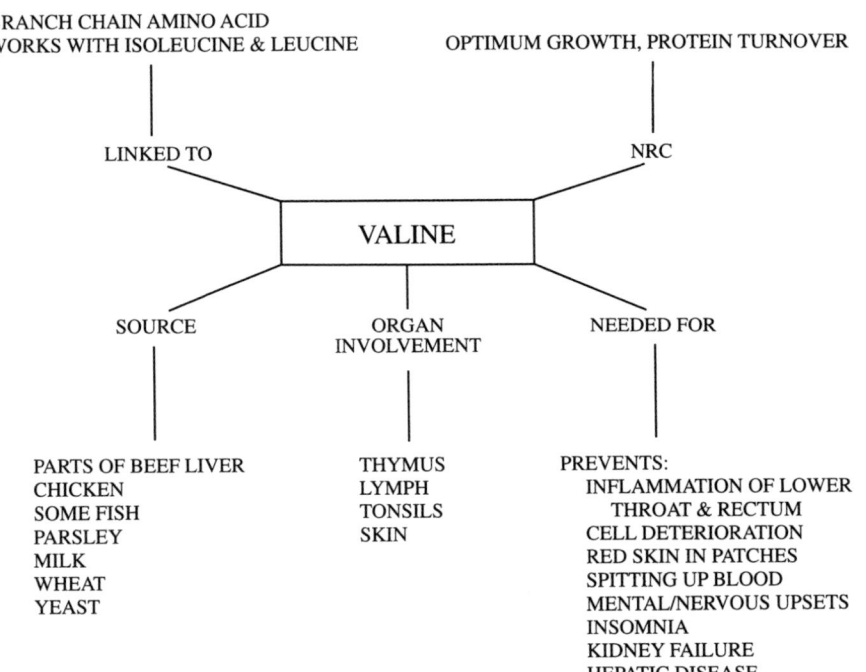

BRANCH CHAIN AMINO ACID
WORKS WITH ISOLEUCINE & LEUCINE   OPTIMUM GROWTH, PROTEIN TURNOVER

LINKED TO   NRC

VALINE

SOURCE   ORGAN   NEEDED FOR
                        INVOLVEMENT

PARTS OF BEEF LIVER   THYMUS   PREVENTS:
CHICKEN   LYMPH   INFLAMMATION OF LOWER
SOME FISH   TONSILS   THROAT & RECTUM
PARSLEY   SKIN   CELL DETERIORATION
MILK   RED SKIN IN PATCHES
WHEAT   SPITTING UP BLOOD
YEAST   MENTAL/NERVOUS UPSETS
                                                   INSOMNIA
                                                   KIDNEY FAILURE
                                                   HEPATIC DISEASE

NON-ESSENTIAL AMINO ACIDS
Alanine
N-EAA

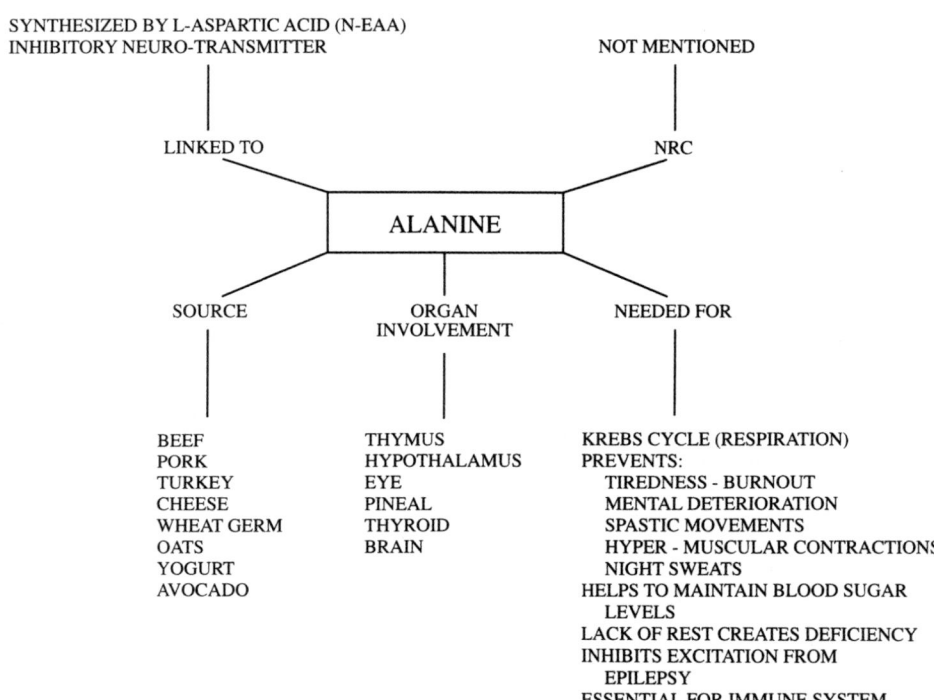

SYNTHESIZED BY L-ASPARTIC ACID (N-EAA)
INHIBITORY NEURO-TRANSMITTER

NOT MENTIONED

LINKED TO

NRC

ALANINE

SOURCE

ORGAN INVOLVEMENT

NEEDED FOR

BEEF
PORK
TURKEY
CHEESE
WHEAT GERM
OATS
YOGURT
AVOCADO

THYMUS
HYPOTHALAMUS
EYE
PINEAL
THYROID
BRAIN

KREBS CYCLE (RESPIRATION)
PREVENTS:
   TIREDNESS - BURNOUT
   MENTAL DETERIORATION
   SPASTIC MOVEMENTS
   HYPER - MUSCULAR CONTRACTIONS
   NIGHT SWEATS
HELPS TO MAINTAIN BLOOD SUGAR
   LEVELS
LACK OF REST CREATES DEFICIENCY
INHIBITS EXCITATION FROM
   EPILEPSY
ESSENTIAL FOR IMMUNE SYSTEM

Asparagine

N-EAA

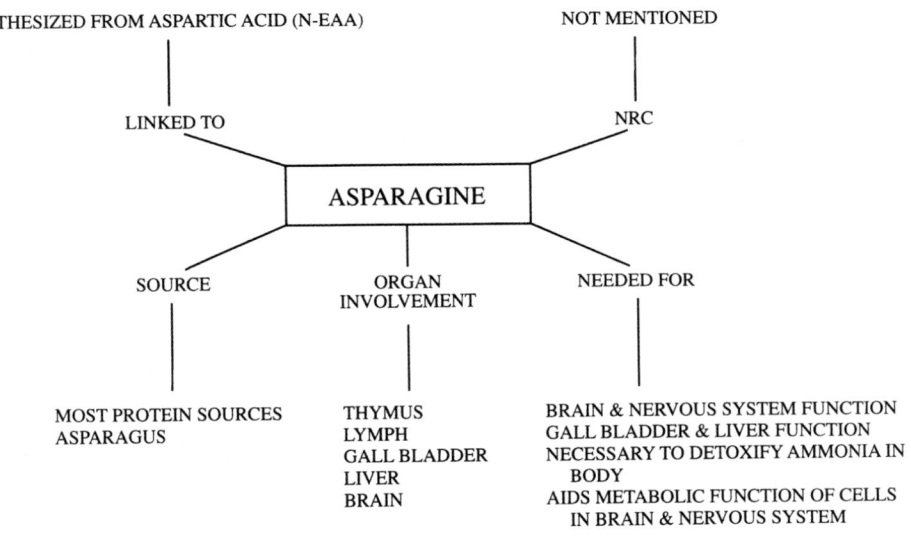

SYNTHESIZED FROM ASPARTIC ACID (N-EAA)

NOT MENTIONED

LINKED TO

NRC

ASPARAGINE

SOURCE

ORGAN
INVOLVEMENT

NEEDED FOR

MOST PROTEIN SOURCES
ASPARAGUS

THYMUS
LYMPH
GALL BLADDER
LIVER
BRAIN

BRAIN & NERVOUS SYSTEM FUNCTION
GALL BLADDER & LIVER FUNCTION
NECESSARY TO DETOXIFY AMMONIA IN
BODY
AIDS METABOLIC FUNCTION OF CELLS
IN BRAIN & NERVOUS SYSTEM

Aspartic Acid

N-EAA

N-EAA

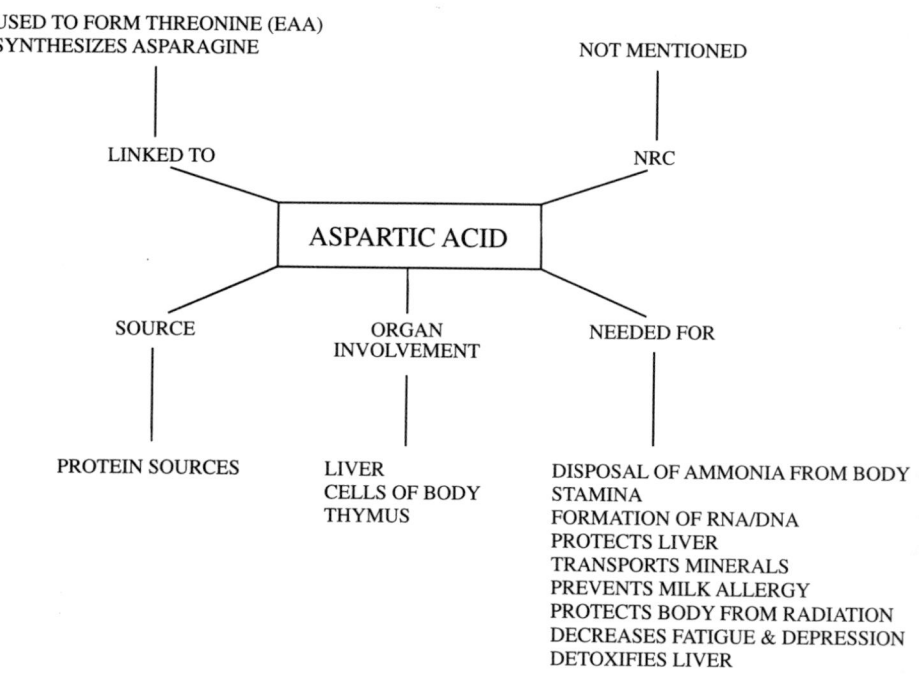

USED TO FORM THREONINE (EAA)
SYNTHESIZES ASPARAGINE
                            NOT MENTIONED

LINKED TO   NRC

ASPARTIC ACID

SOURCE   ORGAN
              INVOLVEMENT   NEEDED FOR

PROTEIN SOURCES   LIVER   DISPOSAL OF AMMONIA FROM BODY
                         CELLS OF BODY   STAMINA
                         THYMUS   FORMATION OF RNA/DNA
                                         PROTECTS LIVER
                                         TRANSPORTS MINERALS
                                         PREVENTS MILK ALLERGY
                                         PROTECTS BODY FROM RADIATION
                                         DECREASES FATIGUE & DEPRESSION
                                         DETOXIFIES LIVER

Carnitine

N-EAA

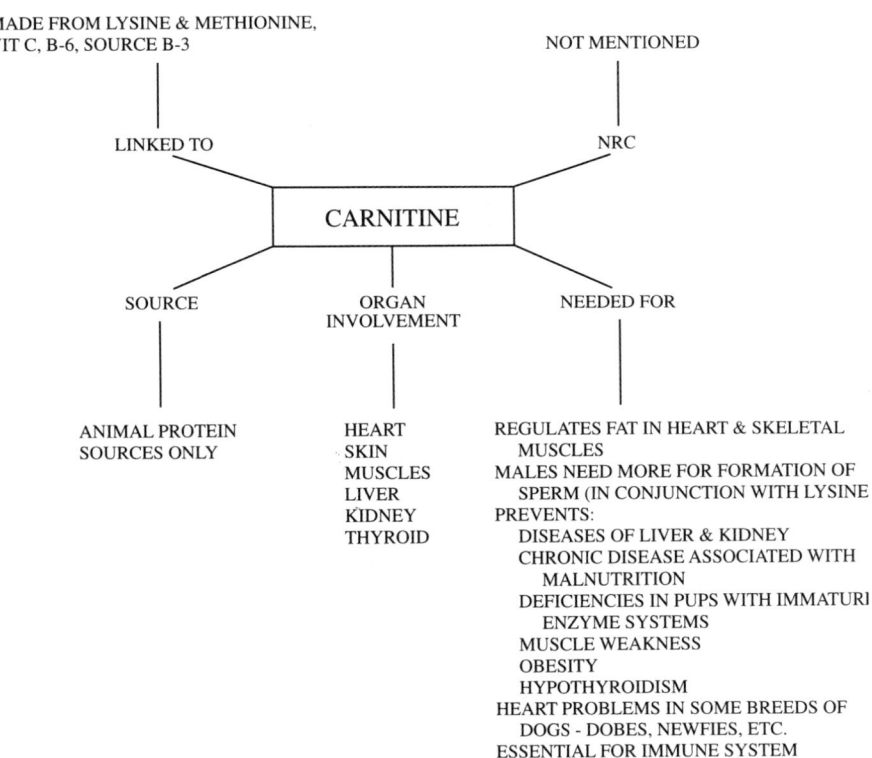

MADE FROM LYSINE & METHIONINE,
VIT C, B-6, SOURCE B-3

NOT MENTIONED

LINKED TO

NRC

CARNITINE

SOURCE

ORGAN
INVOLVEMENT

NEEDED FOR

ANIMAL PROTEIN
SOURCES ONLY

HEART
SKIN
MUSCLES
LIVER
KIDNEY
THYROID

REGULATES FAT IN HEART & SKELETAL
MUSCLES
MALES NEED MORE FOR FORMATION OF
SPERM (IN CONJUNCTION WITH LYSINE
PREVENTS:
DISEASES OF LIVER & KIDNEY
CHRONIC DISEASE ASSOCIATED WITH
MALNUTRITION
DEFICIENCIES IN PUPS WITH IMMATURI
ENZYME SYSTEMS
MUSCLE WEAKNESS
OBESITY
HYPOTHYROIDISM
HEART PROBLEMS IN SOME BREEDS OF
DOGS - DOBES, NEWFIES, ETC.
ESSENTIAL FOR IMMUNE SYSTEM

Citroline

N-EAA

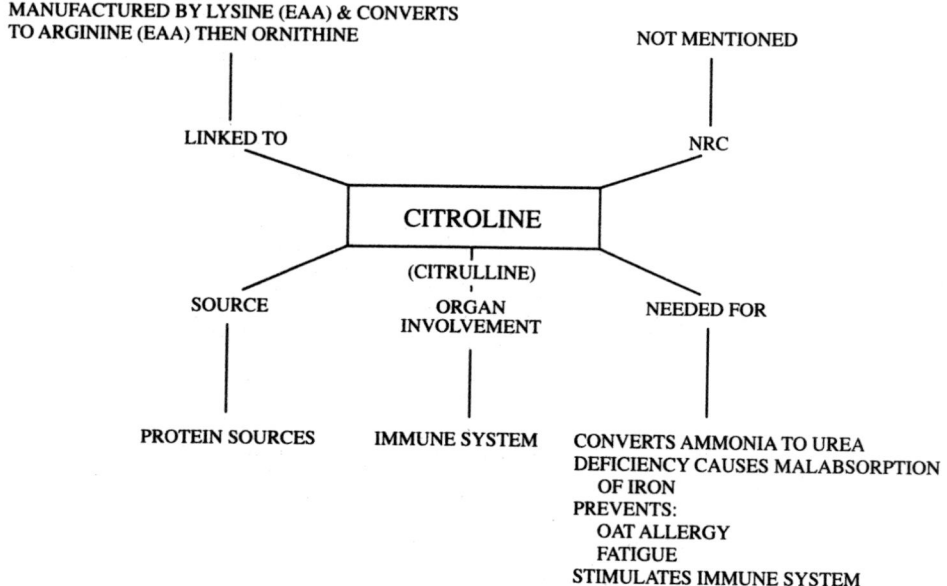

MANUFACTURED BY LYSINE (EAA) & CONVERTS
TO ARGININE (EAA) THEN ORNITHINE

NOT MENTIONED

LINKED TO

NRC

CITROLINE

(CITRULLINE)

SOURCE

ORGAN
INVOLVEMENT

NEEDED FOR

PROTEIN SOURCES

IMMUNE SYSTEM

CONVERTS AMMONIA TO UREA
DEFICIENCY CAUSES MALABSORPTION
OF IRON
PREVENTS:
OAT ALLERGY
FATIGUE
STIMULATES IMMUNE SYSTEM

Cysteine

N-EAA

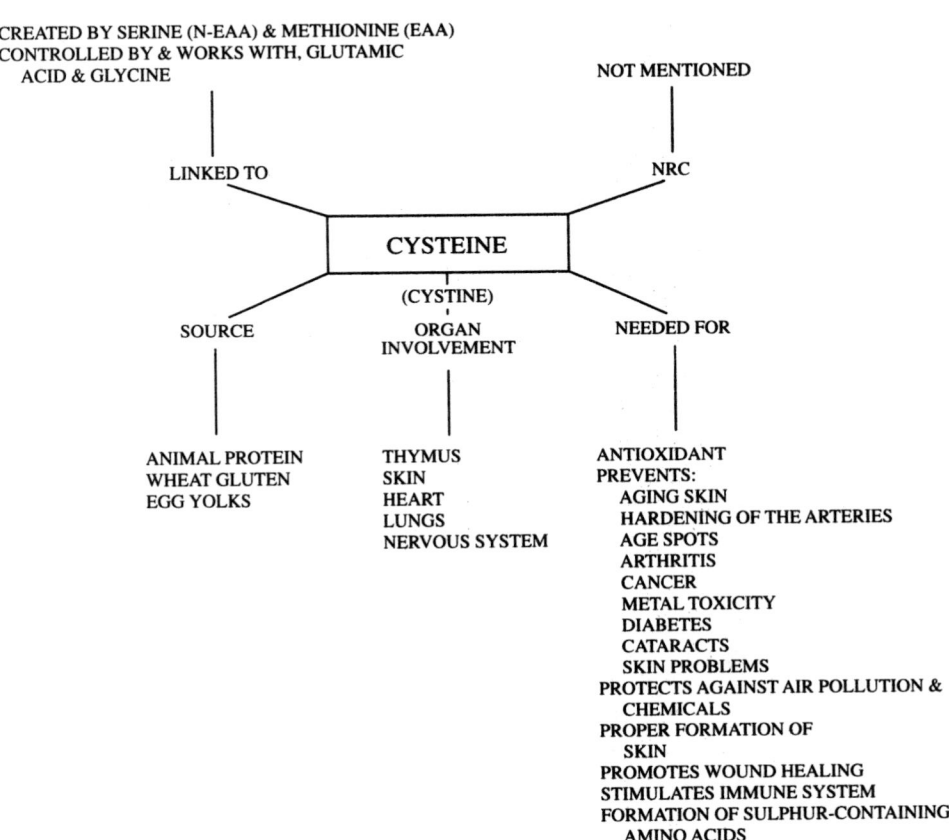

CREATED BY SERINE (N-EAA) & METHIONINE (EAA)
CONTROLLED BY & WORKS WITH, GLUTAMIC
   ACID & GLYCINE

NOT MENTIONED

LINKED TO

NRC

CYSTEINE

(CYSTINE)

SOURCE

ORGAN
INVOLVEMENT

NEEDED FOR

ANIMAL PROTEIN
WHEAT GLUTEN
EGG YOLKS

THYMUS
SKIN
HEART
LUNGS
NERVOUS SYSTEM

ANTIOXIDANT
PREVENTS:
   AGING SKIN
   HARDENING OF THE ARTERIES
   AGE SPOTS
   ARTHRITIS
   CANCER
   METAL TOXICITY
   DIABETES
   CATARACTS
   SKIN PROBLEMS
PROTECTS AGAINST AIR POLLUTION &
   CHEMICALS
PROPER FORMATION OF
   SKIN
PROMOTES WOUND HEALING
STIMULATES IMMUNE SYSTEM
FORMATION OF SULPHUR-CONTAINING
   AMINO ACIDS

GABA
N-EAA

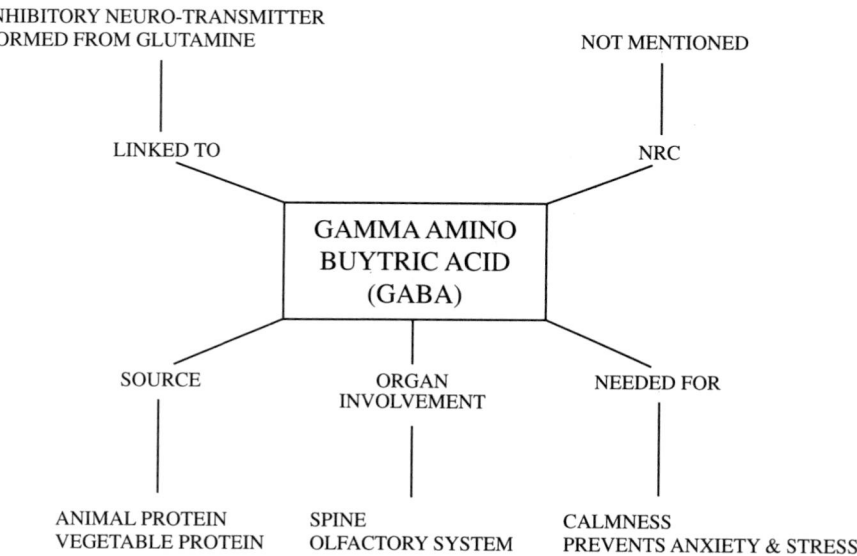

INHIBITORY NEURO-TRANSMITTER
FORMED FROM GLUTAMINE

NOT MENTIONED

LINKED TO

NRC

GAMMA AMINO
BUYTRIC ACID
(GABA)

SOURCE

ORGAN
INVOLVEMENT

NEEDED FOR

ANIMAL PROTEIN
VEGETABLE PROTEIN

SPINE
OLFACTORY SYSTEM

CALMNESS
PREVENTS ANXIETY & STRESS

Glutamic Acid

N-EAA

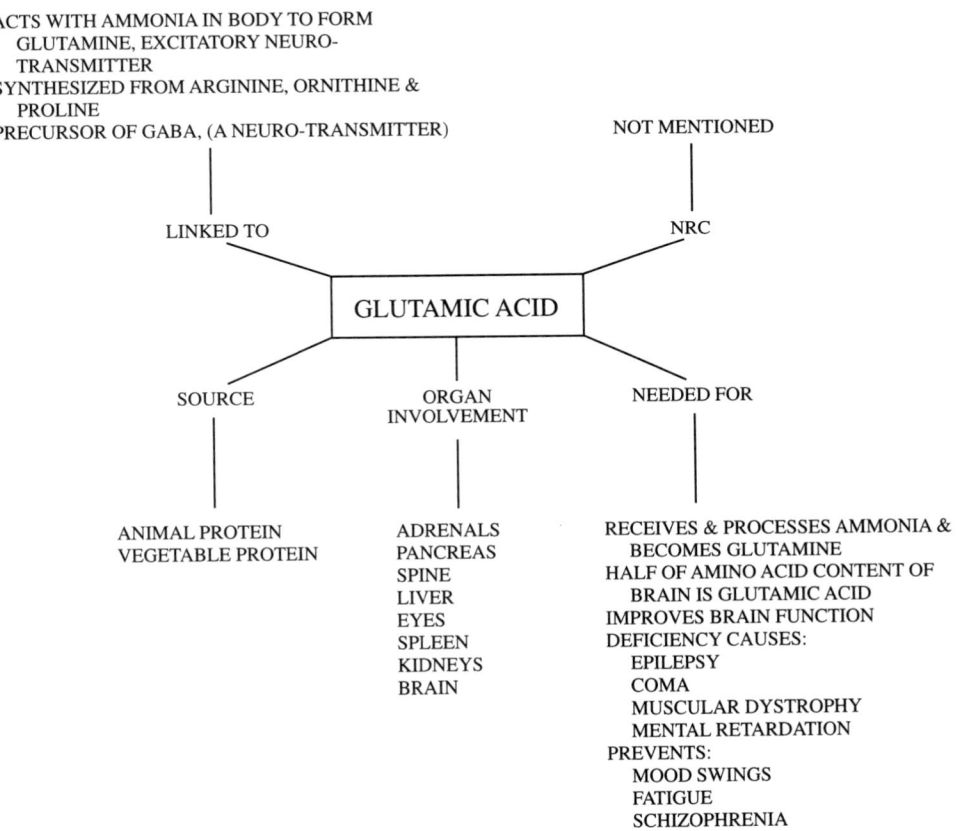

ACTS WITH AMMONIA IN BODY TO FORM
    GLUTAMINE, EXCITATORY NEURO-
    TRANSMITTER
SYNTHESIZED FROM ARGININE, ORNITHINE &
    PROLINE
PRECURSOR OF GABA, (A NEURO-TRANSMITTER)

NOT MENTIONED

LINKED TO

NRC

GLUTAMIC ACID

SOURCE

ORGAN
INVOLVEMENT

NEEDED FOR

ANIMAL PROTEIN
VEGETABLE PROTEIN

ADRENALS
PANCREAS
SPINE
LIVER
EYES
SPLEEN
KIDNEYS
BRAIN

RECEIVES & PROCESSES AMMONIA &
    BECOMES GLUTAMINE
HALF OF AMINO ACID CONTENT OF
    BRAIN IS GLUTAMIC ACID
IMPROVES BRAIN FUNCTION
DEFICIENCY CAUSES:
    EPILEPSY
    COMA
    MUSCULAR DYSTROPHY
    MENTAL RETARDATION
PREVENTS:
    MOOD SWINGS
    FATIGUE
    SCHIZOPHRENIA
    NIGHT-TIME INCONTINENCE

Glutamine
N-EAA

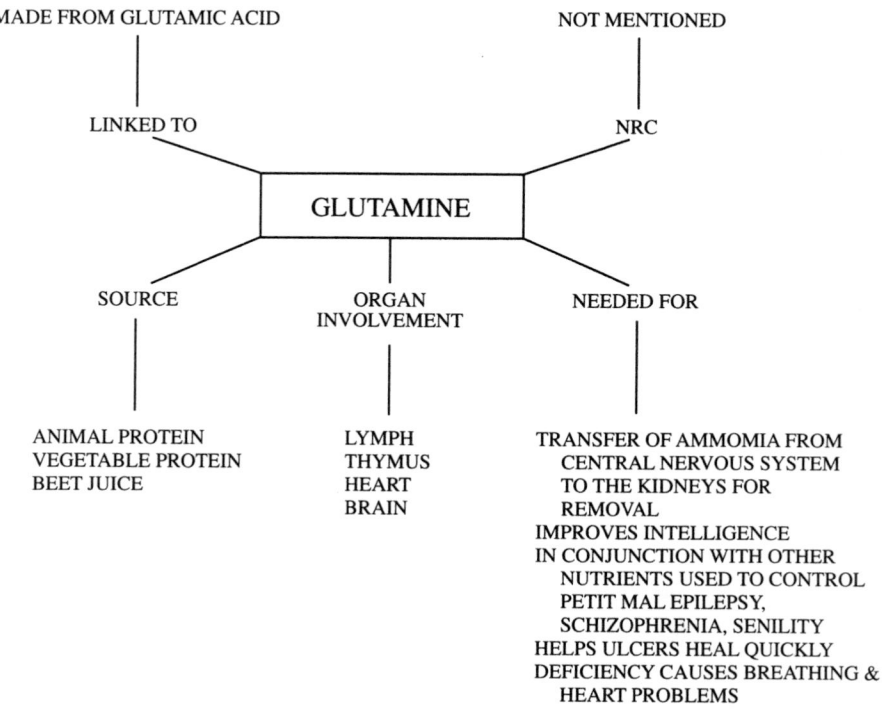

MADE FROM GLUTAMIC ACID

LINKED TO

NOT MENTIONED

NRC

GLUTAMINE

SOURCE

ORGAN
INVOLVEMENT

NEEDED FOR

ANIMAL PROTEIN
VEGETABLE PROTEIN
BEET JUICE

LYMPH
THYMUS
HEART
BRAIN

TRANSFER OF AMMOMIA FROM
CENTRAL NERVOUS SYSTEM
TO THE KIDNEYS FOR
REMOVAL
IMPROVES INTELLIGENCE
IN CONJUNCTION WITH OTHER
NUTRIENTS USED TO CONTROL
PETIT MAL EPILEPSY,
SCHIZOPHRENIA, SENILITY
HELPS ULCERS HEAL QUICKLY
DEFICIENCY CAUSES BREATHING &
HEART PROBLEMS

Glycine

N-EAA

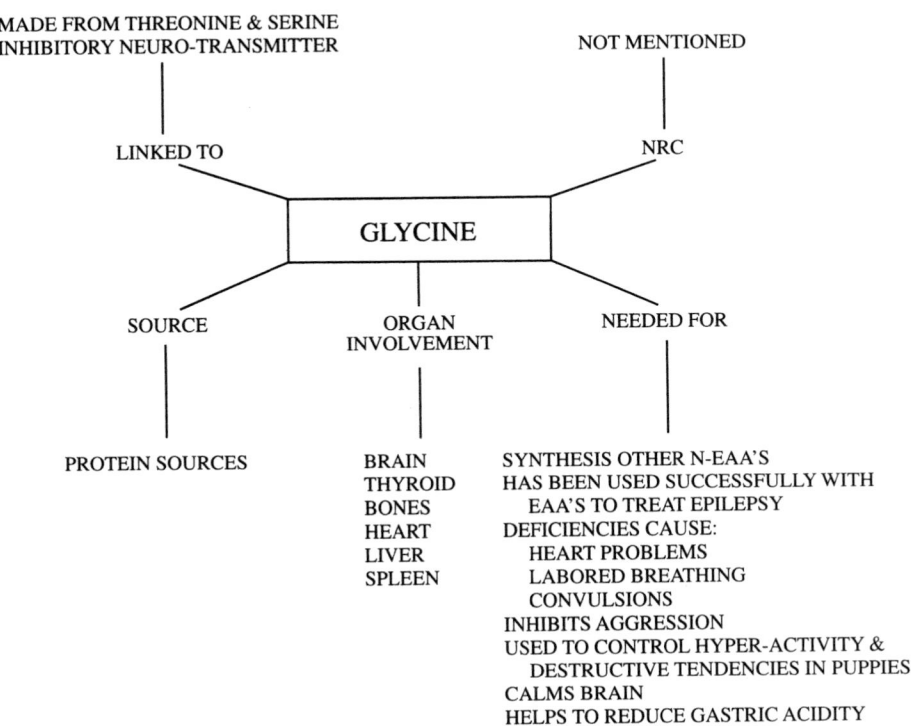

MADE FROM THREONINE & SERINE
INHIBITORY NEURO-TRANSMITTER

NOT MENTIONED

LINKED TO

NRC

GLYCINE

SOURCE

ORGAN
INVOLVEMENT

NEEDED FOR

PROTEIN SOURCES

BRAIN
THYROID
BONES
HEART
LIVER
SPLEEN

SYNTHESIS OTHER N-EAA'S
HAS BEEN USED SUCCESSFULLY WITH
    EAA'S TO TREAT EPILEPSY
DEFICIENCIES CAUSE:
    HEART PROBLEMS
    LABORED BREATHING
    CONVULSIONS
INHIBITS AGGRESSION
USED TO CONTROL HYPER-ACTIVITY &
    DESTRUCTIVE TENDENCIES IN PUPPIES
CALMS BRAIN
HELPS TO REDUCE GASTRIC ACIDITY

Hydroxyproline
N-EAA

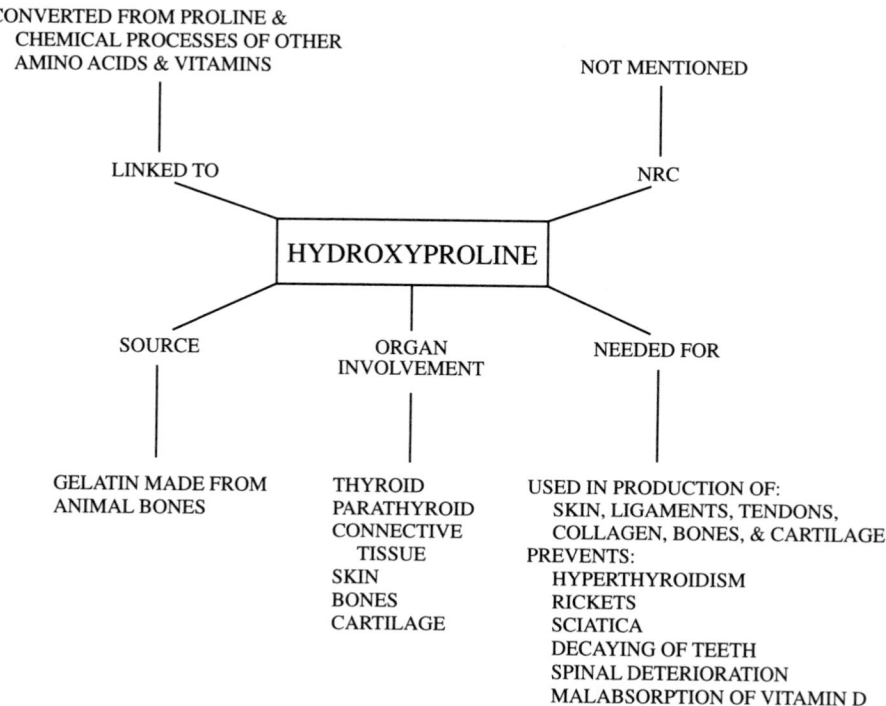

CONVERTED FROM PROLINE &
CHEMICAL PROCESSES OF OTHER
AMINO ACIDS & VITAMINS   NOT MENTIONED

LINKED TO   NRC

HYDROXYPROLINE

SOURCE   ORGAN   NEEDED FOR
                          INVOLVEMENT

GELATIN MADE FROM   THYROID   USED IN PRODUCTION OF:
ANIMAL BONES   PARATHYROID   SKIN, LIGAMENTS, TENDONS,
                          CONNECTIVE   COLLAGEN, BONES, & CARTILAGE
                            TISSUE   PREVENTS:
                          SKIN   HYPERTHYROIDISM
                          BONES   RICKETS
                          CARTILAGE   SCIATICA
                                              DECAYING OF TEETH
                                              SPINAL DETERIORATION
                                              MALABSORPTION OF VITAMIN D

Ornithine

N-EAA

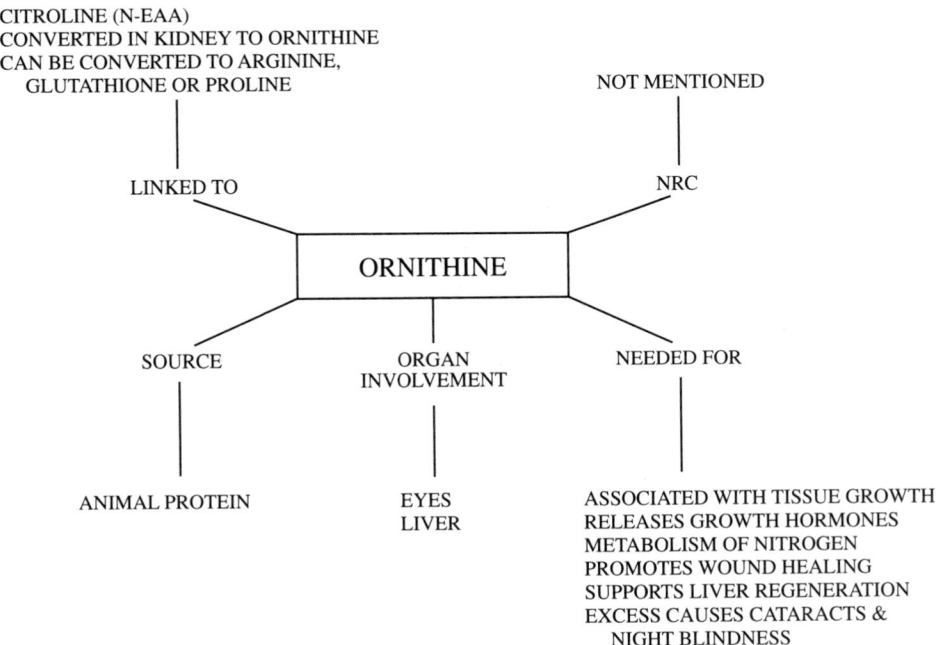

CITROLINE (N-EAA)
CONVERTED IN KIDNEY TO ORNITHINE
CAN BE CONVERTED TO ARGININE,
  GLUTATHIONE OR PROLINE

NOT MENTIONED

LINKED TO

NRC

ORNITHINE

SOURCE

ORGAN
INVOLVEMENT

NEEDED FOR

ANIMAL PROTEIN

EYES
LIVER

ASSOCIATED WITH TISSUE GROWTH
RELEASES GROWTH HORMONES
METABOLISM OF NITROGEN
PROMOTES WOUND HEALING
SUPPORTS LIVER REGENERATION
EXCESS CAUSES CATARACTS &
  NIGHT BLINDNESS

Proline

N-EAA

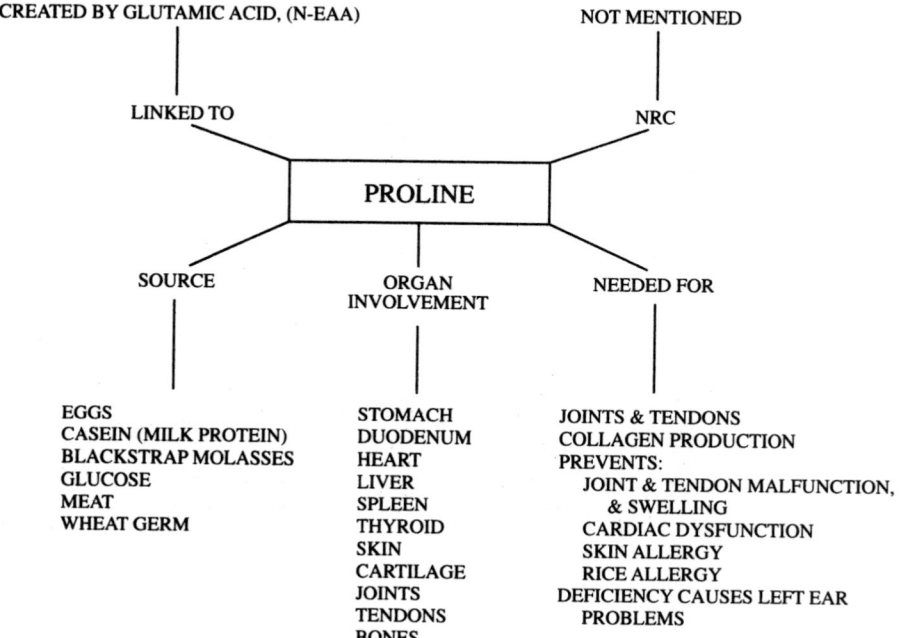

CREATED BY GLUTAMIC ACID, (N-EAA)   NOT MENTIONED

LINKED TO   NRC

PROLINE

SOURCE   ORGAN   NEEDED FOR
                INVOLVEMENT

EGGS   STOMACH   JOINTS & TENDONS
CASEIN (MILK PROTEIN)   DUODENUM   COLLAGEN PRODUCTION
BLACKSTRAP MOLASSES   HEART   PREVENTS:
GLUCOSE   LIVER   JOINT & TENDON MALFUNCTION,
MEAT   SPLEEN   & SWELLING
WHEAT GERM   THYROID   CARDIAC DYSFUNCTION
                            SKIN   SKIN ALLERGY
                            CARTILAGE   RICE ALLERGY
                            JOINTS   DEFICIENCY CAUSES LEFT EAR
                            TENDONS   PROBLEMS
                            BONES

Serine

N-EAA

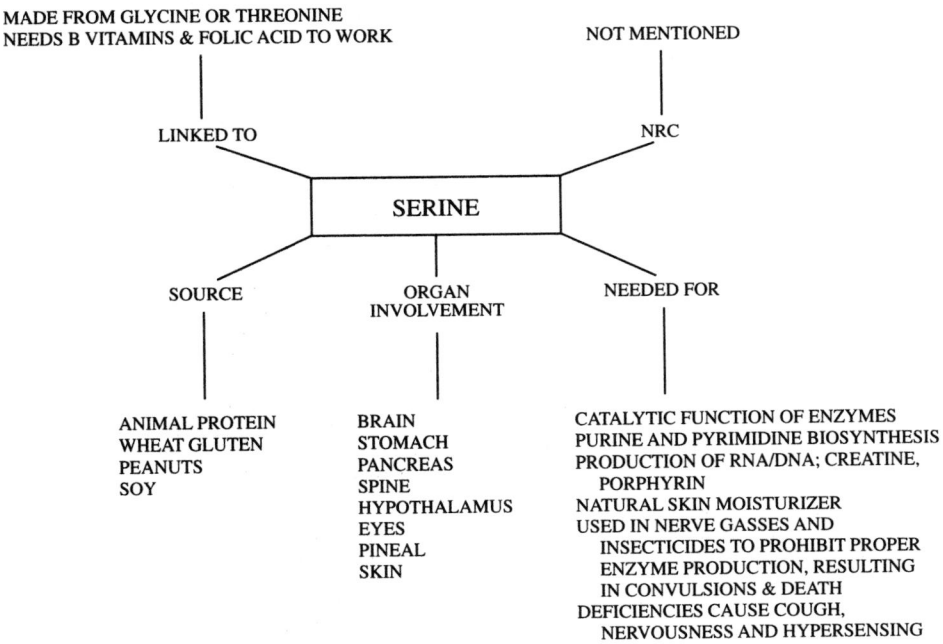

MADE FROM GLYCINE OR THREONINE
NEEDS B VITAMINS & FOLIC ACID TO WORK   NOT MENTIONED

LINKED TO   NRC

SERINE

SOURCE   ORGAN   NEEDED FOR
                    INVOLVEMENT

ANIMAL PROTEIN   BRAIN   CATALYTIC FUNCTION OF ENZYMES
WHEAT GLUTEN   STOMACH   PURINE AND PYRIMIDINE BIOSYNTHESIS
PEANUTS   PANCREAS   PRODUCTION OF RNA/DNA; CREATINE,
SOY   SPINE   PORPHYRIN
                    HYPOTHALAMUS   NATURAL SKIN MOISTURIZER
                    EYES   USED IN NERVE GASSES AND
                    PINEAL   INSECTICIDES TO PROHIBIT PROPER
                    SKIN   ENZYME PRODUCTION, RESULTING
                                            IN CONVULSIONS & DEATH
                                        DEFICIENCIES CAUSE COUGH,
                                            NERVOUSNESS AND HYPERSENSING

Taurine

N-EAA

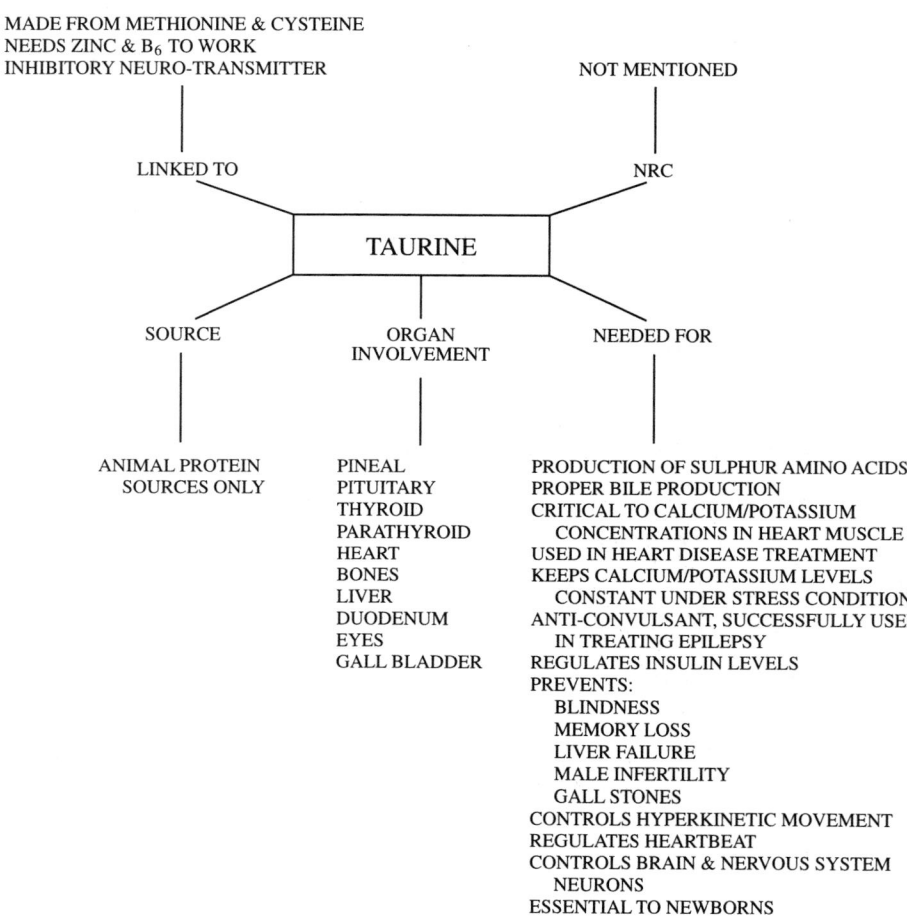

MADE FROM METHIONINE & CYSTEINE
NEEDS ZINC & B$_6$ TO WORK
INHIBITORY NEURO-TRANSMITTER

NOT MENTIONED

LINKED TO

NRC

TAURINE

SOURCE

ORGAN
INVOLVEMENT

NEEDED FOR

ANIMAL PROTEIN
SOURCES ONLY

PINEAL
PITUITARY
THYROID
PARATHYROID
HEART
BONES
LIVER
DUODENUM
EYES
GALL BLADDER

PRODUCTION OF SULPHUR AMINO ACIDS
PROPER BILE PRODUCTION
CRITICAL TO CALCIUM/POTASSIUM
    CONCENTRATIONS IN HEART MUSCLE
USED IN HEART DISEASE TREATMENT
KEEPS CALCIUM/POTASSIUM LEVELS
    CONSTANT UNDER STRESS CONDITIONS
ANTI-CONVULSANT, SUCCESSFULLY USED
    IN TREATING EPILEPSY
REGULATES INSULIN LEVELS
PREVENTS:
    BLINDNESS
    MEMORY LOSS
    LIVER FAILURE
    MALE INFERTILITY
    GALL STONES
CONTROLS HYPERKINETIC MOVEMENT
REGULATES HEARTBEAT
CONTROLS BRAIN & NERVOUS SYSTEM
    NEURONS
ESSENTIAL TO NEWBORNS

Tyrosine

N-EAA

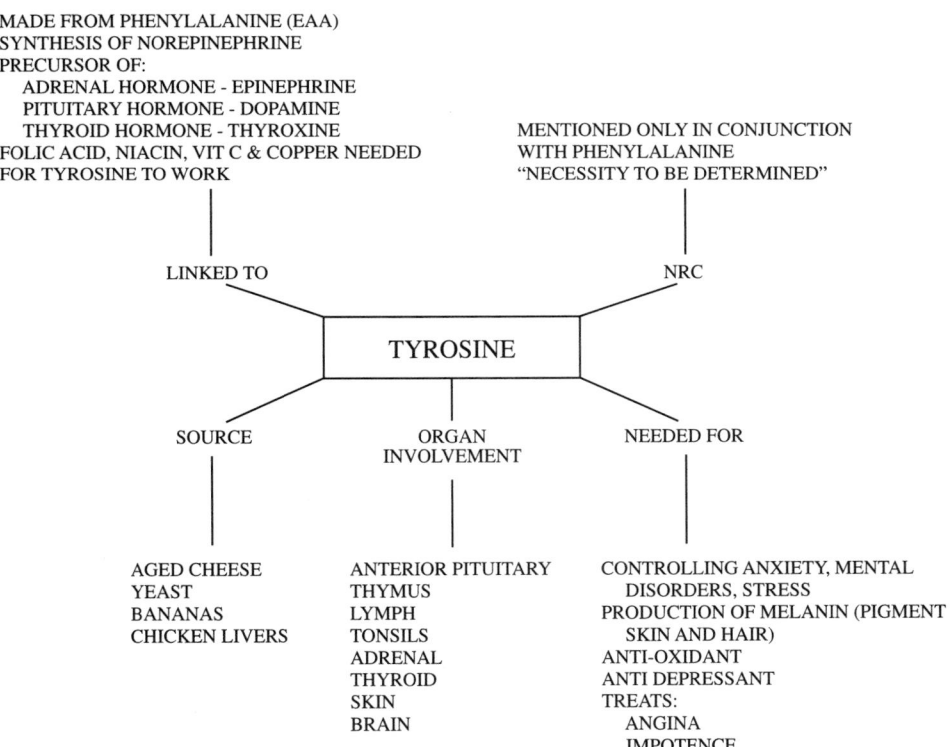

MADE FROM PHENYLALANINE (EAA)
SYNTHESIS OF NOREPINEPHRINE
PRECURSOR OF:
    ADRENAL HORMONE - EPINEPHRINE
    PITUITARY HORMONE - DOPAMINE
    THYROID HORMONE - THYROXINE
FOLIC ACID, NIACIN, VIT C & COPPER NEEDED
FOR TYROSINE TO WORK

MENTIONED ONLY IN CONJUNCTION
WITH PHENYLALANINE
"NECESSITY TO BE DETERMINED"

LINKED TO

NRC

TYROSINE

SOURCE

ORGAN
INVOLVEMENT

NEEDED FOR

AGED CHEESE
YEAST
BANANAS
CHICKEN LIVERS

ANTERIOR PITUITARY
THYMUS
LYMPH
TONSILS
ADRENAL
THYROID
SKIN
BRAIN

CONTROLLING ANXIETY, MENTAL
    DISORDERS, STRESS
PRODUCTION OF MELANIN (PIGMENT
    SKIN AND HAIR)
ANTI-OXIDANT
ANTI DEPRESSANT
TREATS:
    ANGINA
    IMPOTENCE
    TIREDNESS

—Appendix II—

Following is a partial list taken from the 1993 AAFCO Guidelines to Dog Food Manufacturers relating to animal proteins listed on the back of dog food packages.

Meat—The clean flesh of slaughtered cattle, swine, sheep or goats. It may only be striated skeletal muscle, tongue, diaphragm, heart or esophagus. It may include accompanying and overlying fat and the portions of the skin, sinew, nerves and blood vessels that normally accompany the flesh. If a specific type of meat is used, such as lamb or beef, the label may give the type of meat used.

Meat Byproducts—Fresh, nonrendered, clean parts of slaughtered mammals. It does not include meat. It does include but is not limited to lungs, spleen, kidneys, brain, livers, blood, bone, partially defatted low-temperature fatty tissue and stomachs and intestines freed of their contents. It does not include hair, horns, teeth and hoofs.

Poultry Byproduct Meal—The ground, rendered, clean parts of the carcass of slaughtered poultry, such as necks, feet, undeveloped eggs and intestines. It does not contain feathers, except those that are unavoidably included during processing. Byproduct meals are an excellent source of protein, as they are concentrated through rendering (heating).

Meat Meal—A rendered meal made from mammal tissues. It cannot contain blood, hair, hoof, horn, hide trimmings, manure, stomach and rumen contents except for amounts which may be unavoidably included during processing. It can't contain added extraneous materials. The calcium (Ca) to phosphorus (P) ratio must not be more than 2.2:1.

Meat meal may not contain more than 14 percent indigestible materials, and not more than 11 percent of the crude protein in the meal may be indigestible by an animal's stomach.

Lamb meal must be made from lamb parts; meat meal can be from cattle, swine, sheep or goats.

Meat and Bone Meal—Rendered from mammal tissues (meat), including bone. It doesn't include blood, hair, hoof, horn, hide trimmings, manure, stomach and rumen contents except small amounts unavoidably included during processing. It does not contain added extraneous materials. Only 14 percent may be indigestible residue, and no more than 11 percent of the crude protein can be indigestible.

Animal Byproduct Meal—Made by rendering animal tissues that don't fit any of the other ingredient definitions. It still can't contain extra hair, hoof, horn, hide trimmings, manure, stomach and rumen contents, nor any added extraneous materials.

Poultry Byproducts—Nonrendered (fresh) clean parts of carcasses of slaughtered poultry such as heads, feet, and viscera (guts). It must not contain feces or foreign matter, except in unavoidable trace amounts.

Animal Digest—A powder or liquid made by taking clean and non-decomposed animal tissue and breaking it down using chemical and/or enzymatic hydrolysis. It does not contain hair, horn, teeth, hooves, or feathers, except in unavoidable trace amounts. Digest names must be descriptive of their contents: chicken digest must contain chicken; beef byproduct digest must contain beef byproducts.

Dried Whey—The product obtained by removing water from whey. It contains not less than 11 percent protein and not less than 61 percent lactose. (This comes from milk.)

Grains Defined

Fat and Protein Profile

Ingredient	Fat	Protein	Fiber	Carbohydrate
Corn (average)	3.9	9.6	2.1	71.1
Wheat (average)	1.8	14.9	2.5	67.3
Oatmeal	6.5	14.7	4.4	63.1
Rice, ground, rough	1.7	8.4	9.1	65.1
Beet pulp	0.5	8.7	17.9	58.1
Soybean hulls	2.2	11.0	37.3	37.0
Peanut hulls	1.0	6.1	53.9	26.7

Barley—At least 80 percent sound barley and must not contain more than 3 percent heat-damaged kernels, 6 percent foreign material, 20 percent other grains or 10 percent wild oats.

Barley flour—Soft, finely ground and bolted barley meal obtained from the milling of barley. It consists essentially of the starch and gluten of the endosperm.

Barley (Pearl, cracked)—Cracked pearl barley resulting from the manufacture of the pearl barley from clean barley.

Brewers Rice—The dried extracted residue of rice resulting from the manufacture of wort (liquid portion of malted grain) or beer and may contain pulverized dried spent hops in an amount not to exceed 3 percent.

Brown Rice—Unpolished rice after the kernels have been removed.

Corn—Unspecified corn product. (Not complete definition.)

Corn Bran—The outer coating of the corn kernel, with little or none of the starchy part of the germ.

Corn Germ Meal (Dry Milled)—Ground corn germ which consists of corn germ with other parts of the corn kernel from which part of the oil has been removed and is the product obtained in the dry milling process of manufacture of corn meal, corn grits, hominy feed and other corn products.

Corn Gluten—The part of the commercial shelled corn that remains after the extraction of the larger portion of the starch, gluten and germ by the proceses employed in the wet milling manufacture of cornstarch or syrup.

Corn Gluten Meal—the dried residue from corn after the removal of the larger part of the starch and germ, and the separation of the bran by the process employed in the wet milling manufacture of cornstarch or syrup or by enzymatic treatment of the endosperm.

Corn, ground (ground ear corn)—The entire ear of corn ground, without husks, with no greater portion of cob than occurs in the ear corn in its natural state.

Corn, yellow ground—Same as ground corn, except that the corn used is yellow in color.

Corn, kibbled—Obtained by cooking cracked corn under steam pressure and extruding from an expellor or other mechanical pressure device.

Feeding Oatmeal—Obtained in the manufacture of rolled oat groats or rolled oats and consists of broken oat groats, oat groat chips, and floury portions of the oat groats, with only such quantity of finely ground oat hulls as is unavoidable in the usual process of commercial milling. It must not contain more than 4 percent crude fiber.

Rice, ground whole, brown—The entire product obtained by grinding the rice kernels after the hulls have been removed.

Rice bran—The pericarp or bran layer and germ of the rice, with only such quantity of hull fragments, chipped, broken or brewer's rice and calcium carbonate as is unavoidable in the regular milling of edible rice.

Soybean Hulls—Consist primarly of the outer covering of the soybean.

Soybean Meal (Dehulled, solvent extracted)—Obtained by grinding the flakes remaining after removal of most of the oil from dehulled soybeans by a solvent extraction process.

Soybean Meal (Mechanical extraction)—Obtained by grinding the cake or chips that remain after removal of most of the oil from the soybeans by a mechanical extraction process.

Soybean Mill Run—Composed of soybean hulls and such bean meats that adhere to the hulls, which results from normal milling operation in the production of dehulled soybean meal.

Whole Wheat, ground—Ground whole kernel, presumably equivalent to AFFCO's Wheat Mill Run, Wheat Middlings, Wheat Shorts or Wheat Red Dog, whose principal differences are in the percentage of crude fiber.

Wheat Flour—Wheat flour together with fine particles of wheat bran, wheat germ and the offal from the "tail of the mill." This product must be obtained in the usual process of commercial milling and must not contain more than 1.5 percent crude fiber.

Wheat Germ Meal—Consists chiefly of wheat germ together with some bran and middlings or short. It must contain not less than 25 percent crude protein and 7 percent crude fat.

Wheat Mill Run—Coarse wheat bran, fine particles of wheat bran, wheat shorts, wheat germ, wheat flour and the offal from the "tail of the mill." This product must be obtained in the usual process of commerical milling and must contain not more than 9.5 percent crude fiber.

Index

from food, 146
homeopathy, 199
remedies, 193
rhythms (chronobiology), 224-225
English Pointers, protein needs, 7
environmental allergies, 95-99
environmental factors (kinesiology),
   155-156
enzymes (digestive), 70-73, 113, 115
eosinophils (complete blood counts), 130
epilepsy, 193, 204, 207, 235
epithelial cells (urinalysis), 138
esophagus, 110
essential amino acids, 255-265
Ester-C, 29
ethoxyquin preservative, 14
evaluating food, 85
exercise (Natural Diet), 181
exhaustion remedies, 202
exocrine portion of pancreas, 113
Expert Committee on Nutrition, 4
eyes, 236-237
   iridology, 217, 219, 222-223
   remedies, 193, 202-205, 207, 214

F

fabric softeners (environmental allergies),
   95
fasting for Natural Diet, 180
fat, 1, 11-13
   digestion, 112
   grains, 285
fatty acids, 11-12, 41
fear remedies, 193, 202-206, 209-210, 214
fecal analysis, 126, 138-139
Federal guidelines for dog foods, 3-4
feeding amounts, 86
feet remedies, 205-206
females
   brood bitches (Natural Diet), 183-184
   remedies, 205-206
ferrous carbonate, 53
ferrous sulfate, 53
fever remedies, 202
fiber, 86
flea repellents (environmental allergies), 96
fluid retention remedies, 202
fluorescent lighting, 96, 220
fluorine, 57
folacin, 38-39
folic acid, 38-39
food, 83-94
   cravings, 25-29, 31, 37-39, 41
   Dr. Parcell's food cleaning, 221, 225
   effects, 1-4
   energy, 146
   Natural Diet, 167-195
   protein sources, 6
   spoilage, 14, 20-21
   testing (kinesiology), 147-150, 152-155
   undigested material, 138
formaldehyde, 95
free radicals, 80

frozen dog food, 88, 93
fruit
   preparing (Natural Diet), 179-180
full spectrum lighting, 220-221
fundus (stomach), 111

G

GABA (gamma amino buytric acid), 272
gallbladder remedies, 203
garlic, 69-70
gas remedies, 206
gastrin, 111
gastrointestinal (GI) system, 107-116, 204-
   205
German Shepherd Dogs 90, 143-144, 152, 189
giardia, 138
glandular system remedies, 195, 203-204,
   206-207
globulins (Serum Chemistry Profiles), 134
glutamic acid, 9, 273
glutamine (amino acid), 8, 274
glycine (amino acid), 8, 275
Golden Retrievers, food ethnicity, 152
grain
   Natural Diet, 171, 190
graphites, 204
greens, preparing (Natural Diet), 179
gross blood, 139
growth, 2, 12
   see also puppies

H

hair remedies, 195
hard palate, 108
healing crises (homeopathy), 212
heart
   chemical tests, 127
   remedies, 204, 214
heartworm
   medication, 104
   testing for, 139
heat exhaustion remedies, 205
heat stroke, 202, 238
hematocrit (complete blood counts), 128
hemoglobin (complete blood counts), 129
hepatic, 140
hepatitis
   remedies, 205
   vaccine, 102
herbs (Natural Diet), 179, 191-195
hernia remedies, 203, 205
high-performance foods, 89, 92
hindquarters, weak, 246
histidine (amino acid), 9, 257
homeopathic remedies, 201-207
homeopathy, 197-210, 212
honey, 79-8
hookworms, 138
hot spot remedies, 204
humectants, 88
hydrochloric acid, 73-74, 111
hydrophobinum (Lyssin), 205
hydroxyproline (amino acid), 276

mucous membranes, 25, 111, 204
muscle
  chemical tests, 127
  deltoid, testing, 142
  remedies, 202-204
musculoskeletal system remedies, 195
mycotoxicosis, 20

N

National Research Council (NRC), 3-4
natural allergens, 96
Natural Diet, 166-195
natural preservatives, 14, 93
necrosis, 141
nervous system remedies, 195, 204-205
nervousness remedies, 193
neutrophil bands (complete blood counts),
  130
neutrophils (complete blood counts), 129
Newfoundlands, 152, 189, 219
niacin, 32-34
niacinamide, 32-34
nickel, 60
nicotinic acid, 32-34
nitrates, 64
nitrogen (Serum Chemistry Profiles),
  134-135
nonessential amino acids, 255, 266-281
nose remedies, 202, 204-205
nosodes, 208
NRC (National Research Council), 3-4
nursing remedies, 193, 203-204, 206-207
nutrients
  in food, 67-70
  Natural Diet, 169-170
  percentage level analysis for dog foods, 84
  supplements, 70-81
nutrition for working dogs (kinesiology),
  156-157

O

oatmeal (feeding), 286
occult blood, 138-139
occult test, 139
older dogs
  fat needs, 12
  Natural Diet, 180-181
  plant proteins, 6
  remedies, 204-205, 207
oral cavity, 107-109
organ remedies, 202
ornithine (amino acid), 8, 277
orotic acid, 40
owners' lifestyles, choosing food categories
  by, 89

P—Q

PABA (paraminobenzoic acid), 40
pack cell volume (PCV) (complete blood
  counts), 128
pain relievers, 203-204, 209, 214
pancreas, 113, 115, 127

pancreatin, 72
pancreatitis remedies, 193, 205
pangamic acid, 40
pantothenic acid, 34-35
papain, 72
paralysis remedies, 204-205
parasites, 138, 193
parotid gland, 110
Parvo vaccines, 99, 102
PCV (Pack Cell Volume) (complete blood
  counts), 128
pearl barley, 285
penitrem A, 20
pepsin, 72
pepsinogen, 111
performance foods, 83
periodontal disease remedies, 193
peristaltic waves, 111
PH levels (urinalysis), 137
pharyngeal area (oral cavity), 108, 110
phenylalanine (amino acid), 8, 262
phosphatase, 70
phosphorus, 45, 48
physical examinations, 125
plant enzymes, 72
platelet count (complete blood counts),
  129
Pointers (English) cross ref. see English
  pointers
poison control center phone number, 106
poison ivy remedies, 194, 206
poison oak remedies, 205
polydipsia, 141
polyunsaturated fats, 11, 13
polyuria, 141
pork liver, 68-69
potassium, 45, 50-51
potencies of homeopathic remedies,
  197-198
poultry byproduct meal, 283
poultry byproducts, 284
premium foods, 84, 92
preservatives, 14-15
pressure-treated lumber (environmental
  allergies), 98
production codes on labels, 89
proline (amino acid), 8, 278
prophylactics, 210
propylene glycol, 96
protease, 70-72
protein, 1, 5-9
  animal, AAFCO guidelines to listings,
    283-284
  crude, 85-86
  digestion, 112
  grains, 285
  Serum Chemistry Profiles, 134
  urinalysis, 137
proteocytic enzymes, 111
puppies
  growth, 2
  lead poisoning, 98
  plant proteins, 6

raising from seven weeks (Natural Diet), 187
remedies, 203
stress from weaning, 186-187
supplements, 90
vaccinations, 100, 208
weaning (Natural Diet), 184-186
Puppy Stress Formula, 187, 189
purchasing Natural Diet ingredients, 190
pylorus (stomach), 111
pyometra, 141, 205
pyridoxal, 35-36
pyridoxamine, 35-36
pyridoxine, 35-36

R

rabies vaccine, 104, 205
radon, 64
rancid food, 14
raspberry leaf tea, 183
rawhide treats (environmental allergies), 96
recipes (Natural Diet)
  breakfast bars, 188
  treats, 181-183
rectum (large intestine), 113
red blood cells (RBCs)
  CBCs (complete blood counts), 128
  urinalysis, 138
renal, 141
rennin, 72
repetorizing (homeopathy), 198
Rescue Remedy, 208-209
respiratory remedies, 192, 195, 202-205, 207, 214
reticulocytes (complete blood counts), 129
rheumatism remedies, 203, 206
riboflavin, 32
ribonuclease, 113
rice, 285-286
rice bran, 286
ringworm remedies, 194
Rocky Mountain Spotted Fever remedies, 194
Rottweilers, 99, 152
roundworms, 138

S

salivary glands, 110
salt, 51-52
  biochemical cell salts, 210-211
  in semi-moist food, 87-88
saturated fats, 11, 13
scheduling vaccinations, 102-103
sediment (urinalysis), 138
seizure remedies, 194, 204, 214
selenium, 57-58, 80-81
semi-moist food, 87-88
sequestrants, 88
serine (amino acid), 9, 279
Serum Chemistry Profiles (chem scans), 125, 130-136
shedding live virus vaccines, 100
shock remedies, 210

sick dogs, Natural Diet, 181
silicon, 60-61
simple carbohydrates, 17
skin
  fat needs, 11-12
  problems, 243
  remedies, 29, 193, 195, 202-207
small intestine, 112-113
sodium, 45, 51-52
sodium ascorbate, 29
sodium chloride, 51-52, 87-88
sodium fluoride, 57
sodium selenite, 57-58
soft palate, 110
soloxine, 119
sound sensitivity remedies, 204-205, 214
soybean hulls, 286
specific gravity (urinalysis), 137
sphincter (esophagus), 110
spinal misalignment
  effects on humans, 218
  veterinary chiropractic, 213-217
spinal subluxations, 214, 216
splinter remedies, 206
spoiled food, 14, 20-21
sprain remedies, 206
sprayed fruits/vegetables (environmental allergies), 96
staph infection remedies, 194
state regulation of pet foods, 4
stiffness remedies, 206
stomach, 111, 203-205
stool
  analysis, 126, 138-139
  remedies, 203, 205
stress, 3, 90
  effects on kinesiology, 156
  remedies, 194, 204, 210
  weaned puppies, 186-187
stud dogs, Natural Diet, 183-184
sublinguals gland, 110
succussion, 198
sucrase, 70
sulphur, 45, 58-59, 95
super premium I foods, 84
super premium II foods, 84, 89, 92
supplements, 90-91
  fats, 12
  minerals, 44, 46-61
  nutrients, 70-81
  testing (kinesiology), 153, 155
  vitamins, 24-27, 29-41
Supportasode, 186, 208
swelling remedies, 202-204, 206

T

T3, 117-119
T4 (thyroxine), 117-119
taking symptoms (homeopathy), 198
tapeworms, 138
taurine (amino acid), 8, 280
tea tree oil, 194
teas, 183, 191